CONTENTS

LANGUAGE AND DEAFNESS

LANGUAGE AND DEAFNESS

SECOND EDITION

PETER V. PAUL, Ph.D.
The Ohio State University
Columbus

Stephen P. Quigley, Ph.D.
Tucson, Arizona

SINGULAR PUBLISHING GROUP, INC.
SAN DIEGO, CALIFORNIA

Singular Publishing Group, Inc.
4284 41st Street
San Diego, California 92105-1197

© **1994 by Singular Publishing Group, Inc.**

Typeset in 10/12 Times by ExecuStaff
Printed in the United States of America by BookCrafters

Library of Congress Cataloging-in-Publication Data

Paul, Peter V.
    Language and deafness / Peter V. Paul, Stephen P. Quigley.
—2nd ed.
      p. cm.
    Previous edition entered under Stephen P. Quigley.
    Includes bibliographical references and index.
    ISBN 1-56593-108-4
    1. Deaf—Education. 2. Children. Deaf—Language.
3. Deaf—Means of communication—Study and teaching.
4. Deaf—Education—United States. I. Quigley, Stephen P.
(Stephen Patrick). 1927– . II. Title
HV2471.P38 1994
371.91'2—dc20   94-4478
                                          CIP

PREFACE TO
THE FIRST EDITION

The present state of the education of deaf children can be characterized as one of creative confusion. Creative is an appropriate term because the present ferment in the field seems likely to lead to significant changes, which might also be significant advances. Confusion is also an appropriate term since no strongly research-supported directions for educational practice have yet emerged from the ferment. Most of the ferment centers around the languages and the communication modes that should be used initially with deaf infants and children. This book attempts to define the problems and prospects of those languages and communication modes, to discuss elements of the present creative ferment in these areas, to present and discuss much of the data-based research findings pertaining to them, to synthesize the findings and those from other areas (such as bilingualism and English as a second language [ESL]), and to present some conclusions.

The book is seen as being useful to anyone seeking an in-depth introduction to language development in deaf children, but particularly to student teachers and clinicians and practicing teachers and clinicians who bear most of the responsibility for fostering that development both directly and in their training and counseling of parents. The book has much more detail on language than is common in beginning texts, but that is because the authors believe that teachers and clinicians must have a great deal of detailed knowledge about language and communication to promote, through naturally oriented practices, the initial language development of deaf children; and to direct, through analytically oriented practices, more structured development at later ages if the naturally oriented practices do not produce adequate language development. As Russell, Quigley, and Power (1976) have claimed: "It is probably a fair analogy to state that teachers of deaf children should be expected to know as much about language as a teacher of chemistry is expected to know about chemistry" (p. xi). This is not so that teachers can teach language didactically but in order that they have the knowledge and skills to structure situations and construct materials that will allow language to develop in a natural manner or, when necessary, in a more structured manner.

Both natural and structured approaches are seen as playing a role in the language development of deaf children. The preferred approach is the natural approach, in which language is acquired (or absorbed) unconsciously by the child through fluent communicative interaction with the parents in infancy and early childhood and later with teachers. Unfortunately, this early natural development does not always take place (in fact, it rarely takes place), and at some point many teachers feel the need to use more structured approaches to language development. It follows from this, that teachers and clinicians must be familiar with both approaches and know when to use each.

The statement that early language development requires fluent communicative interaction between child and parents and child and teacher raises immediately the question of communication modes, the form in which parent, teacher, and child will communicate. Here again, as with language approaches, no absolute position is taken in the book. All major approaches are described and explored. It is recognized and stated that it is not possible to examine the language development of deaf children apart from the specific communication mode through which it was developed. With hearing children, language is acquired through speech, and spoken language is the primary language on which the secondary language forms of reading and writing are based. Individual variations in IQ, socioeconomic status, educational opportunities, and other factors might alter the degree of language mastery by individual hearing children, but they will not alter the form. All variations are variations on the same basic form, spoken language.

With deaf children the situation is quite different. Any of several communication modes or forms might be used early with them, and language development can be discussed only in relation to the particular form used. That approach is followed here, particularly in Chapter 3 on Primary Language Development and in the concluding chapter. The major communication forms that can be used with deaf children are referred to throughout the book as oral English (OE), manually coded English (MCE), and American Sign Language (ASL). These are described in Chapter 1 on Definitions and Historical Perspectives. Pidgin sign English (PSE) is categorized here as a form of MCE, but it can be regarded also as a separate form. MCE systems are contrived systems (contrived usually by hearing people) which attempt in various ways to conform signs and finger spelling to the structure of English. PSE is a linguistically natural language form developed from interaction or interfacing of the visual ASL with the oral OE.

As with language approaches, it follows from the variety of communication modes and the present support that exists for each, that teachers and clinicians who work with deaf children need to be conversant with, and fluent in, all of them. And since the secondary language forms of reading and writing, at least in our present state of knowledge, have to be related to the child's primary language, teachers and clinicians need to understand the implications of each primary language form (OE, MCE, ASL) for the development of reading and written language. If OE is used exclusively with a deaf child, then perhaps the methods of teaching reading to hearing children (which assume the existence of a spoken language) can be used with that child; but if ASL is the child's primary language, then it is likely that other methods of teaching reading must be sought.

In addition to being skilled in the various language approaches (natural and structured) and the various communication forms (OE, MCE, ASL) that are used with deaf children, teachers and clinicians need to be highly knowledgeable in the language and communication development of hearing children. It is important also that they be familiar with the special problems and techniques used in language development with certain other special populations, especially problems and techniques in bilingualism and the teaching of English as a second language (ESL). All of this amounts to a great deal of knowledge and skill in a large number of areas, but it is difficult to see how a teacher of deaf children can be fully competent without all of it.

This book treats, though only to limited extents, each of these areas of knowledge and skill. References are provided throughout where the reader can obtain more detailed information on the major topic discussed in each chapter. In most chapters, the topic of the chapter (e.g., reading) is discussed first in relation to the hearing population. This is in accord with the stated position that the language development of deaf children can best be examined and understood in the context of language development in general. Each chapter topic is then discussed in relation to deaf children as defined in Chapter 1 and some conclusions and possible applications are presented.

Chapter 1 provides definitions of important terms and historical perspectives on important issues and topics. One of the most neglected issues in the education of deaf children is the differentiation of children who are deaf (visually oriented for purposes of communication even with the best amplification) from those who are hard of hearing (at least partially auditorily oriented). An attempt is made to do this in Chapter 1. In that chapter also, definitions are provided for the various language and communication approaches used with deaf children. Then the historical paths of the various language and communication approaches are traced in an effort to show that most of the present approaches (with the exception of such relatively recent technological advances as amplification) have very long histories. This should not be surprising. The formal teaching and tutoring of deaf children has almost a 400-year history and has involved many very intelligent people. In that lengthy period, it is likely that every conceivable approach has been tried. The fact that none has prevailed, and dissension still reigns, indicates that there is as yet no one "true path" in the education of deaf children.

Chapter 2 deals with language and cognition. Again the topic is discussed in terms of hearing individuals and then in relation to deaf individuals. The position is taken that language is a subset of cognitive abilities and that adequate language development requires adequate cognitive development. It is also accepted that soon after language begins to develop, language and cognition become almost inseparable. Symbolic mediation is discussed in this chapter; the forms of internalized language used by hearing and by deaf individuals as mediators of thought and of the secondary language forms of reading and writing.

Chapter 3 presents current theories of language and traces the development of primary language in hearing and in deaf individuals. As previously stated, the language development of deaf children must be examined in relation to the communication form through which it was developed and given expression. This is done in Chapter 3, with development being discussed within the communication forms of OE, MCE, and ASL. Some implications of the various forms for the later development of reading and written language are discussed. The lack of research based data is stressed.

Chapter 4 presents considerable information on the reading of hearing and of deaf children; Chapter 5 similarly treats written language. The original intent had been to treat these two topics in a single chapter to emphasize their close relationship and the primacy of reading, but the large amount of material available dictated separate chapters. It is recognized, and expounded in the book, that skilled development of reading and written language requires adequate development of a primary language, which in turn is dependent on early fluent communication between parent and child. But the development of literacy is the road to learning and is the primary responsibility of teachers, clinicians, and the schools. Other aspects of the deaf child's development certainly are important. But the failure to develop literacy cannot be compensated for by the promotion of cultural identity or the development of a positive self-image, important as those might be. In fact, it is doubtful that an adult who is semiliterate or illiterate for all practical purposes can have a very positive self-image or find much satisfaction or reward in cultural identity.

Chapter 6 deals with the processes and problems, theories and practices, of bilingualism and the development of English as a second language with minority-culture hearing children, and relates these areas analogically to the language development of deaf children. This is likely to be an area for much fruitful exploration and research with deaf children during the decade of the 1980s. Some of the problems and some of the possible programs and procedures that could be tried with deaf children, based on research with minority-culture hearing children, are discussed. It is emphasized that successful bilingual and ESL programs seem to require that the child come to the program with at least one language already reasonably well established. That, of course, is not the case with many deaf children who often enter school and preschool programs without any well-developed first language. (Some deaf children of ASL-using deaf parents might be exceptions to this.) This reinforces the importance of the family, or some substitute, providing the deaf child with a primary language in infancy and early childhood through some fluent form of communication.

Chapter 7 treats language assessment and some of the major methods used in language development and instruction. Some material in these areas is also presented, where appropriate, in other chapters and much of the other material could have been similarly treated. It was considered convenient for students and teachers, however, to have a separate chapter on these important areas. The material on instructional approaches is related back to the historical treatment of earlier approaches in Chapter 1.

In the final chapter (8), some general summation of the book's topics is provided and some implications for present and future educational practices with deaf children are discussed. If there is a general focus, or unifying theme to the book, it is provided by Chapter 8 and this Preface. The theme is simply that there is as yet no data-based justification for any communication and language approach as the sole means of developing language in deaf children. The teacher and the clinician must master a variety of language approaches (from natural to analytic) and communication forms (e.g., OE, MCE, ASL) to function effectively with a range of deaf children. Fortunately, teachers and clinicians are usually more eclectic and more pragmatic than many textbook writers. They are usually willing to try new approaches on the basis of logical and theoretical arguments, but are also ready to abandon them if they do not seem to work.

A companion text to the present book, *Reading and Deafness,* by Cynthia M. King and Stephen P. Quigley, will be published soon by the same publisher. The topics of the two books, language and reading, are obviously closely related, and the use of a single publisher allows for some overlap of content without the authors having to go through a frustrating rewriting exercise to say the same thing in different words in two different books so as not to violate copyrights held by two different publishers. A major difference between the two texts is that *Reading and Deafness* will provide both a knowledge base and instructional techniques on its topic whereas *Language and Deafness* deals primarily with a knowledge base and treats instructional techniques only generally. This is because the wider scope of the present book makes inclusion of detailed material on instruction impractical. A special chapter on assessment and instruction has been provided for the present book by Barry W. Jones, and a related text on instructional processes and techniques in language development is tentatively planned.

The authors are indebted to many persons for assistance in the preparation of this book. A major debt is acknowledged to the many teachers, clinicians, researchers, and thinkers who provided most of the material on which the book is based. Some, but certainly not all, of this debt is acknowledged by appropriate citation and referencing of the more than 500 authors whose work was used in preparation of the text. Grateful acknowledgment is also made to the graduate students who aided in locating and abstracting the works of those many authors: Jean Andrews, Cheryl Bolebruch, Cynthia King, John-Allen Payne, Stephanie Quigley, Lou Reeves, Marilyn Salter, and Pam Stuckey. And finally, the major and indispensable assistance provided by Ruth Quigley in all phases of the planning, preparation, and completion of the manuscript is gratefully acknowledged and lovingly appreciated.

PREFACE TO THE
SECOND EDITION

All intelligent thoughts have already been thought; what is necessary is only to try to think them again.

(Johann Wolfgang von Goethe, in Beck, 1980, p. 397)

The quote above captures in a nutshell the major intention of the second edition of *Language and Deafness*. With a few exceptions, the second edition adheres to the conceptual framework established by the first edition as described in the first Preface. There are, of course, some notable differences. As much as possible, we have updated the theories and research in a number of areas in almost every chapter. This new source of information did not radically change our original conclusions stated in the first edition. However, it did lead to a refinement of some issues, particularly concerning the interrelationships among language, cognition, and literacy.

This refinement led us to hypothesize that the development of English literacy skills might not be a realistic goal for some, perhaps many, students with severe to profound hearing impairment. We express this concern in our first edition; however, we have become more convinced of this situation. Similar to other scholars, we firmly believe that it is important to develop a first language at as early an age as possible. Unfortunately, we have made little progress since our first edition; that is, there is still not enough evidence on which a firm decision can be based.

Another major change in the second edition is the concept of meta-theory—the driving, conceptual framework which influences the construction of theories, the undertaking of research, the use of specific methods, and, most importantly, the interpretation of results. There should be sufficient background on this concept so that the reader can understand why it is difficult for oral proponents to "agree" with TC proponents, or why each group can offer a different interpretation of the same data. In essence, the notion of metatheory was discussed relative to language acquisition and perspectives on deafness.

As stated in the first edition, this text is useful for preservice personnel and inservice professionals, for example, students, teachers, and clinicians in programs for deaf individuals. As will be seen, there is a much heavier emphasis on the knowledge base of language development. This necessitated the elimination of some information that can be found in other texts. This change is in keeping with the growing movement of teachers-as-scholars (or, clinicians-as-scholars). In essence, teachers or clinicians can no longer be viewed as the personnel who only apply knowledge. They are being encouraged, in some cases, required, to evaluate and provide "support" for their techniques and materials. Teachers and clinicians probably realize that there is, or should be, strong interrelations among theories, research, instruction, curricula, and assessments.

Chapter 1 of the second edition provides an overview of the broad domains of language and deafness. This chapter presents more background information than the first chapter of the first edition on the functions and structure of language. Although both editions provided descriptions of deafness and the communication modes, the second edition elaborates on these issues and discusses the metatheoretical framework of clinical and cultural perspectives.

Chapter 2 is a new chapter that contains both old and new information. The old information involves basically the same theoretical frameworks as discussed in the first edition. It is our hope, however, that the new information provides a better understanding of the foundations of these theories—that is, the metatheoretical foundations. As stated in the chapter, one of the functions of metatheorizing is to understand extant theory. This tool enables us to discuss, in one sense, the "levels" of theoretical adequacy, proposed by Chomsky. More important, the reader should obtain a sense of the growing tension in the field between "child language researchers" (mostly, psycholinguists and psychologists) and "language researchers" (primarily linguists). The information in this chapter should shed more light on the theories and research in the subsequent chapters.

In many ways, Chapter 3 of the second edition is similar to Chapter 2 of the first edition. However, there is additional information on the relationship between language and thought, as can be seen in the discussion of language-based and cognitive-based hypotheses. The new information concerns what can be labeled a fourth stage of intelligence tests—the process paradigm. We also feel that the chapter offers a more efficient framework for understanding the relationships among language, cognition, and intelligence. In fact, this framework builds on the well-stated information in an earlier text (Quigley & Kretschmer, 1982). For example, there is sufficient information to make some strong inferences about the short-term working memory capacity of deaf individuals and about the relationship between short-term working memory and literacy skills. We also felt that there was sufficient information to address the controversial long-standing question: Is there a psychology of deafness? Obviously, there is no simple *yes* or *no* answer.

Chapter 4 of the second edition is very similar to Chapter 3 of the first edition. Unfortunately, this is a reflection of the little research that continues to be undertaken in this area, relative to deafness. Nevertheless, we have improved somewhat in our understanding of the manually coded English systems, especially in relation to the representation of English. There is much more research on American Sign Language (ASL) than there was 10 years ago, and this research has started to unravel some of the mysteries surrounding the development of this language. There is still some debate on the nature of its syntax and nonmanual aspects and its use among deaf people.

Chapter 5 fulfills our original intention of the first edition. That is, we decided to treat the two topics, reading and writing, in a single chapter because of their similar underlying processes. In this chapter, we tried to show that the development of English literacy skills is heavily dependent upon existing conversational language skills in English. This reciprocal relationship is discussed within the framework of interactive theories of reading. In the section on writing, we not only provided a conceptual framework for the consideration of writing, but also included some of the more recent studies on writing as a process approach. As will be seen, viewing writing as a process approach does not mean excluding important lower-level skills such as spelling and grammar. Similar to the process of reading, it is important for the writer to have automatic lower-level skills so that they can engage in the higher-level composition activities such as organization and intent.

Chapter 6 of the second edition contains a great deal of new information, reflecting not only the growing developments in second-language learning, but also the influence of first-language theories on understanding second-language development. The exemplar is the influence of interactive theories of reading, which have essentially replaced the linear bottom-up and top-down models (e.g. Bernhardt, 1991; Grabe, 1988). In the first edition, we predicted that bilingualism would become a major theoretical and research activity in the field of deafness. Our prediction was only partly confirmed. On one hand, there has been a growth in the development of bilingual education models. However, many of these models are not based on theory and research; at least, the description of the theoretical and research foundation is not always explicit. We have proposed a bilingual model based on our critical reflections. This model has evolved somewhat since its original appearance (e.g., Paul & Quigley, 1987b, in press). Although much more theorizing and modeling need to occur, there is also a need for empirical research, which, to our surprise, has been very limited. In addition, some of the more recent investigations seem to be heavily influenced by earlier research.

Chapter 7 provides definitional and historical background for the major language-teaching approaches in the education of deaf children and adolescents. The new information concerns our treatment of what is becoming "the great debate" relative to language acquisition: the learnability/teachability dichotomy. The outcome of this debate has important implications for future research and instruction in language and deafness. Other new additions include examples of instructional strategies or lessons based on the social-cognitive interactive perspective of language comprehension.

As in the first edition, Chapter 8 covers language assessment, including a discussion of some language tests. The second edition of the chapter, however, offers more basic information on language and assessment, for example, types and purposes, and a more detailed discussion on validity. The second edition also offers some insights into the issues of assessment and bilingualism. This information is important if there are attempts to establish bilingual education programs for deaf students. The focus of this chapter is on the knowledge base of language, particularly language assessment, which is critical for the "teacher-as-scholar" movement discussed previously.

In Chapter 9, we present our reflections regarding the development of language and literacy in deaf individuals. This chapter is organized around two questions, based on the ones proposed by King (1981): (1) How do deaf students learn the conversational form of a language? and (2) How well do deaf students learn both (a) the conversational forms of English and American Sign Language and (b) the written form of English? If we have done our work in the earlier chapters, the reader will be able to anticipate our conclusions. In addition, we hope our provocative remarks regarding the development of literate thought stimulate additional theorizing and research in this area. Similar to the first edition, we still firmly believe that there is no "true path" in the language development of deaf students; however, it is critical to develop a first language at as early an age as possible.

The authors are indebted to the many scholars who provided most of the theoretical and research thinking on which this text is based. We want to state also that some of the information in Chapters 7 and 8 was based on the framework and work of the late Barry W. Jones in the first edition. With our brand of "metatheorizing," we hope that we have not only articulated the major findings but also have added to the knowledge base.

As usual, we thank our wives, Mary Beth Pilewski Paul and Ruth Quigley, for putting up with us and putting up without us.

C H A P T E R   1

OVERVIEW OF
LANGUAGE AND
DEAFNESS

The really interesting concepts of this world have the nasty habit of avoiding our most determined attempts to pin them down, to make them say something definite and make them stick to it. Their meanings perversely remain multiple, ambiguous, imprecise, and above all unstable and open—open to argument and disagreement, to sometimes drastic reformulation and redefinition, and to the introduction of new and often unsettling concept instances and examples. . . . therefore we would be wise not to expend too much of our time and energy trying to fix them in formal definition. (Flavell, 1985, p. 2)

With the caveats above in mind, the main purpose of this chapter is to provide a brief, broad overview of two concepts: language and deafness. Relative to language, the chapter covers areas such as function, structure, and medium. The function of a language refers to the many roles that language performs. Language roles can be described as cultural, social, and personal (Cairns, 1986; Crystal, 1987; Goodluck, 1991; Whitehead, 1990). These roles define the individual and social identities of the language users. The structure of a language includes various components or dimensions of a language, for example, grammar, semantics, pragmatics, and discourse. These components underlie all forms or mediums of language—spoken, signed, and written—which are also discussed in this chapter and the rest of the text.

Much of the chapter is devoted to discussing the concept of deafness, particularly as it relates to that of language. Within this purview, the chapter describes deafness from the framework of two broad philosophical perspectives: clinical and cultural. The main intent is to define the population with which this text is primarily concerned, namely, students with severe to profound hearing impairment. It is not possible to cover adequately all of the subgroups within the population of individuals with hearing impairment. In addition, the chapter provides a brief overview of the three major categories of language/communication systems used in the education of deaf students: oralism, total communication, and American Sign Language. The language/communication systems entail a number of approaches, which are some combination of form (oral and/or manual) and language (English and/or American Sign Language).

FUNCTION OF LANGUAGE

Language has several functions or uses. The most commonly recognized function of a language is the communication of ideas (Cairns, 1986; Crystal, 1987; Goodluck, 1991; Whitehead, 1990). However, there are other recognized usages which include social interaction, a tool for thought, expression of identity, emotional expression, recording of information, special effects, and the control of reality (Cromer, 1988a, 1988b; Crystal, 1987; Rice & Kemper, 1984).

Communication of Ideas

The communication of ideas refers to the function of language that is also labeled *referential*, *propositional*, and *ideational*. This involves any spoken, signed, or written interaction between participants in which there is an exchange of ideas, opinions, facts, and other types of information. This function of language has been referred to in a commonly used definition of language as "a code whereby *ideas* about the world are represented by a conventional system of signals for *communication* (Bloom & Lahey, 1978, p. 4; emphasis added).

Communication of ideas can occur in two broad contexts, everyday communicative contexts and decontextualized academic situations, which include education, business, law, and government (Cummins, 1979, 1980, 1984). These two contexts demand different levels of language proficiency. Decontextualized situations (e.g., the teaching of academic courses, literacy skills) incorporate the skills for everyday communicative contexts and additional skills unique to the situations. For example, reading requires knowledge of spoken language as well as other knowledge related to the decontextualized text. This issue is also applicable to the discussion of bilingualism and second-language learning (Cummins, 1984).

The crux of the discussion above is that the communication of ideas function is affected by levels of language proficiency as well as by other factors. It is important to add that this language function is foremost in the minds of many individuals. However, it is wrongly assumed that "communication of ideas" is the only or major use of language.

Social Interaction

The social interaction (or social) function pertains to the use of language to establish and maintain a rapport between the language users (Cairns, 1986; Crystal, 1987). In some cultures, for example, English-speaking cultures, certain stereotypical, automatic phrases are used as "conversational openers" or "conversational fillers." Examples include "How are you?" "Good morning," "Hello," "Is it hot enough for you today?" and "Bless you" (after someone sneezes). The main intent of these phrases is not to communicate or exchange ideas. Rather, the intent is to signal friendship or a nonthreatening or comfortable encounter. Interesting, the lack of acknowledgment (e.g., being silent after meeting someone for the first time or after someone sneezes) may be interpreted as aloofness, alienation, or a threat.

Pragmatics, a component or dimension of language, and discourse analyses are concerned with the social interaction function of language (Bates, 1976; Bohannon & Warren-Leubecker, 1985; Goodluck, 1991; Whitehead, 1990). One of the prominent groups of language theories is labeled social interaction. Social interaction theorists argue that children acquire language via a complex array of communicative interactions within the social milieu, particularly the home environment involving significant others. Social interaction is also one of the viewpoints for describing the relationship between language and thought (e.g., Cromer, 1988a, 1988b; Vygotsky, 1962). Finally, the influence of the social interaction function of language can be seen in theories and methods associated with reading and writing, for example, the Whole Language Approach and both Social and Social-Cognitive Theories (Bernhardt, 1991; Bloom & Green, 1984; Samuels & Kamil, 1984).

A Tool for Thought

One of the most controversial, long-standing issues has been the role that language plays in the development of thought (cognition). Indeed, the relationship between language and thought has been debated since the inception of philosophical inquiry (Cromer, 1988a, 1988b; Rice & Kemper, 1984; Snyder, 1984). As remarked by Snyder (1984):

The Platonic school of thought held that principles such as one finds in language are immutable and unaffected by man's mortal mental structures. By contrast, Aristotelians felt that such principles were affected and defined by the constraints or limitations of the organism that must use them. (p. 108)

Snyder's remarks reflect the two strong, bipolar positions concerning language and thought (cognition): language dominates thought and thought dominates language. If language dominates thought, then specific linguistic factors account for the development of thought. The developmental influence is unidirectional; that it, it flows from language to thought. If thought dominates language, then language is a mapping out of cognitive prerequisites. In other words, language is used to express the pre-existing cognitive structures (knowledge). In this view, development is also unidirectional. The flow of effects proceed from thought to language.

There are also variations between these two extremes. These variations are often considered "weaker" forms of the bipolar positions. To obtain a better understanding of the language/thought debate, some theorists take into account the role of social interactions as well as the influences of the cognitive-biological factors associated with the two strong positions (Cromer, 1988a, 1988b; Vygotsky, 1962).

It is not likely that the language/thought debate will be resolved soon. Nevertheless, insights gained along the way have important instructional implications, especially for students with hearing impairment. For example, it might be the case that some specific language structures (e.g., syntax) develop separately from or are not influenced pervasively by the development of specific cognitive structures. Thus, it is important for students either to learn or be taught the structures. The crux of the issue is that there is no one-to-one correspondence between language and cognitive development. Specific language and cognitive skills must be acquired or taught.

Expression of Identity

Language can also be used to express the identity of the language user (Crystal, 1987; Goodluck, 1991; Muma, 1986; Whitehead, 1990). Individuals have several identities, for example, personal, social, and political. The language that speakers/signers use can reveal information about their background, education, vocation, age, sex, and other personal characteristics.

A good illustration of political identity can be seen in the following example:

In the 1992 presidential primaries, Jerry Brown, a Democratic candidate, took his place on the podium. Before he could speak, several individuals from the audience shouted one of his favorite slogans: "We must take back America!" Hearing these words brought a smile to Mr. Brown's face.

Rather than communicate ideas, these words reflect the individuals' sense of political identity.

It is not difficult to find examples of the expression of social identity, particularly the use of language which unites the group. These include the shoutings that occur at sporting events, the bursts of affirmation that accompany religious sermons, and the appreciative sounds from family members on seeing a Thanksgiving turkey dinner. These remarks represent "the signalling of who we are and where we 'belong'" (Crystal, 1987, p. 13).

The expression of identity is one of the most complex functions of language. In many instances, it is difficult to differentiate between the communication of information and the expression of an identity. This situation is probably most often found in political debates in various arenas such as government, business, and education.

The expression of identity is important for understanding a movement that can be labeled as the "depathologizing of deafness" (Lane, 1988; Padden & Humphries, 1988; Reagan, 1990). This movement has been fueled by the establishment of American Sign Language (ASL) as a bona fide linguistic system and the recognition of Deaf culture. The expression of social, political, and personal identities are evident in statements such as "Deaf is Beautiful," "Deaf Power," and the "Use of Sign Language is the Native Right of All Deaf Children." The call for the establishment of bilingual education programs for deaf students has also been motivated, in part, by the use of language in the expression of identity.

Table 1–1 contains part of a poem that exemplifies the social and personal identities of members of the Deaf culture via the importance of using signs or ASL for communication purposes.

Recording of Information

One of the most important functions of language is the recording of information. Both the primary form of a language (i.e., speech and/or signs) and the secondary form (i.e., written language) can be used to record information. For example, information can be recorded via print (i.e., written language in books and other printed materials), media (e.g., speech on tape recorders, and speech, signs, and captions on films, videotapes), and computers (storing speech, signs, graphics, and captions). One of the foci of this text is on the language of print.

The ability to read and write is one of the most complex skills that humans learn (Adams, 1990; Just & Carpenter, 1987). Progress in

TABLE 1-1. Examples of Social and Personal Identities of Deafness

The Deaf: "By Their Fruits Ye Shall Know Them"

Nature hates force. Just as the flowing stream seeks the easiest path, so the mind seeks the way of least resistance. The sign-language offers to the deaf a broad and smooth avenue for the inflow and outflow of thought, and there is no other avenue for them unto it. —G.M. Teegarden

You Have to be Deaf to Understand

What is it like to comprehend
Some nimble fingers that paint the scene,
And make you smile and feel serene
With the "spoken word" of the moving hand
That makes you part of the world at large?
You have to be deaf to understand. —Willard J. Madsen

Source: Adapted from Gannon (1981).

understanding the process of literacy has dispelled one of the most persistent myths, that print is "speech written down." It has been remarked that:

> when language is used for the purposes of recording facts, it is very different from that used in everyday conversation—in particular, it displays a much greater degree of organization, impersonality, and explicitness. (Crystal, 1987, p. 12)

Adams (1990) and others (e.g., Crain, 1989; Liberman, Shankweiler, & Liberman, 1989) argued that more is required of the reader than the listener. To put it another way—because students can comprehend speech does not mean that they can understand the written equivalents, even if they have good word recognition skills. Listeners receive information from the speakers (e.g., context, prosodic clues, redundancy) which enables them to understand the spoken message. This information is not available to them during the process of reading. In essence, it should be underscored that literacy depends on many types of knowledge, for example, orthography, lexicon, grammar, conventions of discourse, culture, subject matter, and logical inference rules (Anderson & Pearson, 1984; Grabe, 1988; Nickerson, 1986; Rayner & Pollatsek, 1989).

The discussion above should not undermine the importance of an internalized spoken language, including a knowledge of the alphabetic system (i.e., vowels, consonants, and their combinations) for developing literacy skills. This presents problems for deaf students, many of whom do not have access to the "sound system" of the language of print (Hanson, 1989). On a deeper level, it is critical to understand the relationship of written language to the primary form that it represents, in this case, speech. Relative to deafness, it is necessary to understand the relationship of the signed systems to print.

Other Language Functions

The remaining language functions to be discussed are emotional expression, "special effects," and control of reality (Crystal, 1987; Muma, 1986; Whitehead, 1990). That language is used as the expression of emotions can be "heard" in phrases such as "wow," "ouch," and "whoopee." The use of obscenities is also a form of emotive language. The emotive function of language can be expressed alone (e.g., Damn screwdriver!) or in social interactions (e.g., He's a jerk!).

Typically, "special effects" refer to the "power of sound." Children's nursery rhymes and games are good examples of this language function. For example, the rhyming function helps children to "control" the game. "Special effects" are not restricted to spoken languages; they can also be found in sign languages. Instead of "the power of sound," the effects are due to the "power of hand movements."

Perhaps, the most common examples of the control of reality are those associated with religion, the use of magic, and the occult. One of the reasons for the litany of prayers, sounds, and other words directed at supernatural beings and objects is for the individual to gain control over a particular situation. From another perspective, it seems that this type of language is also communicative in nature. However, the response of the supernatural being or object is acknowledged only in the mind of the individual.

THE STRUCTURE OF LANGUAGE

The structure of language refers to the various components, whose names and descriptions are influenced by the prevailing linguistic theories (Bohannon & Warren-Leubecker, 1985; Crystal, 1987; Goodluck, 1991; Ingram, 1989). The language components discussed in this text are phonology, morphology, syntax, semantics, and pragmatics. From one perspective, all but pragmatics constitutes the "grammar" of the language. The lexicon (i.e., words) falls between morphology and syntax; however, the meaning of a word is within the purview of semantics. A better understanding of word identification, an important skill in reading, depends, in part, on an understanding of phonology and morphology. A brief description of each language component is provided in the ensuing paragraphs.

Phonology

Phonology pertains to the sound system of a particular language. Specifically, "phonology concerns the regularities and rules governing pronunciations of words, phrases, and sentences" (Goodluck, 1991, p. 6). Humans are capable of producing a range of sounds with their vocal apparatus; however, only a small, arbitrary sample of those sounds is meaningful for a particular language. The sound system of English refers to the 40 or more distinctive sound units, labeled phonemes, which guide the pronunciation of "words" (see Table 1–2 for a list of consonants and vowels).

It is possible to analyze words as sequences of discrete phonemic aspects. Referring to the information in Table 1–2, the following words are divided into phonetic segments:

TABLE 1–2. List of Selected Consonants and Vowels of English.

Consonants	Vowels
/b/ as in bat	/a/ as in mass
/d/ as in dunk	/e/ as in mate
/dz/ as in jet	/i/ as in beat
/f/ as in fish	/I/ as in hit
/g/ as in give	/u/ as in mood
/h/ as in hat	/U/ as in book
/k/ as in cat	/o/ as in boat
/l/ as in lake	
/m/ as in moon	
/n/ as in noon	
/p/ as in pet	
/r/ as in bar	
/s/ as in some	
/t/ as in time	
/v/ as in van	
/w/ as in wad	
/wh/ as in what	
/z/ as in zip	

Source: Adapted from Creaghead & Newman (1985) and Ling (1976).

B = Books .

```
me    = /m/  /i/
hit   = /h/  /I/  /t/
food  = /f/  /u/  /d/
```

A more detailed discussion of the anatomy and physiology of speech sounds can be found elsewhere (e.g., Crystal, 1987; Goodluck, 1991).

The phonological system also consists of prosodic features such as stress, intonation, and pause, which are critical for the perception of speech (Crystal, 1987; Goodluck, 1991; Ingram, 1989). These features are considered as suprasegmental phenomena. Rules associated with the construct of stress enable listeners to perceive a particular syllable that is emphasized over the others. An adequate knowledge of the phonological system of English includes an intuitive knowledge of rules relating to the production of both segmental and suprasegmental aspects. As mentioned previously, and in greater detail in the chapter on literacy, this knowledge seems to be important for the development of adequate, high-level literacy skills (e.g., Liberman, Shankweiler, & Liberman, 1989).

It is also possible to discuss the phonology of "soundless" languages such as sign languages (Liddell, 1980; Lucas, 1990; Wilbur, 1987). For example, in ASL, there are distinctive manual (i.e., referring to the hand) units such as shape, movement, placement, and orientation (see Table 1–3).

TABLE 1–3. Examples of a Notational System for American Sign Language Signs

Tab Symbols (Hand Location)	Dez Symbols (Hand Shape)
○ Face or whole head	B Flat hand
∩ Forehead or brow, upper face	C Curved hand; like c
∪ Chin, lower face	5 Spread hand; like 5
[ ] Trunk, body from shoulders to hips	F Three-ring hand
✓ Elbow, forearm	O Tapered hand; like o

Sig Symbols (Hand Movement)

∧ upward movement
∨ downward movement
∿ up-and-down movement
> rightward movement
< leftward movement
⊤ movement away from signer
⊥ movement toward signer

Source: Adapted from Stokoe, Casterline, & Croneberg (1976).

Similar to spoken languages, ASL and other sign languages also contain prosodic features. In addition to manual aspects, there are nonmanual aspects which have linguistic functions (e.g., syntactic). Some of the nonmanual (i.e., other than the hands) aspects of ASL are movements of the tongue, cheeks, lips, eyebrows, shoulders, and upper torso.

Morphology   *Smallest segment of speech*

Morphology is the study of morphemes, which can be described as the smallest segment of speech that carries meaning (Goodluck, 1991; Matthews, 1991). In this sense, morphology is related to phonology and is concerned with the structure of words. Morphology is also influenced by and related to syntax, the order of words (Brown, 1973; Crystal, 1987; deVilliers & deVilliers, 1978; Russell, Quigley, & Power, 1976).

This text is concerned with two major divisions of morphology, inflectional and derivational. Inflectional morphology is the study of word variations, or inflections, such as plurality (girl, girls) and tense (walk—present; walked—past). Thus, inflections refer to changes in the root or base word (i.e., uninflected, citation form) to express syntactic functions and relationships. These changes do not affect the meaning of the root or base word.

Derivational morphology deals with the construction of new words, typically via additions of word parts (e.g., in-, re-, -ment, -ness). Derivational morphemes may change the meaning of a word as in clear and unclear or indicate the "part of speech" (form class) of a word, for example, noun suffixes such as -ance in tolerance and -dom in freedom (Deighton, 1959).

The study of morphology is also important for understanding the development of signed systems (e.g., Signed English, Signing Exact English) used with deaf students. The various signed systems are based on the morphosyntactical properties of standard, written English. However, the signed systems have different rules for executing signs, including the use of inflectional signs as well as the construction of new signs via sign markers (similar to word parts) (Paul & Quigley, 1990; Wilbur, 1987). It is also critical to stress that the morphology of the signed systems is different from that of ASL. This issue is undertaken later in this chapter.

Syntax   *Grammar of a language.*

Syntax refers to the order or arrangement of words. This arrangement reveals meaningful relationships within and between sentences. Most syntactic investigations have focused on the relations expressed at the sentence level (i.e., sentence comprehension). This is "where the most important grammatical relationships are expressed" (Crystal, 1987, p. 94).

It is feasible to divide syntactic relations into two major categories: linear and hierarchical. Although descriptions of these terms vary (e.g., see Crystal, 1987), linear structures are defined here as being fairly simple constructions that can be interpreted in a left-to-right fashion (e.g., Subject-Verb-Object [SVO]) as exemplified in the following sentences:

1. The boy hit the ball.
2. Mary read a book.
3. John gave Mary a rose.
4. The man smoked a pipe.
5. The woman drove the truck.

Hierarchical structures are complex and cannot be interpreted in a "simple" SVO fashion. Consider the following sentences as examples.

1. The boy who kissed the girl ran away.
2. The light on the blue police car turned.
3. The girl was mauled by the pit bull.
4. Visiting professors can be boring.
5. That the man was sad was perceived by the woman.

The competent language user understands that the "subjects" of sentences 1 and 2 above are *The boy who kissed the girl* and *The light on the blue police car*, respectively. In sentence 3, *the pit bull* is the performer of an action whereas *the girl* is the recipient. Sentence number 4 is ambiguous; that is, there are at least two interpretations: *Professors who visit* can be boring and *[The act of]* Visiting professors can be boring. In sentence 5, the woman is the person who performs the act of perception. In addition, it is clear to the native user that it is not *sadness* nor the *man* that is perceived; rather it is *the sadness of the man*. As discussed later in the text, deaf students have had enormous difficulty comprehending "hierarchical" sentences, especially on a sentential level (e.g., Russell, Quigley, & Power, 1976).

Chomsky (1957, 1965, 1975, 1988) has revolutionized the field of linguistics via his study of the syntactic component of a language. Chomsky's notion of transformational generative grammar, which has gone through several revisions, is typically a syntax-based grammar. In other words, Chomsky asserts that syntax plays a major role in explaining the grammar of a language. Reactions to Chomsky's views have catapulted two other components of language, semantics and pragmatics, into the limelight.

Semantics   *(Study of meaning)*

In one view, language form refers to phonology, morphology, and syntax, and language content pertains to semantics (Bloom & Lahey, 1978). Semantics is the study of meaning *in* language (Bohannon & Warren-Leubecker, 1985; Crystal, 1987). Meaning can occur at several levels: word, phrase, sentence, and beyond the sentence.

Contemporary linguistic theories of semantics have been influenced by the thinking of philosophers, logicians, and cognitive psychologists (Baars, 1986; Crystal, 1987; Goodluck, 1991; Johnson-Laird, 1988; Steinberg, 1982). The focus is on the study of the way words and sentences are used in specific contexts within a language. The semantics theorists argue that semantics is primary and syntax secondary; that is, semantics determines syntactic representation. Steinberg (1982) provided one description of these theorists' objections to Chomsky's grammar. Semantics theorists:

> argue that syntax cannot be done independently of semantics. Furthermore, they see little need for two levels of syntax. They advocate abandonment of Deep Structure and Base rules, holding that what a grammar must do is to relate the semantic level of structure . . . to a syntactic level of structure, Surface Structure. They posit that this be done with a set of transformational rules and a lexicon. Transformational rules might usefully be regarded as constituting the "syntactic" component of their grammar. The Transformational rules and the Lexicon are viewed as continually interacting so as to produce a final structure, Surface Structure. This view sharply contrasts with that of Chomsky where lexical items are inserted all at once into an already completed tree structure (Deep Structure). (Steinberg, 1982, pp. 48–49)

One of the most interesting aspects of the study of semantics is to determine how "words," or more precisely, lexemes or lexical items, are organized in the mind (Crystal, 1987). Several semantics models have been proposed, for example, networks, frames, and scripts (see brief review in Shadbolt, 1987; see also Anderson & Bower, 1973; Johnson-Laird, 1988; Rumelhart, McClelland, & the PDP Research Group, 1986). In essence, the focus is on how "knowledge" is organized in the mind, and this focus has also influenced current theories of reading (e.g., Samuels & Kamil, 1984). In addition, the study of semantics has provided additional insights into the thought/language debate.

Pragmatics

Pragmatics is the study of the use of language (Bates, 1976; Bloom & Lahey, 1978; Crystal, 1987). Austin (1962), a British philosopher, was one of the first scholars to focus attention on functions of speech utterances in social interactions. He noticed that such utterances do not convey information. These utterances are considered actions (i.e., *performatives*). Examples include statements which contain the words, I believe . . . , I promise . . . , and I apologize . . . .

Searle (1976) studied the effects of the utterances on the behavior of both speaker and listener. His theory of speech acts, particularly his classification of illocutionary acts (the act performed after the speaker's utterances), has influenced research on pragmatics.

A number of pragmatics behaviors have been identified in the communicative interactions of young children, for example, *requesting, showing off, labeling, repeating, negating*, and so on (Thompson, Biro, Vethivelu, Pious, & Hatfield, 1987). Descriptions of some of these behaviors are as follows (Thompson et al., 1987):

Requesting: Solicitation of a service from a listener.

Repeating: Repetition of part or all of previous adult utterance. Child does not wait for a response.

Negating: Denial, resistance to, or rejection by child of adult statement, request, or question. (pp. 11 & 13)

There is some overlap between pragmatics and other language components or areas of language inquiry. For example, both pragmatics and semantics are concerned with the intentions of the language user and the background knowledge about the world of both speakers and listeners as they interact. There are also overlaps between pragmatics and areas such as psycholinguistics and discourse analysis (Crystal, 1987). The analysis of conversations is within the purview of both pragmatics and discourse analysis.

Pragmatics is not considered a part of language structure in the same way as syntax and semantics. A good illustration of this assertion can be seen in the fact that pragmatics errors do not affect the rules of the other language components—phonology, morphology, syntax, and semantics. Nevertheless, pragmatics is intricately connected to the other language domains.

There is some research on the development of some pragmatics aspects in students with hearing impairment. As discussed previously, pragmatics has been influenced by and has in turn influenced the development of social-interaction theories of language acquisition. The roots of social-interaction theories can be found in the writings and research of Vygotsky (1962).

More research on the development of pragmatics in children is needed. It is still true that:

Pragmatics is not at present a coherent field of study. A large number of factors govern our choice of language in social interactions, and it is not yet clear what they all are, how they are best interrelated, and how best to distinguish them from other recognized areas of linguistic enquiry. (Crystal, 1987, p. 120)

PHILOSOPHICAL PERSPECTIVES ON DEAFNESS

Language theories, research, and interventions/practices are influenced by philosophical perspectives on deafness. There are two broad perspectives that affect descriptions of deafness: clinical and cultural. These perspectives are similar in nature to the metatheories of language that are discussed in Chapter 2. Hitherto, the clinical view has dominated the thinking of metatheorists, theorists, researchers, and practitioners in disciplines that focus on the study of deafness (Lane, 1988; Moores, 1987; Paul & Jackson, 1993).

In reading the following descriptions of the two broad viewpoints, the reader should keep two major points in mind. One, the descriptions represent extreme, bipolar positions. There are a number of variations on a continuum between these two extreme views. Research and program models have been influenced by variations that combine tenets from both perspectives (Liedel & Paul, 1991; Paul, 1990, 1991), even though some scholars have argued that these two bipolar views are incompatible (Crittenden, 1993; Lane, 1988; Reagan, 1990; cf. Paul & Jackson, 1993).

Two, it has been argued that if the two bipolar perspectives are incompatible, they may be considered metatheories (Paul & Jackson, 1993). Thus, it is not possible to determine, by using the scientific method, which view is the "better" description of reality. However, it is feasible to refine or improve theories, research, and practices within each viewpoint. Incompatibility is not necessarily a criterion of the existence of two metatheories. Even variations that combine principles from two opposite viewpoints can be considered metatheories (Ritzer, 1991; Turner, 1991).

Clinical Description of Deafness

Relative to deafness, the clinical view has been labeled as a medical or pathological view (Baker & Cokely, 1980; Lane, 1988; Reagan, 1990). However, most of these descriptions are negative and thus are not accurate according to the notion of metatheory (Ritzer, 1991). Perhaps, a better description of the clinical view is to label it as a "mainstream" view (Gliedman & Roth, 1980). In other words, deaf children are described relative to the characteristics of typical children (i.e., normal-hearing) in mainstream society (e.g., schools). Some of the pertinent differences between these two broad groups are the ability to use speech, hearing, and English language skills.

Clinical proponents study the impact of deafness on cognitive, linguistic, and psychosocial developments, typically within the purview of "mainstream" theories and research on nondisabled children. The focus is on remedying the "deficiencies" or improving the skills of deaf children in these areas. One of the main goals is to enable deaf children to participate in mainstream society on social, political, and economical levels. For example, the "prevention" or "cure" of "deficiencies" associated with deafness, and perhaps, even deafness, itself, should lead to an improvement in the low academic achievement levels, which have been documented since the inception of formal, standardized achievement tests (Quigley & Paul, 1986).

Clinical or mainstream theories should not be applied indiscriminately to children with disabilities (Gliedman & Roth, 1980). However, they may be sufficient starting points, especially in the absence of other established theories (Paul & Jackson, 1993). Adequate clinical research on deaf individuals requires the documentation of salient, long-standing demographics and characteristics that have affected the development of English language skills. These include degree of impairment, age at onset, etiology (cause), location of the impairment, parental hearing status, and the condition of additional disabilities (Myklebust, 1964; Quigley & Kretschmer, 1982).

Dimensions of Hearing Impairment

Dimensions of hearing impairment include degree, age at onset, etiology, and location. Age at onset is a linguistic dimension whereas the others are audiological in nature. The focus here is on two of the major dimensions—degree and age at onset—particularly in relation to the development of spoken language.

Hearing impairment is a general, audiological term which pertains to all degrees of losses, regardless of etiology and location. Hearing acuity is measured in decibels across a range of frequencies, typically from 125 to 8000 hertz, or cycles per second (see Davis, 1978 and Meyerhoff, 1986 for a complete description of the measurement and types of hearing losses). The acuity is reported as the average threshold level of pure audiometric tones (pure-tone average—PTA) in the better unaided ear across the speech frequencies, that is, 500, 1000, and 2000 hertz. Table 1–4 illustrates three examples of computed PTAs.

There are five audiological categories that correspond to degrees of hearing impairment (Acoustical Society of America, 1982). There is some debate on what should constitute the "slight" category (e.g., Ross, 1986,

TABLE 1–4. Three Examples of Pure-Tone Average (PTA)

Frequency

	125	250	500	1000	2000	4000	8000
–10							
0							
10							
2							
30			CX				
40			CO				
50			BX BO	CX			
60				BX CO			
70			AO	AO BO	AO BX CX		
80			AX		CO		
90				AX	BO		
100					AX		

Example 1: Left Ear AX = 80, 90, 100, PTA = 90 dB; Right Ear AO = 70, 70, 70, PTA = 70 dB; PTA for better ear = 70 dB

Example 2: Left Ear BX = 50, 60, 70, PTA = 60 dB; Right Ear BO = 50, 70, 90, PTA = 70 dB; PTA for better ear = 60 dB

Example 3: Left Ear CX = 30, 50, 70, PTA = 50 dB; Right Ear CO = 40, 60, 80, PTA = 60 dB; PTA for better ear = 50 dB

1990). The five categories are as follows: slight (27 to 40 dB), mild (41 to 55 dB), marked or moderate (56 to 70 dB), severe (71 to 90 dB), and extreme or profound (91 db or greater). The educational implications of groups of students with these characteristics have been reported in a number of sources (Moores, 1987; Paul & Quigley, 1990; Quigley & Kretschmer, 1982).

Traditionally, students with slight to moderate hearing impairment have been classified as "hard-of-hearing" individuals. One of the most robust findings in the research literature on these groups of students is that even a slight impairment can negatively affect language, literacy, and academic achievement (Paul & Quigley, 1987a, 1989; Ross, Brackett, & Maxon, 1982). With early intervention and an adequate management program that includes a comprehensive array of support services, most students with slight to moderate losses can achieve a high level of competency in English language skills (see discussions in Paul & Quigley, 1990; Ross, 1990; Ross et al., 1982). The overwhelming majority of these students, many of whom are not identified, are enrolled full-time in general-education programs.

Students with severe impairment have constituted a "grey" area. That is, some of these students perform in a manner similar to that of traditional "hard-of-hearing" students. However, others may have difficulties similar to those of students with extreme or profound impairment. It has been argued that poor classroom management conditions have led to the underdevelopment of these students' academic skills (e.g., Ross, 1986; Ross et al., 1982). In addition, placing these students in Total Communication programs (discussed later) or labeling them as *deaf* has resulted in an exposure to a lower quality of oral communication aspects such as training in speech, speech reading, and the use of residual hearing (e.g., Ross & Calvert, 1984).

In our view, students in the extreme or profound category are the only ones who should receive the label, *deaf.* That is, *deaf* refers to individuals who, with or without amplification, are either receiving a fragmented, incomplete auditory message or no message at all. Most—but not all—of these students are connected to a world of vision, in which they are dependent on some form of signing in order to receive and express information. Some students with profound hearing impairment use their eyes (and other skills) to receive information by speech reading a speaker's lips. However, these students are essentially connected to a world of audition, even though they may not hear the sounds adequately (Paul & Quigley, 1990; Ross, 1990). There are also a few students in this category who are able to use their residual hearing, along with their speech reading skills, to achieve high levels of both speech and language development (Connor, 1986; Ling, 1984, 1989).

A better understanding of the language achievement levels of students with hearing losses can be obtained when degree of loss is considered in conjunction with the age at onset factor. Age at onset refers to the age at which the hearing impairment occurred. The time of occurrence of the impairment has a pervasive effect on the development of spoken language.

Because of this notion, age at onset is a linguistic factor. In this conceptual framework, the hearing impairment may be prelinguistic or postlinguistic. A prelinguistic impairment occurs prior to or at the age of 2 years whereas a postlinguistic impairment occurs after the age of 2 years. Birth to 2 years is considered an important period for prelinguistic development; however, a severe to profound hearing impairment disrupts this process (Moores, 1987; Paul & Quigley, 1990; Rodda & Grove, 1987).

Considering both degree and age at onset of impairment together, researchers have reported significant impacts on the development of language and literacy skills (King & Quigley, 1985; Paul & Quigley, 1990; Webster, 1986). For example, a postlinguistic, severely hearing-impaired student may have a higher English language achievement level than a prelinguistic counterpart. The more severe the impairment and the earlier the age at onset, the more significant the impact on language and literacy acquisition.

Degree and age at onset of hearing impairment are highlighted here because of their combined effects. As mentioned previously, it is also important for researchers to consider other factors such as etiology, location of impairment, and the presence of additional disabilities. For example, it has been reported that about one third of students with hearing impairment have additional disabilities (Wolff & Harkins, 1986). That these additional disabilities affect academic achievement is not debatable. However, it is still difficult to detect the presence of some disabilities such as learning disabilities due to the lack of appropriate assessments for students with hearing impairment (Bradley-Johnson & Evans, 1991).

One of the most widely researched factors is parental hearing status. This factor pertains to the hearing acuity of the parents/caregivers, that is, whether the parents/caregivers have normal or impaired hearing. A number of studies have compared the achievement of deaf children of deaf parents (DCDP) with that of deaf children of hearing parents (DCHP). Parental hearing status, similar to socioeconomic status, is not a causative factor. That is, hearing status, by itself, is not the major reason for the differences in achievement in children. Other variables associated with this factor, for example, level of acceptance and quality and form of communication, should be considered (Moores & Meadow-Orlans, 1990; Paul & Quigley, 1990).

Cultural Description of Deafness

At the other end of the spectrum is what can be described as a cultural metatheory or perspective of deafness (e.g., Baker & Cokely, 1980; Lane, 1988; Paul & Quigley, 1990). Only a few remarks are made here. A more detailed discussion of this entity can be found elsewhere (e.g., Gannon, 1981; Neisser, 1983; Padden & Humphries, 1988).

Cultural proponents view deafness as a natural condition, not as a disease or disability that needs to be cured or prevented. It is argued that Deaf individuals do not want to be "like" hearing individuals. That is, the ability to speak and hear are not desirable goals; in fact, they are unrealistic goals for most Deaf people. In essence, the role models for deaf children are Deaf adults, especially those individuals who use ASL and are members of the Deaf culture.

An eloquent anecdote that illustrates the feelings of culturally Deaf individuals is as follows:

A short time ago some members of Congress discussed the establishment of a research institute to identify deafness early and to prevent and cure it. Several deaf activists protested that because they are an ethnic group, the government shouldn't seek to cure their ethnicity. "If I had a bulldozer and a gun," a Gallaudet student leader was quoted as saying, "I would destroy all scientific experiments to cure deafness. If I could hear, I would probably take a pencil and poke myself to be deaf again." (Kisor, 1990, p. 259)

The depathologizing of deafness and the emergence of Deaf culture proceeded in tandem with the growing recognition of ASL as a bona fide language. In addition, it was argued that the use of ASL is not a "compensatory" endeavor as implied by Myklebust (1960, 1964) and other clinical proponents. Rather, ASL, similar to any other language, is used to express many functions of Deaf individuals. For example, one of the most important language functions is identity—personal, social, and political.

The use of a sign language, such as ASL, is thought to be a reflection of Deaf individuals' predisposition toward the acquisition of a visual language. As noted by Neisser (1983), this predisposition is different from the one for hearing individuals, who possess the ability to acquire and use a spoken language:

> The hearing world is deeply biased toward its own oral language, and always prefers to deal with deaf people who can speak. But speech is always difficult for the deaf, never natural, never automatic, never without stress. It violates their integrity; they have a deep biological bias for the language of signs. (Neisser, 1983, p. 281)

COMMUNICATION SYSTEMS

The mode, or form, of communication that should be used to instruct students with hearing impairment is one of the most controversial, long-standing issues in the education of these students (Conrad, 1979; Lou, 1988; Moores, 1987; Paul & Quigley, 1990). There are two modes, or communication philosophies: oralism and total communication (TC). Although the TC philosophy permits the use of ASL as one approach, ASL has not been widely used or systematically investigated in classroom settings since the advent of TC (Lou, 1988; Paul, 1990; Quigley & Paul, 1984; Reagan, 1990). Thus, it might be the case that there is or should be a third communication philosophy—the use of ASL.

Prior to discussing the two major modes and their various approaches, as well as ASL, it is important to clarify the use of other related terms that might cause some confusion. *P.T.O.*

First, it should be stressed that mode of communication does not refer to a specific, language-teaching method. In general, a mode reflects the manner in which a language is *represented*, not taught. Language-teaching method is concerned with the use of structural, natural, or combined approaches in the teaching of a language, specifically English (for an extensive review, see McAnally, Rose, & Quigley, 1987, in press).

The notion of "representing" a language such as English should be highlighted, especially in reference to the use of signed systems within TC programs. As is discussed later, each signed system is purported to represent the structure of written, standard English. The rules for representing certain aspects of English such as past tense and plurality varies across the systems (Paul & Quigley, 1990; Wilbur, 1987). Deaf students are not taught, but rather exposed to a particular system or some form of signing as a medium of instruction. The assumption is that the students either know English or will internalize the rules of a specific system and the language that it represents—English.

On the basis of the discussion above, it should also be clear that the modes of communication are *not* specific methods of instruction. That is, the modes are not methods for teaching reading, mathematics, or science. A specific communication mode might be used as a *medium* of instruction, namely, to convey information. Within this framework, ASL as a "medium of instruction" is most likely to occur in English-as-second-language or bilingual education programs. The use of ASL in these programs has not been extensively documented in the research literature (Paul, 1990; Quigley & Paul, 1984; Strong, 1988a; Woodward & Allen, 1988).

Relative to representing English, the oral communication philosophy has incorporated speech, or the oral form, and TC has used both speech and some form of signing simultaneously. Within the oral philosophy, there are three broad categories of approaches: unisensory, multisensory, and cued speech. There are also variations of these approaches. The TC approaches consist of several manual or signed systems, which can be labeled manual English codes. Many signs in these codes are taken from the lexicon of ASL. However, as is discussed later, this is misleading. Because it differs substantially from both English and the English-based signed systems, ASL is discussed separately from the framework of total communication. The inclusion or discussion of ASL within the TC philosophy is the cause of several misconceptions on the nature and use of ASL (e.g., Woodward & Allen, 1988).

Oralism

In the United States (and other English-speaking countries), the major thrust of oralism is the use of English in the oral form, that is, speech (Connor,

1986; Ling, 1984, 1989). Proponents of oralism stress that "speech" is the medium of instruction for typical normal-hearing students in regular-education programs and the medium of communication for the majority of people in mainstream society. One of the major goals of oral education programs is to enable deaf students to develop oral communication skills in order to participate fully with a majority of English-speaking individuals. The strength of this focus is so strong that a quote from 25 years ago is still applicable today:

> The oral philosophy has a powerful appeal to parents of young deaf children. More than anything else, they want their deaf child to talk and to understand others through lip reading. This is particularly true of parents who have guilt feelings regarding their deaf child. If the child can be taught to speak and read lips well, somehow some or all of the guilt is relieved. (Hester, 1969, p. 154)

Historical perspectives on oralism and its approaches may be found elsewhere (Lou, 1988; Moores, 1987; Paul & Quigley, 1990).

The three major common features of all oral approaches are speech, speech reading, and residual hearing. The use of touch, or taction, is also important, particularly for the development and reception of speech. Speech training focuses on intelligibility, that is, the ability to be understood by listeners. Speech reading refers to the "reading" of lips and other facial cues in order to understand the speaker's message. Residual hearing (aural aspects or audition) is the remaining, usable hearing that can be exploited for the reception of speech via auditory training/learning or amplification devices. In discussing the emphasis of the features within oralism, it has been remarked:

> Some proponents . . . have emphasized or even isolated differing inputs of sensation and information. For example, Pollack . . . has concentrated on the aural or auditory aspects . . . while Ling . . . is known for his speech emphasis, Cornett . . . for his cued speech, and Levitt . . . for his tactile aids. But each of these are acceptable elements . . . and must be included in the definition of oralism. (Connor, 1986, p. 119)

Unisensory Approaches

In unisensory approaches, the primary emphasis is placed on *one* sense, typically, audition; however, vision or taction may also be stressed primarily. Approaches dealing with the development of residual hearing, or audition, have been known as primarily auditory, aural-oral, aural, acoupedic (Pollack, 1984), acoustic (Erber, 1982), and auditory global (Calvert & Silverman, 1983). There is also an approach called the unisensory approach (Beebe, Pearson, & Koch, 1984). In these approaches, deaf children engage in activities designed to encourage them to use their hearing only. Early amplification and proper auditory management (i.e., use of hearing aids) are also essential features. Although the use of speech reading (or vision) is minimized initially, it will be developed or motivated as a result of the intense, earlier focus on audition.

The use of touch primarily, or the tactile-kinesthetic approach, is important for deaf students who do not benefit much from the traditional oral approaches that focus on audition and/or vision (Calvert, 1986; Calvert & Silverman, 1983). The tactile-kinesthetic approach is based on a motor theory of speech production. It incorporates oral communication features such as speech reading, auditory training, and intensive speech training. As in all other approaches, reading and writing are also included.

Multisensory Approaches

Moores (1987) labels the multisensory approach as a "balanced" approach. The "balance" refers to the equal stress on and development of the two primary senses, audition and vision. Similar to the unisensory approaches, early amplification and adequate auditory management are important features. For some students with hearing impairment, the combination of audition and speech reading has been shown to be more effective for understanding speech than the use of audition alone (e.g., Novelli-Olmstead & Ling, 1984). The multisensory approach may also include the use of a tactile component. This variation has been known as the auditory-visual-tactile technique (e.g., Messerly & Aram, 1980; Moores, 1987).

Cued Speech

It is difficult to classify cued speech. According to its creator, cued speech is considered a multisensory oral approach (Cornett, 1967, 1984). However, many educators placed this system within the domain of Total Communication. In this text, cued speech is discussed as one form of Oralism.

In cued speech, eight contrived handshapes are used in four positions either on or near the face (see Figure 1–1). These hand cues supplement the spoken signal. Each handshape represents a group of consonants (i.e., consonantal phonemes) such as /h/, /s/, and /r/. Each group of consonants looks similar on the lips of the speaker. The listener can distinguish between them by observing the lips of the speaker in conjunction with the "consonant" cues. Unlike the use of signs in the signed systems, the use of hand cues without accompanying speech is meaningless.

Each of the four positions represents the "vowels," that is, the vocalic phonemes. The combinations of the hand shapes and "vowel"

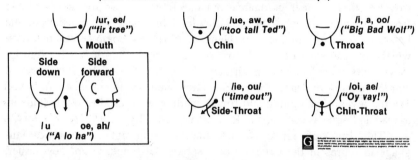

CONSONANT CODE & CUESCRIPT CHART

1 /zh, d, p/ ("je dupe")
2 /tH, k, v, z/ ("the caves")
3 /h, r, s/ ("horse")
4 /b, hw, n/ ("By when?")
5 /m, f, t/ ("miffed")
6 /w, l, sh/ ("Welsh")
7 /j, g, th/ ("joggeth")
8 /ch, y, ng/ ("Chai Yung")

VOWEL CODE & CUESCRIPT CHART
(note: vowels alone are cued with OPEN handshape)

/ur, ee/ ("fir tree") Mouth
/ue, aw, e/ ("too tall Ted") Chin
/i, a, oo/ ("Big Bad Wolf") Throat

Side down   Side forward
/u   oe, ah/ ("A lo ha")

/ie, ou/ ("time out") Side-Throat
/oi, ae/ ("Oy vay!") Chin-Throat

FIGURE 1-1. Cued Speech Symbols. (From the Cued Speech Team, Department of Audiology & Speech-Language Pathology, Gallaudet University, Washington, DC. Reprinted by permission of the publisher.)

positions produce consonant-vowel pairs. Thus, by placing a handshape at any of the four positions, it is possible to represent the consonantal and vocalic sounds of a word in a number of spoken languages. Vowel diphthongs (e.g., *oi* as in *boy*) are executed by a sequence of two different vowel locations. In short, the cued-speech user speaks and represents his or her speech phonemically.

Research on Oralism

Despite its long, illustrious, and contentious history, there has been little research conducted on the effectiveness of the oral approaches since the beginning of formal measures (e.g., Quigley & Paul, 1986, 1989). In addition, few students with severe to profound impairment have been exposed to what can be described as intensive, comprehensive oral programs. More recently, there have been documentations of the effects of cued speech, especially in countries other than the United States (*Cued Speech Journal*, 1990).

Much of the debate on the merits of oralism has centered on the development of intelligible speech and of speech reception abilities. There is growing support for the importance of speech for the development of literacy skills. In this case, the focus is on the awareness of the alphabet code or, in other words, cognitive awareness of the phonological system of the spoken language (e.g., Hanson, 1989).

Manual English Codes

Roy Holcomb, a deaf graduate from the Texas School for the Deaf and from Gallaudet College (now Gallaudet University), is considered the Father of Total Communication (Gannon, 1981). Holcomb coined this term which advocates the use of all forms of communication to teach language to students with hearing impairment. However, the use of simultaneous communication or manual communication methods is not new. Historical records reveal that signing and finger spelling were used to teach students to read and write as early as the 15th century (McClure, 1969; Moores, 1987).

The notion of signed systems, that is, using signs from a sign language to represent the structure of a spoken language, is not new either. During the 18th century, Abbe de l'Epee (1712–1789) and his successor, the Abbe Sicard (1742–1822), attempted to adapt the sign language of their students to conform to the structure of the French language. This novel endeavor to create a French-based signed system was the precursor to the English-based signed systems developed in England and the United States during the 1960s and 1970s. A more detailed account of these events can be found elsewhere (McAnally et al., 1987, in press; McClure, 1969; Moores, 1987; Paul & Quigley, 1990).

The manual English codes refer to the various English-based signed systems and finger spelling that were designed to reflect the morphosyntactic structure of written, standard English in a visual, manual (use of hands) manner. Because the systems are morphologically based, the "signs" represent the English morphemes of *written* words (Raffin, 1976; Wilbur, 1987). As discussed previously, morphology is related to and affected by phonology; however, written language is an abstract representation of spoken language. Thus, knowledge of "spelling-to-sound" correspondence rules, at least, is also necessary for understanding the written word.

From the discussion above, it can be inferred that the signed systems, with their focus on English morphology, are quite different from cued speech, with its focus on English phonology. For example, the first vowel sound in the word, *coffee*, may be "cued" at least two different ways, depending on the dialect of the speaker. In connected discourse (i.e., running sentences), individuals may also pronounce *coffee* with slight differences, and these differences are reflected in cued speech. Typically, the signed systems will execute only one sign for *coffee*. This sign remains the same; that is, it is used in all situations, regardless of the contexts or dialects of the speakers. If individuals are primarily dependent on signing within the signed systems, they are not likely to receive important suprasegmental information such as intonation, stress, and pause.

The crux of the foregoing discussion is not to debate the merits of cued speech versus those of the signed systems. Rather, it is to highlight briefly the relationship of the systems, including cued speech, to the representation of English. Specifically, it is important to focus on the nature and use of the various manual English codes and to present a brief discussion of ASL. The presentation reflects the theoretical placement of the manual codes on a continuum from most representative to least representative of written English. That is, the placement of the codes depends on their representations of a written word. The Rochester method, which represents all of the letters of any word is considered to be most representative of written, standard English. The least representative of the manual English codes has several labels, which have caused considerable confusion in the research and scholarly literature. The term used in this text is English-based signing. Several other systems in between the two extremes—seeing essential English (SEE I), signing exact English (SEE II), and signed English (SE)—are also described. It should be emphasized that all manual English codes are supposed to be executed simultaneously with speech.

Rochester Method

Historically, the Rochester method originated at the Rochester School for the Deaf in New York during the late 1870s (Quigley, 1969; Scouten, 1967). The method entails the use of finger spelling and speech simultaneously. Finger spelling refers to the use of hand shapes that represent alphabetic and numerical systems. In the United States, there are 23 distinct handshapes that correspond to the letters of the alphabet. The movement of three hand shapes represent two different letters each (e.g., *g* and *q*; *k* and *p*; *i* and *j*). Both the sender and the receiver need to have an intuitive knowledge of English, its alphabet system, and the relationship between finger spelling and the alphabet to communicate effectively with each other (see Figure 1–2).

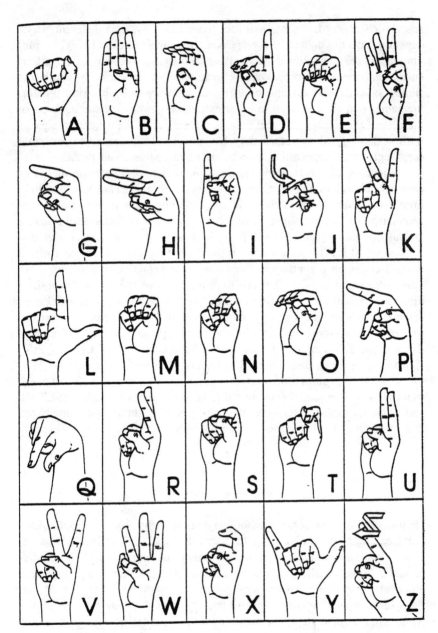

FIGURE 1–2. Finger Spelling—the Manual Alphabet. (Illustrations from *A Basic Course in American Sign Language* [p. 235] by Humphries, T., Padden, C., & O'Rourke, T. J. [1980]. T. J. Publishers, Inc., Silver Spring, MD. Reprinted by permission of the publisher.)

The SEE Systems

The SEE systems refer to two signed systems: seeing essential English (SEE I) (Anthony, 1966) and signing exact English (SEE II) (Gustason, Pfetzing, & Zawolkow, 1980). Because of the overlap in sign-formation principles and historical background, it is feasible to discuss the two systems together. SEE II is covered in greater detail because of the widespread use of its signs (not the entire system) (Gallaudet Research Institute, 1985; Jordan & Karchmer, 1986).

A group of professionals, parents, teachers, and administrators met in California in 1969 to discuss the problem of representing English manually, as described below:

> The main concern of the original group was the consistent, logical, rational, and practical development of signs to represent as specifically as possible the basic essentials of the English language. This concern sprang from the experience of all present with the poor English skills of many deaf students, and the desire for an easier, more successful way of developing mastery of English in a far greater number of such students. (Gustason et al., 1980, p. IX)

This meeting resulted in three signed systems, which were originally similar but now are different: SEE I, SEE II, and Linguistics of Visual English (Wampler, 1972).

Both SEE systems categorize English words into three broad groups: basic (e.g., *girl*), compound (e.g., *butterfly*), and complex (e.g., *runs*). The selection or use of a "sign" to represent a word and its parts is based on a two-out-of-three rule involving sound, spelling, and meaning. For example, consider a word such as *run* in the following sentences:

1. The girl hit a home *run*.
2. There is a *run* in my stocking.
3. I like to walk not *run*.

The same sign is used for *run* in all three sentences above because two of the three criteria are met; sound and spelling. This situation is similar for many English words with multiple meanings.

One of the major differences between the two SEE systems is their treatment of a basic word. This difference results in the use of more contrived inflectional and derivational markers and more "signs" by SEE I to represent a word. For example, in SEE II, the word, *butterfly*, is represented by one sign whereas in SEE I, this word has two "signs," one for *butter* and one for *fly*. In addition, SEE II tends to rely more on "existing" signs, especially from the lexicon of ASL.

In addition to the concepts of basic, compound, and complex words, there are several other important principles of SEE II. As stated by Gustason et al. (1980, pp. XIII and XIV):

1. English should be signed in a manner that is as consistent as possible with how it is spoken or written in order to constitute a language input for the deaf child that will result in his mastery of English.
2. A sign should be translatable to only one English equivalent.
3. When the first letter is added to a basic sign to create synonyms, the basic sign is retained wherever possible as the most commonly used word (e.g., basic sign for MAKE is retained whereas the sign

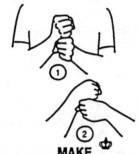

MAKE
Side of S touches on side of S; lift off, both twist to palm-in and touch again

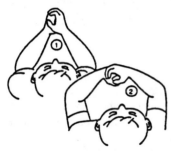

CREATE
Horizontal C's, right on left, both twist to palm-in
(see MAKE)

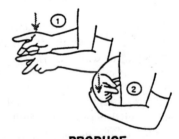

PRODUCE
Touch right P on left, twist hands to palm-in and touch again
(see MAKE)

FIGURE 1-3. SEE II Signs: MAKE, CREATE, and PRODUCE. (Gustason, G., Pfetzing, D., & Zawolkow, E. [1980]. From *Signing Exact English*, published by Modern Signs Press, Inc., Los Alamitos, CA. Reprinted by permission of the publisher.)

is made with C-hands for CREATE and P-hands for PRODUCE (see Figure 1–3).

4. When more than one marker is added to a word, middle markers may be dropped *if* there is no sacrifice of clarity (e.g., the past tense sign is added to BREAK to produce BROKE, but BROKEN may be signed as BREAK plus the past participle or -EN).

5. While following the above principles, respect needs to be shown for characteristics of visual-gestural communication.

Finally, Gustason et al. (1980) also listed suggestions for the development of new signs, that is, signs for English words that are not contained in the SEE II dictionary. The suggestions are as follows (p. XV):

1. Seek an existing sign. Check other sign language texts. Ask skilled signers in your community, especially deaf native signers.

2. Modify an existing sign with a similar or related meaning. Generally, this means adding the first letter of the word to a basic sign.

3. Consider finger spelling. This depends, of course, on the age and perceptual abilities of the child, and the length and frequency of use of the word in question.

4. If all else fails, and you must invent, try to stay as close as possible to ASL principles.

At present, signing exact English is undergoing revisions and another edition of the dictionary will be published soon. An in-depth treatment of the manner in which SEE II handles the pronouns and verbs of English as well as the formation of new words can be found in Wilbur (1987).

Signed English

The rationale of SE is similar to that of the other systems discussed previously. According to Bornstein, and his colleagues:

> Signed English is a reasonable manual parallel to English. It is an educational tool meant to be used while you speak and thereby help you communicate with deaf children.
>
> Here is the basic reason for developing a manual system parallel to speech: Deaf children must depend on what they see to understand what others say to them. (Bornstein, Saulnier, & Hamilton, 1983, p. 2)

There are two groups of signs in SE: "sign words" and sign markers. The SE dictionary contains more than 3,100 sign words. These "words" were compiled from lists of normal-hearing children's spoken language and from vocabulary lists used with young deaf children in homes and class-rooms. A number of signs are ASL-like signs; however, there are signs that are contrived and signs that are borrowed from other signed systems (Wilbur, 1987).

In general, the use of a sign is based on its entry (i.e., bold face type) in a dictionary of standard English (no specific dictionary is named). Despite the exceptions discussed in the dictionary (Bornstein et al., 1983), there are other "exceptions" that exist because of (1) numerous English multimeaning words with several lexical entries, and (2) disagreements among lexicographers on what constitute a lexical entry and what mean-ings should be included in a specific lexical entry.

The 14 sign markers represent the most common inflectional and derivational morphemes in the language of young children. The SE mark-ers are illustrated in Figure 1–4.

SE signs plus markers are executed in an English word order, that is, paralleling the exact spoken utterances. Some basic rules with excep-tions include:

> One sign for each English word: There are a number of phrases, proper nouns, and compounds, of two or more words, in this dictionary which are represented by a single sign word. These exceptions are, for the most part, idiographic, unam-biguous ASL signs. Some examples are: *after a while, of course, Santa Claus, . . .* and *yo-yo.*
>
> One sign word for a separate English dictionary entry: There are two or more signs for a number of single English dictionary entries such as back, blind, brush, fall, glass, right, watch. The various signs represent different meanings of the same English word. For example, the noun *fall* and the verb *fall* are etymo-logically related; however, the common and well-established signs for these words are too ideographic to be used interchangeably.
>
> Thus the two words will be represented by two different sign entries.
>
> One sign word plus only one sign marker: Because use of the agent marker does not preclude a noun form further assuming a plural or possessive form, we permit the use of two sign markers in this one instance; for example, work + agent + plural, or speak + agent + possessive. (Bornstein et al., 1983, p. 8)

Figure 1–5 illustrates some of the sign words from SE.

English-based Signing

There is a form of signing that does not adhere to a clear-cut set of prin-ciples, save the following of an English word order. Traditionally, this signed form has been labeled pidgin sign English (PSE); however, it has been known by other names such as signed English, sign English, Sign English (Siglish), American sign English (Ameslish), manual English, simultaneous communication, and total communication (Bragg, 1973;

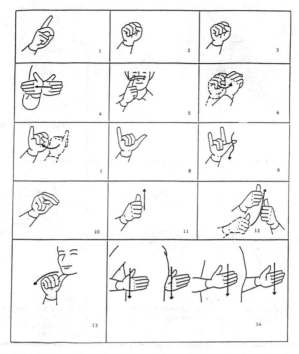

FIGURE 1-4. The 14 Sign Markers of Signed English. (Reprinted by permission of the publisher, from Bornstein, H., Saulnier, K., & Hamilton, L., *The Comprehensive Signed English Dictionary*, [1983]; Inside front cover. Washington, DC: Gallaudet University Press. Copyright 1983 by Gallaudet University.)

NOTE:

1 = regular past verb: -ed—talked, wanted, learned
2 = regular plural nouns: s—bears houses
3 = 3rd person singular: s—walks, eats, sings
4 = irregular past verbs: (sweep RH open B, tips out to the right)—saw, heard, blew
5 = irregular plural nouns: (sign the word twice)—children, sheep, mice
6 = possessive: 's—cat's, chair's
7 = verb form: -ing—climbing, playing, running
8 = adjective: -y—sleepy, sunny, cloudy
9 = adverb: -ly—beautifully, happily, nicely
10 = participle: fallen, gone, grown
11 = comparative: -er—smaller, faster, longer
12 = superlative: -est—smallest, fastest, longest
13 = opposite of: un-, im-, in-, etc. (made before the sign word, as a prefix)—unhappy, impatient, inconsiderate
14 = agent (person and thing): (left picture—sign made near the body)—teacher, actor, artist; (right picture—sign made away from the body)—washer, dryer, planter

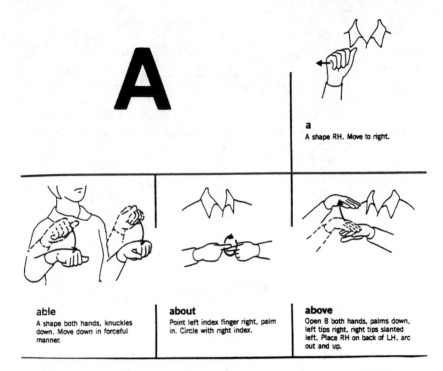

a
A shape RH. Move to right.

able
A shape both hands, knuckles down. Move down in forceful manner.

about
Point left index finger right, palm in. Circle with right index.

above
Open B both hands, palms down, left tips right, right tips slanted left. Place RH on back of LH, arc out and up.

FIGURE 1–5. Examples of Signs from Signed English. (Reprinted by permission of the publisher, from Bornstein, H., Saulnier, K., & Hamilton, L., *The Comprehensive Signed English Dictionary,* [1983]; 29. Washington, DC: Gallaudet University Press. Copyright 1983 by Gallaudet University.)

Quigley & Kretschmer, 1982). This form of signing has also been labeled "sign-supported speech" (Johnson, Liddell, & Erting, 1989).

In this text, we adopt the phrase, English-based or English-like signing to refer to this signed form (Paul & Quigley, 1990). In general, English-based signing is a combination of both English and ASL features executed in an English word order. The use of the features from either language depends on the language proficiency of the signer. For example, if a signer has a high ASL language proficiency and a low English language proficiency, many of the features incorporated in the signing will be taken from ASL. As a result, English-like signing may vary substantially from signer to signer.

Another major source of variation is the sign communication competency of educators and practitioners. To suit their needs, some educators may "borrow" signs from other signed systems while using English-like signing. In fact, this is encouraged within reason (e.g., see Gustason et al.,

1980). There are no set rules for "borrowing" signs, either from one signed system or from several systems. The problems associated with the concept of "borrowing" signs is discussed in further detail later in this text.

It is permissible to consider English-based signing a manual English code; however, it cannot be labeled a pidgin as in Pidgin Sign English (PSE) (Cokely, 1983; Paul & Quigley, 1990; Wilbur, 1987). The term PSE refers to a "pidginization" of ASL and English. Typically, a pidgin involves two languages with the same *form*, that is, speech or sign. A pidgin develops when two speakers or two signers are unfamiliar with the other's language. For example, in a English-French spoken pidgin, some words are English, some French, and some may be a blend of English and French. The syntax is that of the majority language, which is typically listed first in a pair (e.g., English in English-French). Analogically, the same is true for a ASL-FSL (i.e., French Sign Language) signed pidgin. That is, some signs are ASL, some FSL, and some may be a blend of ASL and FSL.

It is not clear how pidginization occurs when the forms of the two languages, for example, ASL and English, are not similar. However, if a particular signed system meets all the requirements of a bona fide *language*, it is possible to have a pidgin comprised of both ASL and that particular signed system. It should be remembered that a pidgin requires that the two languages be of the same form. Thus, in our example, the pidgin entails the signs of ASL and the *signs* of the particular signed system, which is representative of English.

American Sign Language

The study of ASL began with Stokoe (1960) and descriptions of the grammar were published in the late 1970s (Baker & Cokely, 1980; Klima & Bellugi, 1979; Lane & Grosjean, 1980). ASL entails both manual and nonmanual features. The manual features pertain to the shapes, positions, and movements of the hands whereas the nonmanual features refer to the movements of the cheeks, lips, tongue, eyes, eyebrows, shoulders, and the body (e.g., for body shifts). ASL is suited to the motor capacities of the body and the visual capacities of the eyes.

ASL is a visual-gestural language, and, like other sign languages, does not involve the use of speech sounds. That is, instead of speech, native signers express their ideas using manual and nonmanual body features simultaneously. In addition, like other visual-gestural sign languages, there is no standardized, literate form of ASL. Native signers do not read or write their messages in ASL. Information is presented and received via the primary form of ASL, namely sign, which is analogous to speech for this purpose. Examples of ASL are illustrated in Figure 1–6.

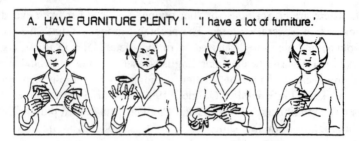

A. HAVE FURNITURE PLENTY I.   'I have a lot of furniture.'

HAVE PLENTY FURNITURE I.   'I have a lot of furniture.'

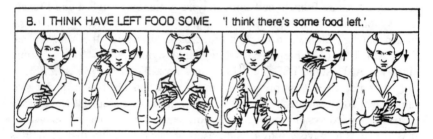

B. I THINK HAVE LEFT FOOD SOME.   'I think there's some food left.'

I THINK HAVE LEFT SOME FOOD.   'I think there's some food left.'

FIGURE 1–6. Examples of American Sign Language Signs. (Illustrations from *A Basic Course in American Sign Language* [p. 132] by Humphries, T., Padden, C., & O'Rourke, T. J. [1980]. T. J. Publishers, Inc., Silver Spring, MD. Reprinted by permission of the publisher.)

ASL and English

Not only is the grammar of ASL different from that of English, but also it is different from that of the various signed systems designed to represent English (Lou, 1988; Paul & Quigley, 1990; Wilbur, 1987). Despite the overlap of "signs" between ASL and some signed systems, there are important differences in the various components such as phonology, morphology, syntax, and semantics. For example, the phonological system of ASL is rule governed, permitting a finite number of features such as the number of allowable hand shapes. Some hand shapes that correspond to the "initialization" of signs in, for example, the SEE systems are not allowable in ASL. That is, these hand shapes violate "phonological" principles.

To provide examples of some other differences between ASL and the signed systems, consider that in ASL:

1. Space may be used to designate and distinguish individuals (pronouns). The area in front of the signer is reserved for second person pronouns; the areas to the sides for third person pronouns.

2. Questions are signalled by the use of eyebrow movements and head tilts.
3. Reduplication (repeated movements) is used to express notions such as plurality, degree, or emphasis.
4. Grammatical boundary is marked by the use of pause between signs or sign sequences.
5. The spatial area can be varied to correspond to "louder" or "quieter" signing.

More recent research on the grammatical features above and other features of ASL can be found elsewhere (Baker & Cokely, 1980; Liddell, 1980; Lucas, 1990; Wilbur, 1987).

FINAL REMARKS

This chapter provided an overview of two major concepts, language and deafness. Specific language areas include function, structure, and medium. Relative to deafness, the chapter covered the two broad philosophical perspectives, clinical and cultural, and the three major language/communication systems used in the education of deaf students, oralism, total communication, and American Sign Language. Finally, it was highlighted that this text is mainly concerned with students who have severe to profound hearing losses, not with all students with hearing impairment.

In our view, the effects of an early onset of deafness on language development is most evident for students with severe to profound hearing impairment. The ongoing debate can be expressed in, but not limited to, the following questions:

1. Should the manual or oral form (or both) of English be developed in deaf children during their preschool and early childhood years?
2. How well do deaf children learn English through exposure to the various forms?
3. Should ASL or some form of English be developed initially in deaf children?
4. Is it possible to learn English literacy skills in ASL/English bilingual programs?
5. What is the relationship of the language or language form to the development of cognition?

There is no debate that there are a number of factors to consider in addressing the questions above as well as their implications. In addition to providing background on theories of language, the thought/language debate, theories of literacy, bilingualism, and language assessment, this text attempts to provide insights into the impact of deafness on language development.

FURTHER READINGS

Campbell, J. (1982). *Grammatical man: Information, entropy, language, and life*. New York: Simon & Schuster.

Fromkin, V., & Rodman, R. (1978). *An introduction to language* (2nd ed.). New York: Holt, Rinehart, & Winston.

Keyser, S., & Postal, P. (1976). *Beginning English grammar*. New York: Harper & Row.

Scheetz, N. (1993). *Orientation to deafness*. Boston, MA: Allyn & Bacon.

Scouten, E. (1984). *Turning points in the education of deaf people*. Danville, IL: Interstate Printers & Publishers, Inc.

Van Cleve, J., & Crouch, B. (1989). *A place of their own: Creating the Deaf community in America*. Washington, DC: Gallaudet University Press.

C H A P T E R 2

LANGUAGE ACQUISITION: METATHEORIES, THEORIES, AND RESEARCH

I t all started with an ape that learned to speak. Man's hominid ancestors were doing well enough, even though the world had slipped into the cold grip of the ice ages. They had solved a few key problems that had held back the other branches of the ape family, such as how to find enough food to feed their rather oversized brains. Then man's ancestors happened on the trick of language. Suddenly, a whole new mental landscape opened up. Man became self-aware and self-possessed. He broke free of the grip of the present—the moment-to-moment life lived by all other animals—and became master of his own memory. Language allowed man to relive his past, plan for the future, and step back to consider the fact of his own existence. Through speaking, man rapidly developed a self-conscious mind. (McCrone, 1991, p. 9)

As revealed by this passage, the emergence of language had pervasive implications for the social and cognitive development of humans. The study of language—particularly how it is acquired, what is acquired, and the time frame in which it is acquired—has intrigued scholars for centuries. A number of current language scholars (e.g., Cairns, 1986; Chomsky, 1975) have stated that the remarkable achievement of language acquisition is part of the general puzzle of human knowledge acquisition, as expressed in a quote by the philosopher, Bertrand Russell (1948): "How comes it that human beings, whose contacts with the world are brief and personal and limited, are nevertheless able to know as much as they do know?" (p. 5).

This chapter presents several prevailing perspectives on the answer to Russell's question. Specifically, we discuss some highlights of the major theories of language acquisition and their general aspects such as innateness, maturation, functionalism, competence/performance dichotomy, and research methodology. Most of the current language theories are essentially "mental models" due to the influence of the cognitive revolution. However, some theorists, notably Searle (1992), have questioned the notion of building and testing mental models for language or other cognitive activities. Nevertheless, relative to language theories, a better understanding of the models requires an adequate description of their metatheoretical foundations. Thus, the chapter begins with a description of the notion, metatheory, and the three major types of metatheorizing.

After discussing metatheories and theories, we provide background information on the manner in which language acquisition has been approached. That is, the chapter describes the concepts of prescription, description, and explanation. These concepts correspond to the various theories of language and have influenced the development of language-teaching methods, especially in the education of deaf students.

The chapter ends with a brief overview of the research on language and deafness. Additional information on the research studies on primary (i.e., speech, sign), secondary (i.e., reading, writing), and bilingual development is presented in the ensuing chapters. The intent here is to show how research has been influenced not only by the metatheories affecting the development of language, but also by those concerning the perspectives on deafness, namely clinical and cultural views.

METATHEORY

In science, a metatheory is a framework, or perspective, that determines how one should do science (Baars, 1986; Bunge & Ardila, 1987). Indeed, a metatheory ascertains whether a particular discipline is a science or not. For example, there have been several debates on whether psychology belongs to the sciences or to the humanities (Bunge & Ardila, 1987). Although the term metatheory is related to others such as paradigm (Kuhn, 1970) and philosophy (Baars, 1986; Bunge & Ardila, 1987; Ritzer, 1991), these three terms are not synonymous.

Within a scholarly field, a metatheory directs the compositions of theories and the types of research methodologies. Within this framework, theories are tested and refined, and the ones that are the most predictive (or aesthetic!) survive the test of time. Thus, a metatheory can be an overarching framework for the scholarly activities within a particular discipline (Ritzer, 1991).

Because of its nature, it is not possible to evaluate an overarching metatheory as "accurate" or "inaccurate." It is also difficult to compare one overarching metatheory with another overarching metatheory. This situation is similar to the notion of paradigm, discussed by Kuhn (1970). Regis (1987) provided an eloquent, readable rendition of this problem:

> For example, if a given scientific community accepts the idea that nature is alive, the notion that there's an *elan vital* at work in the universe, then those scientists will be inclined to interpret natural phenomena teleologically. They'll see events happening for purposes, and view them as if they're all part of a master plan. But another group, one which holds to a philosophy of mechanism (according to which events occur in strict "billiard-ball" cause-and-effect sequences), those scientists will perceive the world quite antithetically. As to whose picture of reality is *correct,* well . . . that's not a question we ask, Kuhn said. At least we don't ask such a question as scientists. (p. 213)

Ritzer (1991) describes three general types of metatheorizing in sociology; these descriptions are also applicable to metatheorizing in other scholarly fields. One type of metatheorizing is undertaken to obtain a better, deeper understanding of extant theory. A second type of metatheorizing focuses on the study of extant theory in order to develop a new theory. The third type, which is somewhat similar to our discussion of metatheory above, "is oriented to the goal of producing a perspective, one could say *a* metatheory, that overarches some part or all of sociological (*or psychological or other disciplinary*) theory" (Ritzer, 1991, p. 6; emphasis and words added). It should be highlighted that these three types of metatheorizing involve the study of theory and occur after theory has been well developed within the field. There is another type of metatheorizing, which acts as an overarching metatheory and is proffered prior to the development of a theory (or even research within a theory). However, this type is considered a weak form of "metatheorizing" and has been shown to cause numerous, unproductive philosophical problems (Ritzer, 1991).

Language and Metatheory

Theories of language development have been influenced by three broad metatheories of psychology, as well as sociocultural perspectives from sociology and anthropology. The three broad metatheories are introspectionism, behaviorism, and cognitive science. Each metatheory is distinguished by its approach to the study of the mind, or what is commonly known as the oldest problem in philosophy—the mind/body problem (Baars, 1986; Eacker, 1975; see Bunge & Ardila, 1987 and Priest, 1991 for in-depth discussions of the various perspectives on the mind/body problem). A brief introduction to the three broad metatheories is presented in the ensuing pages. It is important to emphasize that these are broad types based on one conceptual framework (i.e., Baars, 1986). There might be variations or combinations of these major categories, which are beyond the scope of this chapter.

Introspectionism

Introspectionism can be defined as the process of examining one's mind, specifically the contents, thought process, or sensory experience. It is related to the notion of metacognition (e.g., Baker & Brown, 1984) and to that of mentalism (e.g., see discussions in Baars, 1986, and Steinberg, 1982). According to introspectionism, psychologists (and related scholars) should focus on conscious human experiences. The systematic investigation of human consciousness should lead to a complete understanding of humanity (i.e., human behavior or conduct). The research methodology can be described as systematic or analytic self-observation. It was hypothesized that thoughts could be analyzed or, rather, reduced to substructures or elements (Baars, 1986; Medin & Ross, 1992).

The appeal of this approach to the study of the mind can be seen in the following passage:

> It would seem that we are all potential experts on how the mind works because we have a lot of firsthand experience with our own thoughts and other people's behavior. We often make inferences about other people's beliefs, desires, and intentions and we seem to have privileged, direct access to our own thoughts. Therefore, what better source of information about the mind than introspection? (Medin & Ross, 1992, p. 23)

The use of systematic or analytic self-observation has provided data for the development of linguistic theories (discussed later), particularly those influenced by the mentalistic, rationalistic thinking of Chomsky (1957, 1975). Nevertheless, one major reason that introspectionism as a metatheory is not in vogue is due, in part, to the influences of the unconsciousness on human behavior, which is not considered in the introspectionism metatheory (e.g., Medin & Ross, 1992).

Behaviorism

As a metatheory, behaviorism was a reaction to the notion of introspectionism (Baars, 1986; Medin & Ross, 1992). In general, behaviorists assert that psychology should focus on the study of observable behavior.

Influenced by the work of John B. Watson, behaviorism dominated the field of psychology, particularly experimental psychology, in the United States from about 1913 to the late 1940s (Baars, 1986; Medin & Ross, 1992). In contrast, European psychologists were influenced by movements such as Gestalt psychology, psychoanalysis, and Piagetian theory. Watson, who is considered to be the "Father of Behaviorism":

> argued that behavior is objective and observable and that the agenda for psychology consists of formulating laws relating stimulus conditions to behavior. Consciousness, introspection, and the mind were to play no role in this science of behavior. His views were reinforced by the logical positivist movement in philosophy. Logical positivism emphasized operational definitions tied to specific operations or observations. (Medin & Ross, 1992, p. 24)

The views of Watson and other radical behaviorists, notably B.F. Skinner, represent the most extreme anti-mentalist position relative to the mind-body problem (Baars, 1986; Priest, 1991; Steinberg, 1982). At least four behaviorist positions on the mind/body phenomenon have been delineated (Steinberg, 1982). Regardless of the differences among the positions, the common area of agreement is that the focus of investigation should be on the "body" (i.e., observable behaviors). In one sense, this is interpreted to mean that psychology is not fundamentally different from physiology.

The decline of behaviorism began during the late 1940s (Medin & Ross, 1992). Although behaviorism has declined tremendously since the late 1950s, especially after a scathing review by Chomsky (1959), it still exerts a considerable influence in clinical and animal psychology and in some areas of special education. Perhaps, much of the influence in special education is due to the usefulness of "single-subject" research methodology (e.g., see discussion of special-education reading in McCormick, 1987). In addition, it is possible to see some influence of behaviorism on current language theories, especially those that emphasize the importance of the language-user's performance (e.g., spoken utterances) and the role of the social environment.

To understand this influence, it is important to present the general tenets of behavioristic views of language learning. As is discussed later, the focus is on the view of Skinner (e.g., 1957), who attempted to describe language learning in terms of reinforcement principles. At present, the general principle of behaviorism is thought to have an extremely small role in the language acquisition process (Goodluck, 1991; Medin & Ross, 1992; Steinberg, 1982). Perhaps, the best explanation for this situation is "Behaviorism . . . never got very far in accounting for complex learning" (Medin & Ross, 1992, p. 25).

Cognitive Science

It is difficult to label the cognitive revolution; in psychology, it could be labeled as cognitive psychology (Baars, 1986; Medin & Ross, 1992). However, because the revolution has influenced research and thinking in other fields, notably linguistics, computer science, and philosophy, it could be labeled as cognitive science. Relative to psychology, this metatheory asserts:

> that psychologists observe behavior in order to make inferences about underlying factors that can explain the behavior. They agree with behaviorists that the data of psychology must be public, but the purpose of gathering this data is to generate theories about unobservable constructs, such as "purposes" and "ideas," which can summarize, predict, and explain the data. In particular, cognitive psychologists often talk about the *representations* that organisms can have of themselves and of their world, and about the transformations that these representations undergo. "Transforming representations" is sometimes called *information processing*. Using this kind of theoretical metaphor, cognitive psychologists can interpret commonsense psychological terms in a rather straightforward way. Thought, language, knowledge, meaning, purpose, imagery, motives, even consciousness and emotion-all the commonsense vocabulary inherited from our culture becomes scientifically useful again. (Baars, 1986, pp. 7–8)

As indicated by the passage above, the grand aims of cognitive science seem to focus on resolving long-standing, controversial epistemological issues, namely, those that deal with the nature, extent, and development of knowledge (Baars, 1986; Shadbolt, 1988). One of the most controversial areas is the nature of mental representation. That is, is knowledge represented by symbols, which are, in turn, manipulated (e.g., organized) by an information-processing system? Are there some other forms of mental representation, besides symbols? Is mental representation necessary?

Another area of immense importance, related to the problem of knowledge, is labeled the levels hypothesis (Marr, 1982). Marr (1982) posited three level accounts. Level 1 account can be considered the computational level. At this level, researchers/scholars specify what it is they are attempting to solve (i.e., goals such as letter recognition, syntactic knowledge, etc.), why they are solving it (i.e., appropriateness of the goal), and how they expect to arrive at a goal of computation (i.e., strategy). Level 2 account deals with the implementation of Level 1. Specifically, this concerns the representation of input/output phenomena and the algorithm (i.e., step-by-step procedures) for the transformation process, that is, the transformation of the sensory data to representations (e.g., mental representations). Level 3 account involves the hardware implementation. It describes the intricate apparatus of the physical structure or device (e.g., the brain) in which the aspects of Level 2 are housed.

Each level has a role to play in contributing to a comprehensive, complete explanation of the cognitive process. Relative to language development, Chomsky (e.g., 1975) has argued that Marr's Level 3 account is not important for developing a comprehensive theory of human language acquisition (for an opposing perspective, see Rumelhart, McClelland, & the DP Research Group, 1986). For example, understanding the physiological processes (e.g., theory of neurons, brain mapping techniques) of the language" area of the brain will not explain the language competence (i.e., intuitive knowledge) of the language user.

The theories discussed in this chapter can be labeled predominantly a Level 1 account. In addition, these theories have been influenced by the behavioristic and cognitive science metatheories. The goal of most current theory and research on language acquisition is to arrive at a Level 2 account.

As discussed in the next section, there is also what can be called a "social" component in one group of theories. At present, the social component is not well developed; however, the underpinnings can be traced to the work of Vygotsky (1962) and the thinking of others in social literary criticism and the sociocultural fields, notably sociology and anthropology (see discussions in Lemley, 1993; Wagner, 1986). A summary of the major points of the three metatheories of psychology can be found in Table 2–1.

THEORIES OF LANGUAGE ACQUISITION

In the first edition of this book (Quigley & Paul, 1990 reprint edition of the original 1984 book), we described four major categories of language acquisition theories: behaviorism, transformational generative grammar (TGG), cognition, and socioculture. These four categories are still applicable. For example, Whitehead (1990) categorizes language theories as behaviorist, nativist (similar to TGG), cognitive, and social-interactionist (identical to socioculture). Bohannon and Warren-Leubecker (1985) used three broad groups: behavioristic, linguistic, and interactionist. In this framework, both cognitive and social approaches are considered interactionist.

In our view, Bohannon and Warren-Leubecker's (1985) framework is most useful because it underscores major differences among the groups relative to two controversial issues: innateness versus empiricism (similar to nature/nurture) and competence versus performance. The competence/performance issue, in particular, has engendered two seemingly distinct camps in the study of language: child language (or child language development) and language acquisition (Ingram, 1989; Whitehead, 1990).

TABLE 2-1. Summary of Major Points of the Three Metatheories of Psychology

Introspectionism

- This is the process of examining one's mind, specifically the contents, thought processes, or sensory experiences.
- The focus is on conscious human experiences.
- The research methodology is systematic or analytic self-observation.

Behaviorism

- The focus is on the study of observable behavior.
- Psychology is not fundamentally different from physiology.
- Language learning is described in terms of reinforcement principles.

Cognitive Science

- The main reason for observing behavior is to make inferences about underlying factors that can explain the behavior.
- The grand aims seem to focus on resolving long-standing, controversial epistemological issues, namely, those that deal with the nature, extent, and development of knowledge.
- One of the most controversial areas is the nature of mental representation.

Source: Adapted from Baars (1986) and Shadbolt (1988).

Behavioristic Theories

Behavioristic theories have been influenced by the behaviorism metatheory, which posits that only the body (i.e., observable behaviors) of the mind/body phenomenon is worthy of study. The intent here is to discuss the general tenets of behavioristic theories, relative to language development. Because of the emphasis on observable data, behaviorists are interested in the associations or connections between environmental stimuli (empiricism) and the language behaviors of the child (performance).

Two general processes describe these associations or connections: classical conditioning and operant conditioning (Skinner, 1957). Typically, classical conditioning is used to account for the development of receptive language (mostly vocabulary) and an additional learning principle, that is, operant conditioning, accounts for productive speech. These two processes assume that all behaviors are learned and that there is little or no need for the concept of "innate structures."

Bohannon and Warren-Leubecker (1985) have provided a good example of the process of classical conditioning. This example focuses on the acquisition of the meaning for the word, *milk*.

> Milk (the unconditioned stimulus, or UCS) fed to a hungry infant usually results in physiological responses in the infant (the unconditioned response, or UCR). When the infant's mother says the word *milk* prior to or during feeding, this word (the conditioned stimulus, or CS) becomes associated with the primary stimulus, the milk, and gradually acquires the power to elicit a response (the conditioned response, or CR) in the child that is similar to the response to the milk itself. (Bohannon & Warren-Leubecker, 1985, p. 180)

To account for the child's production of speech, the principle of operant conditioning entails the notions of imitation and reinforcement used by parents. The parents provide a language model for the child. The child is rewarded after a successful imitation of the model, moving from simple sounds to more complex speech. This process is called shaping, which results in the acquisition of the desirable behaviors.

In light of current thinking on language development, the notions of imitation and reinforcement play a very small role in the child's production of language. From one perspective, it does not account for the child's playing with the language, that is, the child's inventiveness, even when the child seems to know the meaning of a word. Probably, the most convincing evidence of the limited role of behaviorism in child language development can be seen in children's uses of words or phrases. Examples include *All gone cookie* and *He goed*. At first glance, these examples are ungrammatical and are not spoken (or reinforced) by typical parents or adult users of the language. However, these utterances and others are understood better in the light of the child's progress toward linguistic maturity. That is, these statements represent intermediate steps (i.e., hypothesis testing) in the child's acquisition of the grammar of language.

Linguistic Theories

Prior to the recognition of the work of Chomsky, the behaviorism metatheory, as well as the logical postivistic movement in philosophy, exerted a marked influence on linguistic theorists (Baars, 1986; Medin & Ross, 1992; Whitehead, 1990). This is most evident in the works of structural linguists, including those who focused mainly on the phonological component of languages. With its focus on description, one of the major shortcomings of structural linguistics was its difficulty (or, rather, inability) to explain how language users understand the ambiguity of sentences, for example: *The chicken is ready to eat* and *Visiting linguists can be dangerous.*

Despite their differences, current linguistic theories have been influenced by the cognitive metatheory and the views of Chomsky (1957, 1965, 1975, 1980). It has been remarked:

> that by studying language we may discover abstract principles that govern its structure and use, principles that are universal by biological necessity and not mere historical accident, that derive from mental characteristics of the species. A human language is a system of remarkable complexity. To come to know a human language would be an extraordinary intellectual achievement for a creature not specifically designed to accomplish this task. A normal child acquires this knowledge on relatively slight exposure and without specific training. . . . For the conscious mind, not specially designed for the purpose, it remains a distant goal to reconstruct and comprehend what the child has done intuitively and with minimal effort. Thus language is a mirror of mind in a deep and significant sense. It is a product of human intelligence, created anew in each individual by operations that lie far beyond the reach of will or consciousness. (Chomsky, 1975, p. 4)

The information in the passage above provides the background for the discussion of Chomsky's major principles: theoretical adequacy, innate capacity, and the notion of competence.

Chomsky (1957, 1965) has proposed that the road to theoretical adequacy consists of three broad levels. For the first level, the linguist needs to describe (or catalogue) all behaviors that are a part of language. These language behaviors must be distinguished from nonlanguage behaviors. To reach a second level of adequacy, the linguist needs to identify a finite number of connective principles which account for (and predict) the appearance of the language behaviors. These two levels of Chomsky constitute the Level 1 hypothesis of Marr (1982), discussed previously. The third and final level of theoretical adequacy is reached when linguists can identify a finite set of principles which accounts for the *actual* rules and mechanisms used by children, relative to the observed language behaviors. The third level corresponds to the Level 2 hypothesis of Marr (1982). Thus, in Chomsky's view, a complete theory of language development must account for both the language behaviors and the processes used by children during the entire language development period.

Because of the limited, albeit adequate, exposure to language and the time frame in which language is acquired, Chomsky has championed the idea of innate knowledge. In general, Chomsky believed that humans are born with minds that contain innate knowledge of a number of different areas (Chomsky, 1975; Steinberg, 1982; for another interesting perspective, see Fodor, 1983). The faculties of mind are independent of one another. Thus, the faculty containing an innate knowledge of language is independent of that containing an innate knowledge of mathematics. In essence, the language innate knowledge is responsible alone for the development of language; knowledge of mathematics or logic is not necessary.

The innate knowledge, relative to language, has been labeled the LAD, or the Language Acquisition Device [also referred to as Universal Grammar] (Bohannon & Warren-Leubecker, 1985; Steinberg, 1982). This knowledge becomes functional or operational when it interacts with the linguistic environment. In Chomsky's view, the environment does not "shape" linguistic knowledge; rather, it activates the innate linguistic knowledge. With this perspective, Chomsky (1975) offered a compelling answer to Russell's question that was discussed previously:

> We can know so much because in a sense we already knew it, though the data of sense were necessary to evoke and elicit this knowledge. Or to put it less paradoxically, our systems of belief are those that the mind, as a biological structure, is designed to construct. We interpret experience as we do because of our special mental design. We attain knowledge when the "inward ideas of the mind itself" and the structures it creates conform to the nature of things. (Chomsky, 1975, p. 8)

It can be inferred that linguistic theories of language are theories of language competence (Stevenson, 1988). These theories attempt to describe the abstract system of rules that account for a person's knowledge of language. This rule system must be sufficient enough to explain a native language user's production and comprehension of a myriad of sentences, many of which she or he has not heard or read previously. According to Chomsky (1957, 1965, 1975), this knowledge is not completely evident in the speaker's performance, that is, utterances. For example, the utterances of speakers are subjected to memory lapses, false starts, and parsimony. Although many speakers can produce and understand complex sentences of "unlimited lengths," they choose to produce shorter sentences. A theory of grammar should describe speakers' knowledge of all possible, permissible sentences, not only sentences that they utter. Only by appealing to speaker's intuitions can linguists arrive at a theory of grammar. Thus, a competence theory "is designed to account for our ability to decide whether or not a sentence is grammatical" (Stevenson, 1988, p. 8).

Chomsky based his notions of innate faculties and the competence/performance distinction on the study of syntactic structures. Many linguists accept the major features of these notions; however, most of the objections (or differences) are due to the emphasis on a syntax-based grammar (Steinberg, 1982). In other words, these theorists object to the primary role being assigned to syntax with a secondary role assigned to semantics.

Semantic theorists argue that semantics is primary and syntax is secondary. It should be reemphasized here that semantics refers to meaning *in language*. The most prominent semantic movements were those associated with the notions of generative semantics, case grammar, and relational

P.T.O

grammarians (see discussions in Steinberg, 1982 and Steinberg & Jakobovits, 1971). Essentially, semantic theorists argue that semantic structures can be specified independently of syntactic structures and that syntax depends on or is guided by semantic underpinnings.

Within the linguistic theoretical framework, Chomsky's notions still dominate, mainly because the work of semantic theorists is not well developed. Linguistic theory has evolved significantly since the beginning of "transformational grammar." The evolution of the theory has proceeded from standard theory to interpretative semantics to trace to government and binding, leading to the more recent notion of head movement (Chomsky, 1981, 1988; Goodluck, 1991; Steinberg, 1982; Stevenson, 1988). For example, government and binding reduces the number of transformations (phrase structure rules) to only one, which is abstractly defined as "move x," and assigns more structure or information to the individual lexical items (i.e., at the word level). A good readable explanation of government and binding theory can be found in Stevenson (1988) and Goodluck (1991).

A heavy emphasis on the notion that language has a grammar that is separate from or independent of its use plus a different perspective on the notion of nativism (e.g., constructionist, discussed later) has created what can be described as "two distinct fields of language acquisition" (Ingram, 1989, p. 27). As discussed by Wasow (in Ingram, 1989):

> There has been, for some years now, a fairly sharp split in the field of developmental psycholinguistics between what I will call researchers in "child language" versus those in "language acquisition." Child language research is concerned primarily with what children say; that is, it focuses on the *data.* The central concern of most child language research is on data collection and classification, with correspondingly close attention to data collection *techniques,* and relatively little concern for abstract theoretical issues. Language acquisition specialists . . . regard child language as interesting only to the extent that it bears on questions of linguistic theory. (Ingram, 1989, p. 27)

Relative to the discussion above, most "language acquisition specialists" are linguists, that is, they have received their formal training in linguistics. In contrast, most "child language researchers" are psychologists, who have received their formal training in psychology with an emphasis on language development (Ingram, 1989). These individuals are also known as psycholinguists. Language acquisition specialists begin with the linguistic theory (i.e., competence model) and then focus on the problems of language acquisition (i.e., performance data). On the other hand, child language researchers tend to engage in what can be called "inductive" theorizing, that is, hypotheses are generated from the patterns observed in the performance data of children.

There are a number of scholars who believe that a complete theory of language acquisition needs to consider both competence and performance (e.g., Ingram, 1989; Stevenson, 1988). Many child language researchers disagree with linguists on the notion of nativism and the role of the social environment. Most child language researchers belong to a third group called interactionist.

Interactionist

Relative to interactionist theories, it has been remarked that:

> If the behavioristic and linguistic approaches can be considered radical comple-
> ments on the ends of each theoretical continuum, then the interactionist might be
> thought of as a moderate compromise between them. (Bohannon & Warren-
> Leubecker, 1985, pp. 187–188)

The interactionist theory (perhaps, a micro-metatheory) incorporates tenets from both behavioristic and linguistic approaches. The term interaction implies that there are a number of factors—for example, cognitive, linguistic, and social—that are critical for the development of an individual. It is important to emphasize the interactive influences of these factors. For example, language factors influence the development of cognition and social development. As another example, cognitive and social factors affect the acquisition of language. The interactionist framework has had a marked influence on the thinking of the relationship between thought and language (Cromer, 1981, 1988a, 1988b).

Within the interactionist framework are two major approaches (Bohannon & Warren-Leubecker, 1985; Whitehead, 1990). One approach labeled, cognitive-interactionist, is concerned primarily with the relationship between cognition and language development. This approach, also called a cognitive approach (Quigley & Paul, 1990; Whitehead, 1990), has engendered several cognitively based thought/language hypotheses. The second major approach, labeled social-interactionist, focuses primarily on the relationship between social development and language acquisition. Although this approach has contributed to the thinking of the relationship between cognition and language, one of its major influences seems to be on theories and research on pragmatics, that is, factors that govern language choices during social intercourse (Crystal, 1987).

Cognitive-Interactionist

The major impetus for the cognitive-interactionist position is the work of Jean Piaget on the development of cognition (see discussions of Piaget's work in Flavell [1985] and Phillips [1981]). Piaget's thinking highlights two important differences—mentioned previously—between the cognitive-interactionist and linguistic positions: competence/performance and nature/nurture (or rather, the innate principle).

Similar to the linguistic advocates, cognitive-interactionists recognize the distinction between competence and performance. However, cognitive-interactionists believe that performance data can provide useful information on the language acquisition process of children (Bohannon & Warren-Leubecker, 1985; Ingram, 1989; Stevenson, 1988). It is argued that the cognitive capacity of children is both qualitatively and quantitatively different from that of the mature adult language user. By observing the performances of children, it is possible to provide a more complete understanding of the road to mature linguistic development. Cognitive-interactionists also believe that the cognitive processes that underlie children's linguistic performance are also the same processes that account for children's linguistic competence.

The innate principle was one of the major topics of a debate by Chomsky and Piaget (Ingram, 1989; Piattelli-Palmarini, 1980). Chomsky's views on the innate principle discussed previously (i.e., LAD or Universal Grammar) have been labeled as maturationism. Succinctly stated, the maturationist position of innateness posits that linguistic knowledge is innate and becomes functional or operational when the individual interacts with the environment (Ingram, 1989; Steinberg, 1982). Thus, environmental stimuli activate this innate knowledge; they do not shape or modify it.

Piaget's views on the innate principle have been labeled as constructivism. The constructivist position assumes that:

> The complex structures of language might be neither innate nor learned. Instead, these structures emerge as a result of the continuing interaction between the child's current level of cognitive functioning and his current linguistic, and nonlinguistic, environment. (Bohannon & Warren-Leubecker, 1985, p. 189)

In this view, language development (as well as other kinds of development) is said to be a part of the overall cognitive development of individuals. Language development may be an independent system; however, its growth depends on the development of cognitive underpinnings. This approach is compatible with Vygotsky's (1962) notion of inner speech (i.e., symbolic speech) in which thinking dominants or regulates language processes. Vygotsky's internalization principle has also influenced the development of the social-interactionist approach.

Social-Interactionist

Perhaps, the compromise between linguistic and behavioral approaches is most evident in the social-interactionist framework. In describing this framework, Whitehead (1990) remarked that many developmental psychologists, who were interested in human (i.e., adult-child) interactions, began to pay more attention to and to reaffirm the roles that these interactions play in the learning process. In particular, there was an emphasis on the language interactions. It was argued that the language-learning process is facilitated by the critical functions of language—for example, for social-communication interactions and making sense of the world in which we live. Thus, developmental psychologists began to support the concepts associated with the linguistic theory of pragmatics. Additional support for the social-interactionist view can be gleaned from the research on the social activity and sensitivity of infants, including the newborn.

Similar to linguistic proponents, social interactionists assert that language has a unique, rule-governed structure. However, they argue that these structures develop (i.e., emerge or result) from the social functions of language as evident in human interactions. The development of more mature linguistic functions permits the growth of more sophisticated human interactions. Social interactionists view language acquisition as a complex, reciprocal, dynamic interplay between the child and the social-linguistic environment.

A better understanding of this dynamic interplay may be seen in the following discussion. Consider that linguists view children as active processors of language. Because of language's specialized nature, children's development is guided by maturation (Bohannon & Warren-Leubecker, 1985; Ingram, 1989; Whitehead, 1990). The input of significant others is important because this input "triggers" (sets in motion) the innate structures.

On the other hand, behaviorists view children as passive processors of language information. Children's development is guided mainly by the stimuli and actions (e.g., reinforcement) of significant others, particularly parents. In essence, the input and actions of significant others are totally responsible for children's language development.

By focusing on turn-taking and other "pragmatic" functions, social interactionists assert that children's utterances elicit a response from parents (particularly mothers) and vice versa. The social interaction is dynamic and enriching because parents provide language stimuli necessary for children's language growth. Relative to the competence/performance issue, social interactionists believe the linguistic competence of children can only be understood by their performance (i.e., understanding and use) within a social context.

It can be inferred from the foregoing discussion that social interactionists believe that both "nature" and "nurture" factors contribute to the child's acquisition of language. The following passage exemplifies this position:

> Social interactionists . . . recognize that humans are physiologically specialized
> as language users and that some language abilities may require the maturation of

physiological systems in order to appear. .... On the other hand, interactionists, like the behaviorists, insist that the environment, particularly the social interactive system, is the place to look for the emergence of language. Proponents of this view insist that some specific types of experience and even training are probably necessary for children's language to develop. The social interactionist argues that innate mechanisms alone cannot explain the children's mastery of language and, moreover, that linguistic competence goes beyond conditioning and imitation to include nonlinguistic aspects of interaction: turn-taking, mutual gaze, joint attention, context, and cultural conventions. (Bohannon & Warren-Leubecker, 1985, p. 193)

A summary of the major points of the three groups of language theories can be found in Table 2–2.

THE STUDY OF LANGUAGE

The study of language acquisition is essentially the study of how the neonate, apparently totally devoid of linguistic skills, develops into an adult who enjoys the full command of at least one human language . . . It is an amazingly rapid process, given the complexity of the acquisition enterprise. (Cairns, 1986, p. 4)

An understanding of the phrase, the study of language, requires some discussion of several other concepts: prescription, description, and explanation. In addition, it is important to relate the study of language to the ongoing debate on the mind/brain problem.

Prescription, Description, and Explanation

The three terms, prescription, description, and explanation, are not always mutually exclusive. For example, prescriptive grammarians are interested in describing (description) the grammar of the language (Crystal, 1987). Descriptive grammarians may also attempt to provide explanations of language acquisition rules (Ingram, 1989). Finally, linguists who are interested in explanatory adequacy do rely on descriptions of the grammar, at least as a starting point (Chomsky, 1965, 1975). Nevertheless, there are some salient characteristics associated with each term. In addition, each term has been influenced, or rather, is the outcome of the prevailing theoretical perspectives of an era, discussed previously in this chapter.

It is argued that much of the focus of language research, including that on deafness, should be placed on description and explanation (Ingram, 1989; Quigley & Paul, 1990). As is discussed later, the goal of language research should be to "explain" language acquisition, specifically how language (and other knowledge) is represented in the mind of the user.

TABLE 2–2. Summary of Major Points of the Three Groups of Language Theories

Behavioristic Theories

- Behaviorists are interested in the associations or connections between environmental stimuli (empiricism) and the language behaviors of the child (performance).
- Two general processes characterize the associations or connections: classical and operant conditioning.
- The two processes, classical and operant conditioning, assume that all behaviors are learned and that there is little or no need for the concept of "innate structures."

Linguistic Theories

- Current linguistic theories have been influenced by the views of Noam Chomsky.
- It can be inferred that linguistic theories are theories of language competence.
- Linguistic theories have evolved from standard theory to interpretative semantics to trace to government and binding.

Interactionist Theories

- These theories incorporate tenets from both behavioristic and linguistic approaches.
- There are two major approaches: cognitive-interactionist and social-interactionist.
- Interaction implies that there are a number of factors—for example, cognitive, linguistic, and social—that are critical for the development of an individual.

Source: Adapted from Bohannon and Warren-Leubecker (1985) and Skinner (1957).

Subsequently, this explanation is the basis on which to develop instructional and assessment techniques.

Prescription

Focusing on the writing of grammars and dictionaries, it is possible to see the influence of prescriptive grammarians, especially in the 18th century (Crystal, 1987; Ingram, 1989). Prescriptivism implies that a specific dialect of a language is more prestigious, or has a higher value, than other dialects. Typically, the dialect that is favored is one associated with the standard, written form of the language, particularly in its literature (i.e., classic works). As a result, this dialect establishes the norms of pronunciation and grammar. "Correct" pronunciation and grammar adhere to this "prestigious" dialect whereas differences (or rather, deviations) reflect an "incorrect" usage.

This notion of prescribing, and even proscribing, the tenets of "correct" usage of the language is still present in modern times. The emphasis is on maintaining "high" linguistic standards. The following description of prescriptivism is illustrative:

> The aims of these early grammarians were threefold: (a) they wanted to codify the principles of their languages, to show that there was a system beneath the apparent chaos of usage, (b) they wanted a means of settling disputes over usage, (c) they wanted to point out what they felt to be common errors, in order to "improve" the language. The authoritarian nature of the approach is best characterized by its reliance on "rules" of grammar. Some usages are "prescribed," to be learnt and followed accurately; others are "proscribed," to be avoided. In this early period, there were no half-measures: usage was either right or wrong, and it was the task of the grammarian not simply to record alternatives, but to pronounce judgment upon them. (Crystal, 1987, p. 2)

Description

The descriptive view was influenced by two major forces in the early 20th century, the logical-positivist school of philosophy and the behaviorist movement in psychology (see previous discussion on behaviorism) (Ingram, 1989; Rodda & Grove, 1987). This view was most evident during the period of 1926 to about 1957 (Ingram, 1989). One result of these influences was structural linguistics. The emphasis on uncovering the facts of language—that is, describing language usage—rather than on establishing standards also has a long history. Crystal (1987) remarked that advocates of this view emerge during the second half of the 18th century (i.e., from 1750 onward).

To obtain a glimpse of the descriptive approach, consider the following example (Crystal, 1987). Prescriptive advocates state that the word, *whom,* instead of *who* should be used in both spoken and written language in sentences such as:

_____ did you give the book to?

Descriptive grammarians argue that:

> *Whom* is common in writing, and in formal styles of speech; but *who* is more acceptable in informal speech. The rules which govern acceptable speech and writing are often very different. (Crystal, 1987, p. 3)

Although there are strengths and weaknesses of any approach, it is relevant here to state some weaknesses of the descriptive approach, which became the springboard for the explanatory movement in linguistics (Crystal, 1987; Goodluck, 1991; Ingram, 1989; Whitehead, 1990). It is more accurate to state that these weaknesses are associated with the large sample studies which constituted child language research from 1926 to 1957 (Ingram, 1989).

One of the prominent weaknesses was the focus on the presence of language structures such as vocabulary, sentence length, and speech sounds (Ingram, 1989). In other words, the descriptive approach attempted to document the number of words, types of words, length of sentences, and type of speech sounds in the language of children at certain stages. The focus on group data yielded the age at which certain structures, for example, relative clauses and passive voice, appear; however, this focus does not "explain" how the rules are acquired. It has been noted:

> Language . . . is much more than vocabulary, sentence length, and speech sounds. It is a system of rules, and insights into the acquisition of these rules is at the core of the study of language acquisition. (Ingram, 1989, p. 16)

Explanation

The emphasis on explanatory adequacy or rule-based descriptions of language acquisition was influenced by the thinking of Noam Chomsky (1957, 1965, 1980, 1988). Some specific tenets of Chomsky's approach have been discussed previously. The intent here is to provide insights into the notion of explanation as expounded by Chomsky.

Chomsky (1965) argued that linguists should focus on describing the competence of the language user (i.e., native speaker; can also be native signer). By competence, Chomsky was referring to the underlying rule system which manifests itself in utterances that are observed in the performance of language users. This rule system is below the conscious level of the individual; that is, it is known intuitively or tacitly. Nevertheless, the competence of the native language user governs the production of utterances that are observed. In essence, Chomsky stated:

> It should be clearly recognized that a grammar is not a description of the performance of a speaker, but rather of his linguistic competence. (Chomsky, 1965, p. 35)

Chomsky's competence/performance view has engendered several reactions, which have stressed, at least, the importance of other language components, notably, semantics and pragmatics. However, to obtain a complete understanding of the explanatory view, it is necessary to highlight briefly Chomsky's view of language study. The main implication of this view is that linguistics is a domain of psychology, specifically cognitive psychology. The underlying rule system of a language or languages reveal more than just the grammar or grammars. It has been stated that:

> By studying the properties of natural languages, their structure, organization, and use, we may hope to gain some understanding of the specific characteristics of human intelligence. We may hope to learn something about human nature; something significant, if it is true that human cognitive capacity is the truly distinctive and most remarkable characteristic of the species. Furthermore, it is not unreasonable to suppose that the study of this particular human achievement, the ability to speak and understand a human language, may serve as a suggestive model for inquiry into other domains of human competence and action that are not quite so amenable to direct observation. (Chomsky, 1975, pp. 4–5)

The major points of the three views of language are summarized in Table 2–3.

LANGUAGE AND THE MIND

With the advent of the explanatory focus of language researchers within a cognitive metatheory, theorists have attempted to build mental models based on the manner in which language (and other types of knowledge) is represented in the mind (Fodor, 1983; Medin & Ross, 1992; Priest, 1991; Searle, 1992). As mentioned previously, the attempt is to provide a Level 2 description (Marr, 1982). One of the most controversial models has been proposed by Fodor (1983).

Fodor (1983) proffered his modularity hypothesis, which was motivated by the notion of Universal Grammar (i.e., the Language Acquisition Device) and which, itself, has influenced a line of research. Fodor's view is that the brain is organized in a vertical manner with separate "modules" to deal with specific, localized information. For example, he argued that the brain deals with visual information in a set of modules. Initially, these modules do not communicate with other areas of the brain. An example of this process is as follows:

> At a magic show we "know" that one thing is taking place before our eyes but we continue to "see" something quite different. It's as if two separate modules are operating independently, each exerting only the faintest influence on each other. (Restak, 1988, p. 253)

Despite the influence of this model, it has been criticized because of its inability to deal with the complex operations of the brain such as self-awareness and memory (Restak, 1988).

TABLE 2-3. Major Principles of Prescription, Description, and Explanation

Prescription

- The notion implies that a specific dialect of a language is more prestigious, or has a higher value, than other dialects.
- The notion of prescribing, and even proscribing, the tenets of "correct" usage of the language is still present in modern times.
- The emphasis is on maintaining "high" linguistic standards.

Description

- The notion is influenced by two major forces: logical-positivist in philosophy and behaviorism in psychology.
- The emphasis is on uncovering the facts of language, that is, describing language usage.
- The focus is on documenting the number of words, types of words, length of sentences, and type of speech sounds in the language of children at certain stages.

Explanation

- The emphasis is on explanatory adequacy or rule-based descriptions of language acquisition.
- The focus is on describing the competence of the language user, that is, the underlying rule system which manifests itself in utterances that are observed via performance.
- With explanation, one "may hope to gain some understanding of the specific characteristics of human intelligence" (Chomsky, 1975, p. xx).

Source: Adapted from Chomsky (1975), Crystal (1987), and Ingram (1989).

Perhaps the most radical counterproposal in recent years is that of Searle (1992), who also was responsible for the theory of speech acts, which contributed to the revolution of pragmatics as a legitimate area of language study. In developing his hypothesis on the manner in which the mind works, Searle focused on resolving the famous mind-body problem, which has baffled philosophers for centuries. In essence, Searle's position is that there is no need for developing mental models or models that explain how the brain processes information. This proposal is a reaction against the thinking of Chomsky, in particular, and other cognitive scientists, in general. That is, Searle argued that there is no psychological reality for the notion of Universal Grammar. In addition, there is no rule following and no language of thought in the brain.

Searle reasoned that mental events are "features" of the brain in the same way that liquidity is a feature of water. For Searle, the important concepts are consciousness and intentionality. Thus, researchers should focus on understanding the parameters of these concepts. This perspective has pervasive implications for theory, research, and instruction relative to language acquisition. For example, it might be debatable whether language can be taught via the presentation of a natural order of structures based on a mental model of how language is acquired. More specifically, the development of mental models is, in Searle's view, a misguided, dead-end endeavor.

It seems that Searle's thinking is an extension of his views on speech acts relative to a social-interactionist view of language development. In our opinion, Searle's remarks are also related to the introspectionist metatheory (discussed previously) with the addition of a strong neurobiological component. A sample of Searle's argument is as follows:

> The brain, as far as its intrinsic operations are concerned, does no information processing. It is a specific biological organ and its specific neurobiological processes cause specific forms of intentionality. In the brain, intrinsically, there are neurobiological processes and sometimes they cause consciousness. But that is the end of the story. All other mental attributions are either dispositional, as when we ascribe unconscious states to the agent, or they are observer relative, as when we assign a computational interpretation to his brain processes. (Searle, 1992, p. 226)

ISSUES IN LANGUAGE AND DEAFNESS

Relative to the information presented in this chapter, this section provides a brief overview on certain issues in language and deafness, such as:

- the interrelationships of theory, research, assessment, and practice
- the study of language and deafness
- the development of language

This information sets the stage for the more detailed discussion of the language development of deaf children in the rest of the text.

Interrelationship

This construct can be posed as a question: Is there or should there be an interrelationship among theory, research, assessment, and practice? It is possible to conduct research to validate aspects of a theory; however, the implications of a theory for assessment and practice are not always clear (e.g., Eacker, 1975; Ritzer, 1991). Nevertheless, in the field of reading and hearing children, it has been argued, for example, that assessment and practice should adhere to the salient principles of literacy theories (Nystrand & Knapp, 1987; Pearson & Valencia, 1986).

In the field of deafness, much of the research and practice seems to be atheoretical or, rather, a trial-by-error process to determine "what works for the child." In addition, there has been little research conducted on deafness and language comprehension, particularly the teaching of language and reading skills. This has led to the remarks by Clarke, Rogers, and Booth (1982), which are still applicable today: "The current state of instructional methodology is one of confused eclecticism . . . (due to) . . . the remarkable lack of empirical data in this critical area" (p. 65). More important, it is difficult to interpret the ongoing research so as to offer implications for practice.

Despite these problems, there are two notable examples, at least, of scholars who have attempted to establish this linkage from theory to practice. For example, the longitudinal work of Quigley and his colleagues (discussed later in the text) was based on linguistic theory, particular on the thinking of Chomsky. Quigley and his colleagues were also influenced by interactive theories of reading. These foci have led to the development of language materials (e.g., the recent publications of the TSA syntax program) and reading materials (e.g., Quigley, Paul, McAnally, Rose, & Payne, 1990, 1991).

The second example is the monograph supplement of the *Journal of the Academy of Rehabilitative Audiology* (Kretschmer & Kretschmer, 1988a). Much of the work in this monograph has been influenced by pragmatics, particularly within the framework of social-interactionist theory of language development. In essence, it is possible to see the linkage of the various strategies for assessment and practices to the belief that:

> The child's development and use of communication, whether spoken, signed, or written, must be seen in a socially interactive context. Children require both communication models and opportunities to communicate in order to construct their own communication competence. (Kretschmer & Kretschmer, 1988b, p. 5)

Study of Language and Deafness

As is evident later, much of the research on the language development of deaf students has focused on "descriptions" of the acquisition of English via the use of the various signed systems. With the acceptance of American Sign Language (ASL) as a bona fide language, there seems to be a reemergence of "prescription" viewpoints, particularly in the domain of linguistic chauvinism. The crux of the matter is that there is very little research that strives for "explanation." That is, there are few ongoing efforts to uncover the reasons why deaf students have difficulty acquiring, for example, complex syntactic structures or multimeanings of vocabulary words and to suggest ways to remedy the situation.

Traditional prescription views of language are the precursors to the more recent view of linguistic chauvinism. Linguistic chauvinism refers to the view that some languages (e.g., English, French) are more prestigious or have a higher value than other languages. This notion has been a part of the discussions on language and deafness. For example, prior to the emergence of a sign language such as ASL, it was not uncommon for researchers and educators to refer to high forms of signing and low (i.e, uneducated) forms of signing (e.g., Baker & Cokely, 1980; Reagan, 1990; Wilbur, 1987). Typically, the high forms of signing refer to the use of signs in an English word order whereas the low forms of signing were described as nonstandard English or low forms of English.

In retrospect, it seems that some high forms of signing resemble the signing in one of the manually coded English systems such as SEE I or SEE II or the attempts to sign in an English word order such as English-based signing. The low forms of signing might have been executed by students who either did not know English well or who knew ASL. In either case, the low forms of signing were not easily understood by classroom teachers and other practitioners. In addition, many teachers of students with hearing impairment do not know or are not proficient in the use of ASL (Woodward & Allen, 1988).

Despite the acceptance of ASL as a bona fide language, it does not have the same level of prestige in an educational setting as English-based signing (e.g., Reagan, 1985, 1990). There are several factors that contribute to this condition—most notably is the persistent debate on whether ASL and other sign language users can receive and express information relative to the wide range of complex topics that are typically available to English and other spoken language users (see discussion in McAnally et al., 1987; Quigley & Paul, in press). This debate is not on the linguistic status of ASL; that status is well accepted (Baker & Cokely, 1980; Klima & Bellugi, 1979; Liddell, 1980; Lucas, 1990). Rather, the focus is on the availability or accessibility of mainstream culture experiences (e.g., books, literature, television) in natural, meaningful situations (e.g., see discussion in Paul, 1993). To simplify, it is meaningless to "translate" a political debate between President Clinton and members of Congress if the participants are not aware of or have not experienced the concepts of politics and government. Whether these kinds of information should be or can be made available to ASL users is discussed in Chapters 4 and 5, especially in the chapter on literacy.

Despite the proliferation and the development of the various signed systems, there is a dearth of "descriptive" research on the merits of these systems. In addition, most school programs do not adhere to a particular system, that is, none of the signed systems is widely used (e.g., Jordan & Karchmer, 1986). Thus, much of our knowledge on language and deafness has come from the results of secondary language measures (Allen, 1986; King & Quigley, 1985).

King (1981) has argued eloquently that there are two foci that need to be recognized and researched further. These can be expressed as questions:

1. How do deaf children acquire language?
2. How well do deaf children acquire language?

From one theoretical viewpoint, we have some information on these two questions relative to development in the English language and, in some cases, ASL. However, there is a great need for additional research on deaf students' reception and expression of information not only in the various signed systems, but also in American Sign Language. Some of the questions that still need to be examined are:

1. What does it mean to represent English manually?
2. Can English be represented manually in a consistent and systematic manner? Is consistency of representation important?
3. Is a manual representation of English *similar* to the type of representation provided by the use of speech?
4. What do we know about deaf children's acquisition of ASL? Is the acquisition of ASL easier than the acquisition of English? What are the implications of this question, relative to the issue of acquiring *any* language at as early an age as possible?

The Development of Language

Perhaps one of the most important issues in language and deafness is to determine whether the English language development of deaf students is qualitatively similar to that of hearing students. That is, it is critical to know whether deaf students proceed through stages, make errors, or use language strategies that are similar to those of hearing students. The outcomes of this research on language, reading, and writing have pervasive implications for theory and instruction. In addition, it might also provide information on whether the development of English is a feasible construct for many students with severe to profound hearing impairment.

Relative to theory, the issue of qualitative (or developmental) similarity is related to the deeper issue of whether it is permissible to use, in part, theory and research on hearing students to understand, do research, or make policy on language and deafness. There is some support that research on deafness should be conducted mainly by Deaf researchers and within the metatheoretical framework of a cultural perspective (Lane, 1988; Reagan, 1990). One of the most radical manifestations of this view is that proposed by Johnson et al. (1989): ASL should be the language of instruction for *all* deaf students, regardless of degree of hearing impairment and parental background.

As discussed later in this text, there is a substantial amount of research that provides some insights into the English language and literacy development of deaf students. This research has kept in mind the caveat expressed elsewhere:

> It is simply not enough to apply mainstream developmental theories to disability. Psychologists must first assess the applicability of these theories to each of the many groups of children with handicaps. (Gliedman & Roth, 1980, p. 59)

More important, there seems to be sufficient information to provide an answer to the question of whether there is a psychology of deafness (i.e., qualitatively different development) relative to language and cognitive development.

FINAL REMARKS

This chapter presented basic information on metatheories and theories of language acquisition. In addition, we described the various ways in which language has been studied. In the last section of the chapter, we related this information to selected, major issues of language and deafness. Our intent was to highlight constructs that are discussed in detail in the ensuing chapters.

One of the most important issues relative to language and deafness concerns the development of language. For example, it is important to know whether the English language development of deaf students is similar to or different than that of typical hearing students. Research on this issue will provide some perspectives on the development of a first language in deaf students at as early an age as possible. In addition, the question of whether English is a feasible language for students with severe to profound impairment will be addressed. Finally, the outcomes of this research might provide some insights into the question of whether mainstream theories of language and literacy should be applicable to deaf students.

FURTHER READINGS

Atkinson, M. (1992). *Children's syntax: An introduction to principles and parameters theory.* Cambridge, MA: Blackwell.

Bloomfield, L. (1933). *Language.* New York: Holt, Rinehart, & Winston.

Hattiangadi, J. (1987). *How is language possible? Philosophical reflections on the evolution of language and knowledge.* La Salle, IL: Open Court.

Lyons, J. (1970). *Noam Chomsky.* New York: The Viking Press

Snow, C., & Ferguson, C. (Eds.). (1977). *Talking to children: Language input and acquisition.* Cambridge, UK: Cambridge University Press.

Watson, J. (1928). *Behaviorism.* Chicago, IL: Norton.

CHAPTER 3

LANGUAGE AND THOUGHT

We would never consider a machine intelligent that repeats a task over and over again without getting bored or learning from its mistakes. The ability to remember and utilize experiences seems central to what we call intelligence. Yet having a large stock of past experiences stored in memory does not necessarily mean that they can be recalled and used when they are appropriate. Experiences need to be organized so as to be useful for understanding and reasoning processes. And even the best organization can become unusable over time, so memory needs to be reorganized as the needs of those understanding and reasoning processes change. (Schank & Farrell, 1988, p. 120)

From the passage above, it can be inferred that two constructs, intelligence and memory, are concerned with organizing, remembering, and using information. Within the cognitive metatheory, the notions of intelligence, memory, and even language are considered cognitive constructs. Relative to language, Chomsky (1975) proposed that linguistics should be a subdiscipline of cognitive psychology. For the purposes of this chapter, it is argued that a better understanding of the organization and application of knowledge is contingent on a better understanding of the relationship between language and thought.

It should be underscored that we are interested in the relationship between some of the major aspects of cognitive functioning, such as memory and perception, and those of language, such as vocabulary and syntax (e.g., sentence comprehension). As we noted in the first edition of this text (Quigley & Paul, 1990) and elsewhere (Paul & Quigley, 1990), the language/thought relationship has pervasive implications for the development of language in individuals with severe to profound hearing impairment. For example, if language and thought are mutually exclusive domains, language deficits cannot be attributed to cognitive deficits or even to adequate cognitive development.

In this chapter, we also examine whether there are quantitative or qualitative differences in cognition between individuals with severe to profound hearing impairment and those with normal hearing acuity. In light of a relationship between language and thought, the resolution of the qualitative issue provides insights into the acquisition of English language and literacy by deaf individuals. That is, if certain differences do exist, they might indicate limitations on deaf persons' abilities to acquire particular cognitive-based skills that are acquired readily by hearing people (such as reading), or they might dictate that in order to acquire those skills different developmental and teaching approaches need to be used with deaf children than are used with hearing children.

Relative to deafness, there is research on both cognitive processes (e.g., Piagetian stages, information processing) and intelligence (e.g., the *Wechsler Intelligence Scale for Children-Revised;* Wechsler, 1974). These two lines of research have caused considerable confusion. Moores (1987) remarked that the confusion is due mainly to the fact that these two research lines have had different agendas and goals.

To clear up some of the confusion, it is necessary to describe the notion of intelligence and its relationship to the broad domain of cognition. In addition, we synthesize the results of a representative sample of research studies on cognition, intelligence, and deafness. It is demonstrated that the interpretation of the research findings have been influenced by the prevailing views of the relationships between language and thought.

The chapter also provides an overview of the current thinking on the relationship between language and thought. In depicting the views on this relationship, it is important to convey whether a high-level development of language is dependent on a high-level development of thought or vice versa. This overview draws from the information on the language theories presented in Chapter 2 and from the research on cognition and intelligence. We also describe the relationship between memory and literacy and the relationship between language and literacy. These remarks should shed light on the English text-based literacy difficulties of deaf students, which is described in more detail in Chapter 5.

The last section of the chapter concerns the integration of the research on cognition, language, and deafness. Specifically, we provide our perspective on the question: Is there a psychology of deafness relative to language and literacy? Also discussed is the importance of learning *a* language at as early an age as possible for the further development of thought.

INTELLIGENCE AND COGNITION

Central to the constructs of intelligence and cognition is the question: What is intelligence? As noted by Sternberg and Detterman (1986) and others (Horn, 1989; Mann & Sabatino, 1985), the answer depends on one's metatheoretical and theoretical perspectives. For example, early developers of Intelligence Quotient (IQ) tests and early thinkers on intelligence, such as Binet, Terman, and Spearman, were influenced by psychometric theories, which in turn were influenced by the behavioristic metatheory. Much of the focus was on developing IQ tests that could predict academic or vocational achievement. These tests have been labeled product-oriented intelligence tests (see reviews in Blennerhassett, 1990; Paul & Jackson, 1993).

Most of the research on the intellectual functioning of deaf individuals has been based on the use of product-oriented tests (Moores, 1987; Quigley & Kretschmer, 1982). In essence, the answer to the question, What is intelligence? depends on factor analyses, that is, analyses of the nature and number of factors to provide the best explanation of IQ test results. In addition, the interpretation of the results of the IQ tests is influenced by the prevailing view on the relationship between language and thought (Conrad, 1979; Moores, 1987; Paul & Jackson, 1993).

From another perspective, the question of intelligence is best considered within the purview of cognitive theories, influenced by the cognitive metatheory. Models of cognition include the contributions of the pioneer giants such as Piaget, Vygotsky, and Luria as well as those of individuals who propose information-processing approaches (see reviews in Horn, 1989; Mann & Sabatino, 1985; Sternberg & Detterman, 1986). Many of these theorists have attempted to deal with epistemological questions such as those posed by Furth:

> From where do general ideas or universally valid concepts derive? Is human knowledge something different from animal knowledge? Is intelligence a fixed disposition transmitted through heredity that largely determines our capacity to behave intelligently? Do we acquire the general knowledge implied in intelligence in the same manner in which we learn any particular skill or fact? Is intelligence mainly a matter of memory? (Furth, 1969, p. 3)

Relative to intelligence and cognition, there have been several outcomes of the cognitive influence. For example, the more recent "intelligence" tests are labeled process-oriented tests because of the focus on understanding cognitive processes. This understanding should lead to an improvement of cognition, which in turn should lead to an improvement of academic achievement. Intelligence and cognitive process should be considered synonymous terms. Several researchers have recommended that the word intelligence be replaced with cognitive process (e.g., see discussion in Naglieri, 1987; Naglieri & Das, 1988). Instead of IQ tests, there would be tests of cognitive processes. Some of the research on the intellectual functioning of deaf individuals has been based on the use of process-oriented tests, including those that are termed "test-teach-test."

RESEARCH ON INTELLIGENCE AND DEAFNESS:
A BRIEF OVERVIEW

This brief overview discusses the tenets of the three major stages of research on intelligence and deafness (Moores, 1987; Quigley & Kretschmer, 1982). It also highlights the existence of a fourth stage, which represents a different way of thinking about intelligence or cognition (Blennerhassett, 1990; Paul & Quigley, 1990). Specifically, the overview addresses whether quantitative or qualitative differences exist between deaf and hearing individuals and examines the results of IQ tests relative to the development and use of a bona fide language system.

The first of the three major stages has been labeled "The Deaf as Inferior" by Moores (1987). Most of the tests used during this period were developed for and normed on individuals with typical or normal-hearing ability. This situation still exists at the present time (Blennerhassett, 1990; Paul & Jackson, 1993).

The work of Pintner and his colleagues is representative of the thinking of this era (e.g., see discussion in Pintner, Eisenson, & Stanton, 1941). Despite the development and use of nonverbal performance tests and the contradictive results of other studies, Pintner argued that deafness leads to intellectual deficiency. Because of the influence of the "language-dominates-thought" paradigm, it is possible to attribute quantitative differences to deaf individuals' difficulty with the acquisition of a language (i.e., a spoken language) (Paul & Quigley, 1990). In fact, Pintner noted that deaf students had difficulty with the tasks on digit-symbol and symbol-digit tests, and this has been attributed to the lack of an internalized, verbal-symbol system, such as a language, and its associated representations of experiences (see discussions in Conrad, 1979; Paul & Jackson, 1993).

The language-dominates-thought paradigm also influenced the thinking of Myklebust (1964), whose work characterizes the second stage of research labeled "The Deaf as Concrete" (Moores, 1987). Myklebust argued that deaf and hearing individuals are quantitatively similar on nonverbal intelligence tests or cognitive tasks, particularly those that contained "concrete" tasks. However, he noticed qualitative differences between the groups on tasks that require "abstract" thinking. Myklebust's organismic-shift hypothesis attempts to explain that deprivation of the hearing sense leads to a different organization of experiences by the other senses. This deprivation also precludes the development of a spoken language, which contributes to deaf individuals' difficulty to engage in abstract thought.

It should be underscored that Myklebust did not considered the signing behavior of his subjects to be part of a rule-governed linguistic system. In fact, in keeping with the thinking of this era, it was thought that only individuals who had internalized a "spoken" language could engage in high-level cognitive or intellectual functioning. The proffering of unique, qualitative differences between deaf and hearing individuals has led to the notion that there is a "psychology of deafness" (see discussions in Paul & Jackson, 1993; Quigley & Kretschmer, 1982).

Bolton's (1978) work serves as a representative study in support of Myklebust's hypothesis. Examining the results of the *Hiskey-Nebraska Test of Learning Aptitude* (HNTLA; Hiskey, 1966), this researcher compared deaf and hearing children, between the ages of three to ten years, inclusive. His conclusion, based on his results and his synthesis of other factor analytic studies, favored Myklebust's organismic shift hypothesis. This hypothesis is stated as follows:

> A sensory deprivation limits the world of experience. It deprives the organism of some of the material resources from which the mind develops. Because total experience is reduced, there is an imposition on the balance and equilibrium of all psychological processes. When one type of sensation is lacking, it alters the integration and function of all of the others. Experience is now constituted differently; the world of perception, conception, imagination, and thought has an altered foundation, a new configuration. Such alteration occurs naturally and unknowingly, because unless the individual is organized and attuned differently, survival itself may be in jeopardy. (Myklebust, 1960, p. 1)

Despite the shortcomings of Myklebust's views, his internalization principle, also shared by Pintner, is still relevant for explaining the English language and literacy problems of many deaf individuals, that is, those with severe to profound hearing impairment (see discussions in Conrad, 1979; Paul & Jackson, 1993). An extension of both Pintner's and Myklebust's views can be found in the research on short-term memory and literacy, discussed later in this chapter (see discussion in Hanson, 1989). In fact, this research, conducted within the purview of an information-processing framework, seems to suggest that "Myklebust's phrase *psychology of deafness* may apply to some individuals with severe hearing impairment and most individuals with profound hearing impairment, especially when the impairment occurs prior to two years of age" (Paul & Jackson, 1993, p. 88).

The third stage of this historical perspective is the one that is in vogue today: "the Deaf as Intellectually Normal" (Moores, 1987). The implication is that deaf individuals are intellectually and cognitively similar to hearing individuals in all important abilities. The third stage has been influenced by the thought-dominates-language paradigm (Paul & Jackson, 1993; Paul & Quigley, 1990). The position espoused by the third stage has been attributed to Furth (1966a); however, there are other strong proponents (e.g., Rosenstein, 1960, 1961; Vernon, 1967). It is argued that differences that exist between deaf and hearing individuals are due to linguistic, cultural, environmental, and task factors, rather than to the condition of deafness.

There is recent research to support this position (e.g., see Braden, 1984; see also the review in Blennerhassett, 1990). The work of Braden (1984) is representative of the viewpoint of the third stage. He conducted a factor analysis of both the performance scale of the *Wechsler Intelligence Scale for Children-Revised* (WISC-R; Wechsler, 1974) and the HNTLA (Hiskey, 1966). His results indicated no major qualitative differences between deaf and hearing individuals on nonverbal intelligence tasks.

After summarizing and synthesizing the findings of the major studies conducted during this stage, Quigley and Kretschmer (1982, p. 51) remarked that the research influences can be categorized as: (1) the inability of the researcher to properly convey the task demands because of language differences or deficits on the part of the subjects, (2) implicit bias within the solution of the task, or (3) general experiential deficits (including verbal language and communication in general) on part of the subjects.

A summary of the major findings and tenets of the three stages of intelligence testing and deafness is illustrated in Table 3–1.

The emergence of a fourth stage of intelligence testing, properly labeled cognitive testing, has been discussed (Paul & Quigley, 1990; Paul & Jackson, 1993). Whereas the first three stages have been based predominantly on psychometric theories, the fourth stage is influenced by the cognitive metatheory. The focus is on process-oriented tests, which are based on the works of major cognitive theorists such as Piaget, Vygotsky, Luria, and those who favor information-processing frameworks.

Process-oriented tests emerged because of the limitations of product-oriented psychometric tests (Blennerhassett, 1990; Paul & Jackson, 1993; Sternberg & Detterman, 1986). The emphasis is not on comparing the "intelligence" or "cognitive processes" of individuals; rather, it is on

TABLE 3-1. Three Stages of Intelligence Testing and Deafness: Major Tenets and Findings

Stage 1

- The first stage has been labeled "The Deaf as Inferior."
- Most of the tests used with deaf individuals were developed for and normed on individuals with normal-hearing ability.
- It is argued that deafness leads to intellectual deficiency.
- Most of deaf students' difficulty is attributed to the lack of an internalized, verbal symbol system, such as a language, and its associated representations of experiences.
- Findings are interpreted within a language-dominates-thought paradigm.

Stage 2

- The second stage has been labeled "The Deaf as Concrete."
- There are qualitative differences between deaf and hearing individuals relative to tasks that require abstract thinking.
- The organismic shift hypothesis asserts that deprivation of the hearing sense leads to a different organization of experiences by the other senses.
- The proffering of unique, qualitative differences between deaf and hearing individuals has led to the notion that there is a "psychology of deafness."
- Findings are interpreted within a "language-dominates-thought" paradigm.

Stage 3

- The third stage has been labeled "The Deaf as Intellectually Normal."
- Deaf individuals are intellectually and cognitively similar to hearing individuals in all important abilities.
- Differences that exist between deaf and hearing individuals are due to linguistic, cultural, environmental, and task factors, rather than to the condition of deafness.
- Deaf norms are established.
- Findings are interpreted within a "thought-dominates-language" paradigm.

Source: Adapted from Moores (1987), Paul & Jackson (1993), and Paul & Quigley (1990).

understanding the notion of cognitive processes and, subsequently, facilitating the improvement of such processes. There has been some research on deaf individuals within the conceptual framework of process-oriented tests (e.g., see the work of Feuerstein discussed in Feuerstein, Rand, & Hoffman, 1979; Feuerstein, Rand, Hoffman, & Miller, 1980; see also Jonas & Martin, 1985; Martin & Jonas, 1987, 1991). One common rendition of this viewpoint is the test-teach-test paradigm (i.e., assessment, training, and reassessment). In essence, the results of process-oriented tests are used to develop ways to improve "cognition," which in turn leads to the improvement of academic achievement.

The critical component of present process-oriented tests is the improvement of cognition—which demands a stronger and closer relationship between the tasks on cognitive tests and those on achievement tests. For example, one of the subtests of the *Planning-Attention-Simultaneous-Successive* cognitive test (PASS, see Naglieri & Das, 1988) involves planning, which entails the use of metacognitive skills (i.e., comprehension monitoring). Metacognitive skills are considered important for the development of fluent, high-level reading skills (e.g., Baker & Brown, 1984). Thus, one way to improve metacognitive skills might be to improve individuals' skills on the planning subtest of the PASS.

The fourth stage seems to be operating on the assumption that there is no psychology of deafness or, rather, that this notion should not be the major focus of cognitive testing. In a recent article, Lane (1988) argued against the use of the phrase, psychology of deafness. He proposed a paternalism metatheory, which states that the phrase reflected the paternalistic thinking of *hearing* experts making these judgments. These judgments do not reflect the actual characteristics of deaf individuals. Lane compared this situation to that which existed between Africans and their European colonizers.

Lane documented his paternalism metatheory with an extensive review and synthesis of the literature involving studies on the "psychology of deafness." He argued that many of these investigations contain serious methodological flaws. His major suggestions for improving this situation include the involvement of *Deaf* researchers and improvement in the research methodology of the investigations.

Recent studies and analyses seem to indicate that the question of whether there is a psychology of deafness is still open to debate. For example, Zwiebel (1991) asserted that the interpretation of his work does not lend itself to a confirmation either of Myklebust's theory nor of those that espouse the thinking of the third stage. Three general remarks on Zwiebel's work should be underscored here:

1. It was observed that differences between deaf and hearing subjects occurred across ages; however, the older deaf individuals were similar to hearing counterparts. This suggested that both groups are identical at the end of development.

2. The contribution of the form of the language (oral or sign) to the development of abstract ability in cognition needs to be further studied.
3. These results are based on research conducted within the purview of psychometric theories, especially via the use of factor analyses.

The research on intelligence and deafness provides some insights into the question of whether qualitative differences exist between deaf and hearing individuals. Although this notion is far from being understood, a clearer picture emerges when the research on cognition and deafness is considered, especially within the purview of an information-processing paradigm. Prior to discussing this research, it is important to provide some highlights of the relationship between thought and language.

THOUGHT AND LANGUAGE

Any discussion regarding the relationship of thought and language is not an exercise in futility or merely an academic debate. If researchers move away from an emphasis on the global comparison of the two entities to a focus on the relationships of specific aspects of each domain, a better understanding of this relationship might surface (e.g., see Cromer, 1981, 1988a, 1988b). For example, our knowledge of the reading difficulties of deaf students has progressed because of studies on the relationship between the processes of short-term memory (specific aspect of cognition) and comprehension of sentences, particularly syntactic constructions (specific aspect of language). This line of research has underscored the importance of using a phonological code in short-term memory (STM). This is controversial and problematic for individuals with severe to profound hearing impairment (Hanson, 1989; Paul & Jackson, 1993).

Our goal in this section is not to present a comprehensive review of the various thought-language models. Rather, we focus on providing some basic tenets of the global views. More important, we emphasize the eventual interactive effects of thought and language. Our reflections on the findings of interactive effects lead to the conclusion that high-level performance in one domain is dependent on a high-level development in the other domain. In addition, it is argued that some knowledge is domain specific and does not always depend on a corresponding level of knowledge in the other domain. For example, the understanding of a relative clause is predominantly a language-specific behavior which does not depend on cognitive prerequisites, other than a basic level of developmental maturity. As discussed later, language-specific knowledge is influenced by the notion of constraints, especially within a modularity hypothesis (e.g.,

Fodor, 1983), which is motivated by Chomsky's concept of innate structures, or Language Acquisition Device (see Chapter 2; see also Chomsky, 1975; Fodor, 1983).

It was noted previously that the works of pioneers such as Piaget, Vygotsky, and Luria have influenced the development of process-oriented cognitive tests. It is also possible to see the influence of these theorists on the study of language. In Chapter 2, we noted that cognitive-interactionism is based on Piaget's model of cognition and that social-interactionism is based, in part, on Vygotsky's model.

Both cognitive theorists and language theorists, for example, Chomsky, Sapir, and Whorf, have influenced the various models concerning the relationship between thought and language (e.g., see Byrnes & Gelman, 1991). Both groups of theorists view language as a window into the intricate operations of the mind. Some language theorists are interested in the linguistic underpinnings of the development of language whereas some cognitive theorists focus on the cognitive underpinnings. These emphases represent what are considered "strong" views of the thought-language relationships (Cromer, 1981, 1988a, 1988b). There is also evidence for "weak" views of this relationship which include the perspective of an interactive relationship, motivated by the work of Vygotsky and the current social-interactionist theory of language development (see discussion in Paul & Jackson, 1993).

Thought-based Hypotheses

The basic premise of thought-based hypotheses is that thought (cognition) influences or accounts for the development of language (Byrnes & Gelman, 1991; Cromer, 1988a, 1988b; Snyder, 1984). That is, language grows out of cognition, or language is a mapping out of cognitive skills. Variations among the hypotheses are related to the interpretation of the strength of the influence of thought on language development.

The strong forms of thought-based hypotheses assert that language is not possible without cognitive underpinnings. This is a unidirectional model in which the direction of influence is from cognition to language. In these versions, the development of language is equal to but does not exceed cognitive development. This implies a one-to-one, or perfect, correlation between thought and language development.

The strong forms of thought-based hypotheses have been influenced pervasively by the work of Piaget (1980; see also Flavell, 1985; Phillips, 1981). Piaget asserted that language has only a modest, albeit important, role in the development of thought. Nevertheless, the role of language has called into question the basic tenets of the strong views. Relative to research on cognition and deafness, some scholars (e.g., Kusche &

Greenberg, 1991; Paul & Quigley, 1990) have argued that discrepancies between hearing and deaf individuals on high-level, abstract cognitive tasks might be due predominantly to the effects of an inadequate development of *a* language in many deaf individuals.

The thinking of Cromer (1974, 1976, 1981) has influenced the "weak" versions of thought-based hypotheses. Weak versions assert that thought does not completely account for the development of language. It is acknowledged that some linguistic knowledge is dependent on language-specific skills. Language development is equal to or less than, but does not exceed, the development of thought. Evidence for the weak thought-based hypotheses has been reported in a number of investigations (see reviews in Cromer, 1988a, 1988b; Johnston, 1985; Slobin, 1979).

Other variations of thought-based hypotheses can be found elsewhere (see discussions in Gelman & Byrnes, 1991; Snyder, 1984). In our view, Harris (1982) proffered some compelling data against the strong thought-based hypotheses. This scholar argued that one possible implication of the strong view is that older second-language learners' acquisition of a language should be qualitatively different from that of first-language learners. For example, the older learners should know concepts (i.e., aspects of thought) that are not known by younger first-language learners. Harris concluded that research has not confirmed this argument. In fact, there is ample research showing that the language acquisition patterns of both first- and second-language learners (of English) are qualitatively similar. That is, both groups proceed through similar stages, make the same errors, and use congruent strategies in the acquisition of a language (e.g., McLaughlin, 1984, 1985).

Additional evidence against a strong view can be inferred from the research on deaf students. For example, Quigley and his collaborators (see review in Quigley, Wilbur, Power, Montanelli, & Steinkamp, 1976) demonstrated that deaf students' acquisition of syntax is qualitatively similar, albeit quantitatively slower, than that of hearing students. Similar arguments have been made for deaf students learning English as a first or second language (King, 1981). In addition, there is some evidence for qualitative similarity in vocabulary development (Paul, 1984; Paul & Gustafson, 1991; Paul & O'Rourke, 1988). The details of some of these major studies are presented in Chapter 5 of this text.

A few general principles of the thought-based hypotheses, including a common variation labeled correlational, are presented in Table 3–2.

Language-based Hypotheses

Similar to the thought-based hypotheses, there are strong and weak versions of language-based hypotheses and variations of these views. The

TABLE 3-2.   General Principles of Thought-Based Hypotheses

All Hypotheses

- Basic premise is that thought influences or accounts for the development of language.
- Language grows out of cognition, or language is a mapping out of cognitive skills.
- Variations among the hypotheses are related to the interpretation of the strength of the influence of thought on language development.

Strong Versions

- Language is not possible without cognitive underpinnings.
- Direction of influence is from thought to language.
- Development of language is equal to, but does not exceed, cognitive development.
- There is a one-to-one correlation between language and thought.

Weak Versions

- Thought does not completely account for the development of language.
- Language development is equal to or less than, but does not exceed, the development of thought.

Correlational Hypothesis

- Thought and language share common underpinnings.
- Relationships between language and cognition are influenced by social interactions and environmental factors.

Source: Adapted from Gelman & Byrnes (1991) and Snyder (1984).

strongest version asserts that language determines thought (i.e., linguistic determinism; Sapir, 1958; Whorf, 1956). There is a perfect, one-to-one correspondence between linguistic and cognitive aspects. However, in this case, the direction of the influence flows from language underpinnings to thought structures. This position is exemplified by the linguist Sapir who remarked that:

> It is quite an illusion to imagine that one adjusts to reality without the use of language and that language is merely an incidental means of solving specific problems of communication or reflection . . . we see and hear and otherwise

experience as we do because the language habits of our community predispose certain choices of interpretation. (Sapir, 1958, p. 162)

Although the evidence on the strong version is equivocal (e.g., see Bloom, 1981, for affirmative data, and Au, 1988, for contrary evidence), it is not a widely accepted hypothesis. The focus seems to be on weak variations or on language-specific hypotheses, which take into consideration the notion of innate structure and one of its major implications—constraints. One view that seems to be gaining proponents is termed the learnability hypothesis (see discussion in Pinker, 1989).

A few major principles of language-based hypotheses, including language-specific hypotheses, are presented in Table 3–3.

There is growing evidence that the relationship between thought and language is bidirectional and interactive. In some variations of this view, language plays an influential role. The interactive viewpoint has been influenced by social-interactionist accounts of language development (e.g., Callanan, 1991; Gleason, Hay, & Cain, 1989; Scholnick & Hall, 1991).

RESEARCH ON COGNITION AND DEAFNESS

In this section, we examine the research on cognition and deaf individuals within the frameworks of commonly used cognitive models. In synthesizing the studies, we relate the findings to our understanding of the importance

TABLE 3–3. General Principles of Language-Based Hypotheses

Strong Versions

- Language determines thought; this is also known as linguistic determinism.
- There is a perfect, one-to-one correspondence between linguistic and cognitive aspects.
- The direction of influence is from language to thought.

Language-Specific Versions

- These versions consider the notion of innate structure and one of its major implications—"constraints."
- Three common forms are little linguist, lexical, and learnability.
- One weak form is labeled the interaction hypothesis, which asserts that the relationship between language and thought is bidirectional and interactive.

Source: Adapted from Gelman & Byrnes (1991) and Snyder (1984).

of language as indicated by the previous discussion of thought-language relationships. Prior to discussing and synthesizing the research findings, it is necessary to provide some brief background on the salient cognitive models, notably those of Piaget and an information-processing model known as a stage-of-processing model. We do not mean to imply that research on other models are either not important or do not have implications for language development. Our focus here is selective, not exhaustive. Good reviews of cognitive research on deafness can be found elsewhere (Greenberg & Kusche, 1989; Martin, 1991; Moores & Meadow-Orlans, 1990).

Piagetian Model

One of the most commonly used models for understanding the cognitive development of children is that of Piaget (1952, 1977, 1980). It seems that Piaget's view on the cognitive development of young children is much more influential than his view on older children, for example, from age 7 on up (Mann & Sabatino, 1985). Until quite recently, most of the cognitive research with deaf children has been motivated by the thinking of Piaget (see reviews in Moores, 1987; Paul & Quigley, 1990).

Piaget portrays the child as progressing through four general stages to the development of mature thinking (see discussions in Flavell, 1985; Phillips, 1981). The first stage is the period of sensorimotor intelligence, which typically occupies the first 2 years of life. During this period, the child perceives and reacts to sensory data as related to basic needs and begins to organize and integrate these data into schemas. The child proceeds through a process of establishing an equilibrium (equilibration) between adapting to the environment (accommodation) and acting upon the environment (assimilation). Interactions between accommodation and assimilation further develop schemas as the child's representations of experience. These schemas are the units necessary for an organized pattern of sensorimotor functioning (Flavell, 1985; Phillips, 1981). For example, the child will organize the schema for face as an integrated pattern of eyes, nose, and mouth in a spatial relationship to each other. Schema theory has become a highly developed cognitive model and is incorporated into modern interactive theories of reading as will be discussed in Chapter 5.

Piaget's second stage is known as the preoperational stage and extends from about 2 to 7 years of age. This represents a period of establishing relationships between experience and action. The child's symbol system is expanding during this period, and language use and perceptual abilities continue to develop well beyond the child's capabilities at the end of Stage 1 (Flavell, 1985; Phillips, 1981). In this stage, egocentrism prevents the child from separating the personal perspective from that of others as manifested in the social interactions of the child. There is an inability to think in a logical manner; thus, the child cannot understand basic Piagetian concepts such as conservation and reversibility. The classic Piagetian example of conservation and reversibility is the ball of clay which when changed into another shape still retains the same mass and can be restored to its original shape. Another example is the volume of water remaining the same when poured from a short wide glass into a tall narrow one and vice versa.

Piaget's third stage is labeled concrete operation and extends from about 7 to about 11 years of age. The child is now capable of distinguishing personal self from others (egocentrism and relativism) and begins to understand concepts such as conservation and reversibility (Flavell, 1985; Phillips, 1981). In essence, the child is able to perform mental operations on objects that are concrete or present.

The fourth and final stage in Piaget's model is labeled formal operation. It extends from about age 11 to about age 15 years. This stage is characterized primarily by abstract thinking and a shift from the need for concrete objects and experiences. During this stage, an individual can think about thinking, that is, engage in metalinguistic or metacognitive behaviors.

A summary of the major principles of the four stages are presented in Table 3–4.

Piaget identifies three time periods at which language might play an important—albeit modest—role in the development of thought. These three time periods are transitions from one stage to the next—for example, from sensorimotor to preoperation, from preoperation to concrete operation, and from concrete operation to formal operation (Byrnes & Gelman, 1991). Piaget also divides the development of children's language into two broad stages. The first stage includes egocentric speech which emerges from noncommunicative thought. This involves monologues and language play where the child repeats simply for the pleasure of talking. The second stage involves socialized speech which develops to include eventually all the forms required for social communication such as information, criticism, commands, requests, questions, and so forth.

It should be underscored that Piaget only assigns a modest role for language in the development of thought. As stated in the following passage:

> Language is thus a necessary but not a sufficient condition for the construction of logical operations. It is necessary because without the system of symbolic expression which constitutes language the operations would remain at the stage of successive actions without ever being integrated into simultaneous systems or simultaneously encompassing a set of interdependent transformations. Without language the operations would remain personal and would consequently not be

TABLE 3-4. Major Principles of Piaget's Stages of Cognition

Sensorimotor Stage

- This stage covers the period from birth to about 2 years of age.
- Six substages have been identified.
- Child perceives and reacts to sensory data as related to basic needs and begins to organize and integrate these data into schemas.

Preoperational Stage

- This stage extends from about 2 to 7 years of age.
- There is an inability to think in a logical manner.
- Egocentrism prevents the child from separating the personal perspective from that of others as manifested in the social interactions of the child.

Concrete Operational Stage

- This stage extends from 7 to about 11 years of age.
- The child is now able to distinguish personal self from others.
- The child is now able to perform mental operations on objects that are physically present.

Formal Operational Stage

- This stage is the final stage and extends from about age 11 to about age 15 years.
- The stage is characterized primarily by abstract thinking and a shift from the need for concrete objects and experiences.
- The individual can engage in metalinguistic and metacognitive activities, that is, she or he can think about language or about thinking.

Source: Adapted from Flavell (1985) and Phillips (1981).

regulated by interpersonal exchange and cooperation. It is in this dual sense of symbolic condensation and social regulation that language is indispensable to the elaboration of thought. (Piaget, 1968, p. 98)

Research on Piaget's Model with Deaf Individuals

Although little research has been conducted on deaf children within the frameworks of Piaget's first two stages, it is generally accepted that little or no differences exist between deaf and hearing children. For example, observations reveal that deaf children progress typically through the sensorimotor stage (Best & Roberts, 1976) and through most of the preoperational stage (see reviews in Furth, 1966a, and Greenberg & Kusche, 1989).

These general findings have been confirmed by more recent studies, using a variety of nonverbal cognitive tasks (e.g., Bond, 1987). Bond (1987) examined the performance of 40 hearing-impaired and hearing preschoolers between the ages of 2 1/2 and 5 years. The children's hearing impairment pure-tone average (PTA) ranges from 65 to 110 dB. Based on their performance on nonverbal cognitive tasks, the researcher reported no significant differences between the hearing-impaired and hearing subjects. Despite differences in the English language ability of the two groups, the researcher argued that the cognitive development of hearing-impaired children was commensurate to that of hearing peers.

Relative to Piaget's model, differences between hearing-impaired and hearing children begin to emerge near the end of the preoperational stage on tasks dealing with seriation and transivity (e.g., see Furth, 1964, 1966a, 1973). On some concrete operational tasks, the performances of deaf and hearing children are equal with respect to the concept of horizontality or of rotation. These tasks seem to require visual-spatial ability, which does not present a problem for deaf children. A number of studies have indicated that deaf children have great difficulty with the notion of conservation, involving the concepts of number, quantity, length, weight, area, and volume (e.g., Chang & Gonzales, 1987; Furth, 1973; Rittenhouse, 1977, 1987). In fact, the differences between deaf and hearing children increase as the children become older. Deaf individuals do not exhibit a "concrete operational" understanding of some aspects of conservation until they are in the middle or late adolescent stage.

It has been argued that earlier studies on conservation were confounded by the language difficulties in the instructions of the tests (e.g., Furth, 1973). Furth (1973) attempted to demonstrate the importance of controlling the nature of the task, the directions, and subject response on the tasks dealing with the conservation of liquid. He found that responses of the subjects became more appropriate as the directions were adapted to the needs of the subjects. This was interpreted as another indication that cognitive differences between deaf and hearing individuals are the result of verbal influences in directions and responses rather than inherent consequences of deafness.

Rittenhouse (1977) examined the situation further relative to the conservation of matter. He hypothesized that the performance of hearing as well as of deaf children might be influenced on such tasks by the verbal instructions and by the subjects' perceptions of the experimenter's expectations of performance. Comparisons were made between the standard instructions of four conservation tasks and parallel sets of instructions designed to focus on task attributes. It was found that modified instructions improved the performance of both the deaf and the hearing subjects. Nevertheless, the deaf subjects still exhibited an average 2- to 3-year delay in performance.

Although modifications of directions and responses reduce differences between deaf and hearing subjects, there are still significant differences, as demonstrated by more recent studies (Chang & Gonzales, 1987; Rittenhouse, 1987). For example, Rittenhouse (1987) investigated the rate and order of conservation in 24 deaf students, ranging in ages from 8 to about 13 years old. The researcher presented the standard Piagetian instructions and procedures in sign language. Results revealed that the oldest students did not possess competency of the conservation concept. These results were interpreted to mean that there might be a cognitive difference in deaf individuals.

Perhaps one of the most pressing problems in these studies is that it is extremely difficult to construct cognitive tasks that are completely nonverbal or not dependent on language. Hearing subjects can almost always verbalize the tasks for internal, silent rehearsal. As is discussed later, language might play a noticeable role in some of these high-level cognitive tasks.

There is even less certainty about comparable performance of deaf and hearing subjects at the formal operational stage. For example, Furth and Youniss (1965) have shown that deaf adolescents and adults can be taught to use very complex logical operation principles (similar to the test-teach-test paradigm discussed previously). Nevertheless, these researchers reported that the deaf subjects did not have the ability to discover these principles spontaneously and consistently.

Influenced by the thinking connected with the third stage (Deaf as Intellectually Normal), most interpretations of the performances of deaf children and adolescents on Piagetian tasks are related to the nature and administration of the tasks (e.g., see discussion in Moores, 1987). Some scholars (notably, Rodda & Grove, 1987) remarked that the inferior performances of deaf children and adolescents are the result of social and psychological factors such as reduced stimulation, restricted educational access, inadequate social and communicative interactions. This is an experiential hypothesis, which might also include language deprivation.

In our view, the effects of language on cognition cannot be overemphasized relative to the current thinking on the thought-language relationship. The interactive effects of language and cognition might have influenced the performances of deaf children on many tasks in the concrete and formal operational stages (see discussion in Greenberg & Kusche, 1989; Paul & Jackson, 1993). The lack of language or a poorly developed language can affect the way information is organized, stored, and retrieved. It has even been speculated that this "language deprivation" prevents a transfer of function from the right hemisphere to the left hemisphere of the brain, which deals with processes that require a highly organized descriptive system or code (e.g., language) (Sacks, 1989).

Relative to deaf individuals' performances on Piagetian tasks, our view concurs with that of Greenberg and Kusche's (1989). Greenberg and Kusche (1989) acknowledged the role of visual-spatial ability for progress through the sensorimotor and much of the preoperational stages. In addition, these researchers asserted that:

> Although Furth . . . has interpreted the literature as evidence that language does not affect thinking, we believe that language has a strong effect on concrete and formal operational modes of thinking, while it has relatively less influence on sensorimotor and preoperational thought . . . With regard to abstract-proportional (or formal operational) thought, it may be that episodic memories which are encoded linguistically and/or symbolically (in speech or in signs) in the hippocampal areas . . . , perhaps through the use of verbal/sign mediation, are more easily translated into propositional concepts or schemes in the association area of the cortex . . . than are visually encoded memories or images. (Greenberg & Kusche, 1989, p. 101)

Memory Research and Deafness

As in previous sections, our focus here is on the importance of memory for language and literacy development. Research on memory has been driven by a particular theoretical memory model (Shadbolt, 1988). Relative to deafness, much of the research has been conducted within the framework of an information-processing model (IP) that contains three general stages of processing, that is, sensory register, short-term memory, and long-term memory (see reviews in Greenberg & Kusche, 1989; Paul & Jackson, 1993).

Much of the research within the information-processing paradigm has focused on the basic processes in short-term memory (STM). This line of investigation has attempted to delineate the nature of short-term memory, to compare the short-term memories of both hearing and deaf individuals, and to relate the type of processing in STM to the acquisition of language or reading. Advances in this area have contributed to a better understanding of the relationship between language and thought (Paul & Jackson, 1993; Tsui, Rodda, & Grove, 1991). In our view, there is enough evidence to provide some insights into the question of whether or not there is a psychology of deafness.

Prior to relating and synthesizing the findings of a sample of research studies on deafness, it is important to provide some background on the three broad stages of information processing. In addition, we discuss the notions of spatial (or simultaneous) and sequential memory. These notions have been operationalized as tasks on several tests of intelligence and cognitive processing, for example, the *Kaufman Assessment Battery for Children* (Kaufman & Kaufman, 1983) and the PASS battery (Naglieri &

Das, 1988). More important, spatial and sequential processing might be related to the acquisition of a sign language or of a spoken language for deaf individuals.

IP Sensory Register

Relative to a separate-storage model (e.g., Atkinson & Shiffrin, 1971), the IP sensory register is also known as sensory store or sensory memory. Supposedly, there is a sensory register for each of our senses. In relation to language and reading development, much attention has been devoted to the stores for vision and audition. Despite the hypothetical large capacity of the sensory register, it can only take in unanalyzed information for about one second (e.g., Sperling, 1963, 1968). This information will disappear unless it receives focused attention and is transferred to the second stage, STM.

Short-Term Memory

On entering STM, the information can remain there for about 30 seconds (e.g., Miller, 1956). This is a temporary storage, and the amount of information that can be held is about seven (plus or minus two) units. A unit is considered to be a chunk of information which is influenced by long-term memory (LTM). For example, an individual with no background in American history might only remember seven (plus or minus two) of the following numbers: 177618121865, whereas an individual with background might process this list of numbers as three units, 1776, 1812, and 1865, leaving room, theoretically, for four (plus or minus two) more.

The research on deafness has been influenced by a model of working memory (WM) proposed by Baddeley (1979, 1990). In this view, WM is considered to be a component of STM (see discussion in Mann & Sabatino, 1985). A model of working memory for congenitally deaf individuals, based on Baddeley's model, has also been proposed (Chalifoux, 1991). Setting controversies aside, it is permissible to use STM and WM synonymously; however, we will use WM in discussing the research on deafness.

Long-Term Memory

Information from WM (or STM) proceeds into LTM, the third and final stage. It can be inferred that the strength and efficiency of the relationship between STM and LTM is markedly influenced by the development of a well-established social-conventional language or, in Vygotsky's terms, the establishment of "inner speech" (e.g., Vygotsky, 1962; see also discussion in Chapter 2). The manner in which information is represented and organized in LTM and retrieved from LTM is the focus of the bulk of the research in cognitive science (Medin & Ross, 1992; Shadbolt, 1988). The LTM of an individual contains that person's knowledge about the world, including knowledge about language and reading. This stored information enables the individual to interpret, understand, and store new experiences.

In general, LTM is considered to consist of two broad types: episodic and semantic (Rumelhart, 1977; Tulving, 1983; Tulving & Donaldson, 1972). Episodic memory is personal, for example, knowledge of one's favorite car, what one had for breakfast, and so on. The other type of memory, semantic, entails general organized structures of knowledge. Relative to language, this might include knowledge of syntax and the lexicon (Chomsky, 1975, 1988). Relative to reading, this might include knowledge of prior experiences (Anderson & Pearson, 1984; Rumelhart, 1980) or metacognition (Baker & Brown, 1984). Another important issue to address is the manner in which knowledge is retrieved from LTM. In relation to deaf individuals, this might be influenced by the relationship between STM and LTM (see discussions in Paul & Quigley, 1990; Paul & Jackson, 1993).

Sequential and Spatial (Simultaneous) Processing

These processes have referred to the nature of the presentation of the stimuli and the nature of the processing of the senses. There seems to be a strong relationship between these two events. Stimuli can be presented in a serial, sequential manner, typically one item at a time. After exposure, each item is removed from sight prior to the presentation of the next item. Because this involves a time element, this type of processing is often referred to as temporal-sequential. Simultaneous (i.e., co-occurring) stimuli are presented in "chunks"; that is, at one time. Because the presentation can involve the use of a certain amount of space, it is often referred to as spatial-simultaneous.

The sense of audition seems to process input in a temporal-sequential manner whereas vision seems to process spatially (simultaneously) as well as sequentially. However, vision might be a less efficient processor of sequential information than is audition. The temporal-sequential/spatial-simultaneous (also known as verbosequential/visuospatial) distinction seems to be related to the properties of languages or to the effects of severe hearing impairment. For example, relative to language properties, English and other phonetic-based languages can be characterized mainly by temporal-sequential properties whereas American Sign Language (ASL) and other sign languages are characterized mainly by spatial-simultaneous properties (however, ASL does have sequential properties; Hanson, 1989; Krakow & Hanson, 1985; Paul & Jackson, 1993). As is discussed later, this situation can be used to explain why many individuals with severe to profound hearing impairment have difficulty acquiring a spoken language and its written representation. In addition, it explains why a sign language might be a "natural" language for these individuals; natural in the sense of matching the processing capabilities of the eye and for enabling individuals to reach a high level of literate thought, that is, critical and reflective thought.

Additional insights into the processing of information can be gleaned from studies that focus on the specialized cognitive functions associated with the left or right hemisphere (e.g., see discussions in Craig & Gordon, 1988; Sacks, 1989). There is evidence that the left hemisphere is specialized for language functions, for example, speech, reading, and writing, as well as for analytic and temporal-sequential processes. On the other hand, the right hemisphere is specialized, or has the far greater role, for areas such as visuospatial skills and in holistic, or gestalt, processing. As discussed later, relative to English and other spoken languages, there seems to be a strong relationship between verbosequential processing and achievement in reading and in other academic areas requiring this type of processing (e.g., Craig & Gordon, 1988).

Working Memory, Verbosequential Processing, and Reading

In this section, we examine the interrelationships among working memory, verbosequential processing, and reading. First, we briefly describe the types of coding that occur in working memories of both hearing and deaf individuals. Next, we discuss the relationship between type of coding and verbosequential properties of a spoken language such as English. Finally, we argue that both cognitive knowledge of the alphabetic system and the use of a phonological-based code in working memory are important for the development of reading ability. There are other important skills for reading, and these are discussed in Chapter 5. In essence, it seems that the use of a phonological-based code is best for handling verbosequential tasks and for facilitating cognitive awareness of the alphabetic system.

Working Memory and Verbosequential Properties

Descriptions of the nature of WM coding strategies are dependent on the similarities between the features of the tasks and the strategies used by individuals. By analyzing the production errors of the individuals or by analyzing the manner in which individuals remember certain segments of information, it is possible to specify their WM strategies. For example, the use of a phonological code can be inferred if individuals produce "confusion" errors based on the similarities between two rhyming sounds in words such as *bill* and *mill*.

Hearing individuals use a phonological-based code in working memory for recalling both spoken and written linguistic stimuli. The use of a phonological-based code seems to be related to the structure of their spoken language, in this case, English, which contains verbosequential properties. This characterization is an abstraction of the phonological and morphophonological structures of English. For example, it has been remarked that:

> Words are composed of sequentially arranged processes, and morphological processes typically add one or more prefixes and/or suffixes (each composed of one or a series of phonemes) to a stem. (Krakow & Hanson, 1985, p. 265)

Research on deaf individuals reveals four major types of coding on either WM tasks or during reading—sign (e.g., Bellugi, Klima, & Siple, 1974/1975; Odom, Blanton, & McIntyre, 1970), dactylic (e.g., Locke & Locke, 1971), phonological-based (e.g., see reviews in Conrad, 1979; Hanson, 1989), visual (e.g., Blanton, Nunnally, & Odom, 1967), and multiple (e.g., Lichtenstein, 1983, 1984, 1985). A brief description of each type is presented in Table 3–5.

The study by Odom et al. (1970) is an example of an investigation that revealed sign coding. These researchers tested deaf students and hearing students on their ability to remember words with sign equivalents and words without sign equivalents. The two groups were matched on reading ability. It was found that deaf students had little difficulty memorizing

TABLE 3–5. Descriptions of Internal Coding Strategies of Deaf Individuals

Internal Code	Brief Description
Sign	Refers to the manual aspects of signs relative to American Sign Language or English-based signed systems
Dactylic	Refers to the manual alphabet; also known as finger spelling
Visual	Refers to the shapes of printed letters, or graphemes
Speech or phonology	Refers to either the subvocalizations or the mental representations of the auditory-articulatory process

Source: Adapted from Conrad (1979), Hanson (1989), and Locke & Locke (1971).

words in signs but greater difficulty memorizing words that did not have sign equivalents. Other studies by these investigators found that deaf subjects could understand connected prose better when the syntax of printed messages had been changed to the syntactic order of ASL.

Another early study that focus on coding strategies was that of Locke and Locke (1971). Using a grapheme recall task, the researchers tested three groups of adolescents: normal-hearing subjects, hearing-impaired subjects with intelligible speech, and hearing-impaired subjects with unintelligible speech. Stimuli were three lists of letters paired either by (1) phonetic similarity, for example, B-V; (2) visual similarity, for example, P-F; or (3) dactylic similarity, for example, K-P. Results showed that the three groups recalled at essentially the same level, but confusion errors differentiated the groups. Overt coding was also observed. One of the conclusions was that deaf individuals do not effectively mediate print with speech.

Deaf individuals' ineffective use of a phonological-based code has been documented in a number of recent studies (e.g., see reviews in Conrad, 1979; Hanson, 1989; Lichtenstein, 1984, 1985; Paul & Quigley, 1990). It seems that most deaf individuals engage predominantly in nonphonological-based coding strategies, for example, visual, dactylic, and sign. As discussed in the next section on reading, interpreting the findings of these studies in light of more recent ones indicates that deaf students' problems with English literacy, particularly reading, seems to be based on processing difficulties, rather than on structural difficulties, for example, knowledge of syntax (e.g., Lillo-Martin, Hanson, & Smith, 1991).

The processing-difficulty hypothesis is influenced by text-based, or bottom-up, models of reading. As will be discussed in Chapter 5, current research on first- and second-language readers of English favors an interactive model, which includes both bottom-up and top-down skills (e.g., Bernhardt, 1991; Grabe, 1988; King & Quigley, 1985; Samuels & Kamil, 1984). Top-down skills refer to knowledge-based aspects such as prior knowledge and metacognitive skills. In fact, one researcher has argued that metacognitive ability is much more important than the use of phonological coding (Gibbs, 1989), implying that the teaching of word decoding skills are not critical for deaf students. We discuss these issues briefly in the section dealing with the notion of a psychology of deafness.

Mediation and Reading

Deaf students who use predominantly a phonological-based code in WM tend to be better readers than other deaf students who use predominantly a nonphonological-based code (e.g., Hanson, 1989; Tzeng, 1993; cf., Gibbs, 1989). As expressed in the following passage:

What makes phonological coding in working memory so important? In reading and listening, individual words of a sentence must be retained while the grammatical relations among words are determined. Evidence suggests that working memory is most efficient for verbal material (including written material) when the processing involves phonological coding. For readers suffering from impaired phonological coding in working memory, processing individual words and putting these words together into phrases and sentences can be computationally overloading, impairing overall reading performance. (Lillo-Martin et al., 1991, p. 147)

The importance of phonological coding for reading and for handling verbosequential information has been documented in a number of studies (e.g., Hanson, 1990; Hanson & Lichtenstein, 1990; Lichtenstein, 1983, 1984, 1985; Tzeng, 1993). In addition, the relationship between verbosequential skills and reading has also been reported by more recent studies (e.g., Craig & Gordon, 1988). We discuss the works of Lichtenstein (1983, 1984, 1985), Craig and Gordon (1988), and Lillo-Martin et al. (1991) as representative of this line of research.

Lichtenstein's (1983, 1984, 1985) work involved students at the National Technical Institute for the Deaf (NTID), all of whom had reading abilities considerably above the average for prelinguistic deaf students. His subjects exhibited a considerable range of competence in English skills and came from a variety of educational and communication backgrounds. Lichtenstein's goals were (1) to study their working memory processes with word and sentence memory tasks; (2) obtain extensive self-reports through questionnaires of their conscious coding and recoding strategies; (3) gather extensive descriptive and performance data on their auditory, intellectual, and linguistic abilities; and (4) analyze the relations among these data in the framework of a series of hypotheses connecting working memory to coding and recoding processes and to psycholinguistic functioning. His detailed investigations produced findings of critical importance to understanding the role of working memory in the development of primary and secondary (reading and writing) language in deaf children.

Lichtenstein reported that individual deaf students typically used two or more codes rather than just one exclusively. The various codes were used with varying degrees of effectiveness. The most commonly used codes were sign and speech.

It was also found that the better readers relied very heavily on speech (phonological-based) coding. In addition, reliance on speech coding was not confined to those deaf students who had intelligible speech. The primary relationships of working memory capacity and coding processes seem to be with syntactic skills. Speech coders tend to be better readers apparently because speech coding can better represent the grammatical structure of English than sign or visual coding. This allows the short-term retention of enough information to decode grammatical structures which often are not linear (e.g., relative clause—The boy *who kissed the girl* ran away; passive voice—The dog *was bit* by the boy). These findings have been confirmed by more recent studies (see reviews in Hanson, 1989; Paul & Jackson, 1993).

Perhaps the most controversial evidence reported by Lichtenstein was the fact that working memory capacity is related to the extent to which students make use of a phonological-based coding strategy. Lichtenstein used a model of working memory involving separate subsystems (Baddeley, 1990; Baddeley & Hitch, 1974). One subsystem, the central processor (CP), performs higher level or control functions but also has a limited amount of processing capacity which can be used for temporary storage of information. A second subsystem, the articulatory loop (AL), is a more peripheral system which maintains coded information by subvocal speech rehearsal. This model proved useful to Lichtenstein's research in suggesting why deaf persons generally have shorter memory spans than hearing persons for linguistically codable materials. He found that the more central cognitive components of working memory in deaf individuals appear to function as effectively as those of hearing individuals. He also found that the more peripheral components of the deaf person's working memory system are not as capable as those of the hearing person's in maintaining English linguistic information in working memory.

Whether Baddeley's model accurately explains the working memory of deaf individuals remains to be seen. It has been argued that a model of working memory for deaf persons should include subsystems for articulatory, sign, and visual coding (Chalifoux, 1991). To the best of our knowledge, research related to this model has not been reported.

In a more recent study, Craig and Gordon (1988) provide another perspective on the interrelationships among verbosequential processing, working memory, and reading achievement as well as other types of academic achievement, for example, mathematics. The researchers administered a series of cognitive tasks to 62 students who were severely to profoundly hearing impaired and between the ages of 15 to 20 years old. The sample was divided into two broad groups: high readers and low readers. The researchers were interested in assessing verbosequential skills, associated primarily with the left hemisphere, and visuospatial skills, associated primarily with the right hemisphere.

Results revealed that the students with hearing impairment performed below average on tasks requiring verbosequential processing and average and above on tasks requiring visuospatial processing. In addition, there was a strong relationship between verbosequential skills (e.g., verbal fluency and serial tasks) and academic achievement, including reading. Weak relationships were found between visuospatial skills and achievement. Finally, it was noted that high readers performed significantly better than low readers on all verbosequential tasks. However, no differences between the groups were reported on the visuospatial tasks. It should be noted that the researchers recommended the teaching of strategies for using right hemisphere skills "to bridge toward and improve left hemisphere performance" (p. 40).

Lillo-Martin et al. (1991) provided additional insights into the interrelationships among phonological coding, working memory, and syntactic comprehension. The researchers were interested in delineating factors that differentiate good deaf readers from poor deaf readers. They focused on the comprehension of one syntactic structure, relative clause, in several modes, for example, written English, signed English, and American Sign Language. The researchers also investigated a long-standing issue discussed previously: the effects of phonological coding in working memory on reading ability.

Subjects were 26 Gallaudet University students with severe to profound hearing impairment who came from homes in which ASL was the major mode of communication. The subjects were divided into two groups: good readers and poor readers. The average reading level of the poor readers was fifth grade and the average reading level of the good readers was about ninth grade. No differences between the IQ scores of the two groups were observed.

The test battery included the *Gates-MacGinitie Reading Test* (1978)- Comprehension Subtest; the *Test of Syntactic Abilities* (Quigley, Steinkamp, Power, & Jones, 1978)-Relativization 1: Comprehension subtest (selected items); American Sign Language relative clause comprehension test; signed English relative clause comprehension test; and a serial recall test. Results revealed no significant differences between the two groups on the written English relative clause test and on all the signed tests. In addition, it was observed that the performance of the groups was similar across sentence types and that there was no group by sentence type interaction. Lillo-Martin et al. (1991) interpreted this latter result as support for their unified-processing deficit hypothesis, rather than for structural deficits, for example, knowledge of grammar. This means that deaf students have adequate knowledge of syntax; thus, differences between the reading ability of the two groups in this study must be due to their processing ability. Surprisingly, the researchers did not find evidence of phonological coding for either group.

IS THERE A PSYCHOLOGY OF DEAFNESS?

In this section, we provide our views on the notion of a psychology of deafness. Because of the focus of this text, the question becomes: Is there a psychology of deafness and language comprehension? The discussion of this question is based on our understanding of the research presented in this chapter on the relationship between (1) thought and language and between (2) working memory and reading. Additional support for our response can be gleaned from the information presented in Chapters 4 and 5.

Despite intense efforts on the part of educators and researchers, there are still significant differences between deaf and hearing individuals on higher-level Piagetian and other cognitive tasks. These differences persist in spite of modifications and adjustments in the instructions and procedures, including the presentation of the tasks in a form of sign language. Artifacts associated with the tests notwithstanding, we tend to side with scholars who argue that the major problem is the lack of a well-developed language for communication and thought.

In considering a language for thought, our view, and those of others, is that a complex mediating system (i.e., internalized language) is necessary for solving complex cognitive tasks. It is difficult to construct complex cognitive tasks that are language-free. Theoretically, there should be little or no significant differences between deaf and hearing individuals, providing the two groups are fairly equal in terms of language development and *experiences and knowledge that typically accompany such development.* In this case, we are arguing that complex cognitive tasks are not and should not be biased toward a particular language, but these tasks do assume a certain level of language sophistication. Thus, it can be assumed that there should be no significant differences among the three following groups: average ASL-using deaf individuals, average English-using deaf individuals, and average English-using hearing individuals.

The notion of a psychology of deafness seems to apply to the acquisition of a language for receptive and expressive communication. In this instance, we are referring to the acquisition of a spoken, phonetic language such as English and its printed representation—reading and writing. The manner and rate of English acquisition is detailed in the next two chapters. The intent here is to argue that many students with severe to profound hearing impairment have extreme difficulty accessing a sufficient amount of information in the major components of English—semantics, syntax, morphology, and phonology—in order to internalize its complex rule system. It should be underscored that this rule system includes the rules associated with *all of the components* of a language. Difficulty with accessing English also affects the acquisition of its secondary forms—reading and writing.

Much of the research on memory and deafness seems to indicate that the problem is one of processing, specifically related to the nature of STM and a phonetic language such as English. In other words, the primary problem is the inability of many deaf individuals to use a phonological code in STM efficiently for handling the relevant verbosequential stimuli of a phonetic language such as English. This problem places a heavy demand on working memory processes which interferes with, and in many cases, prevents the use of higher-level cognitive skills for comprehending larger units such as syntax and other connected discourse.

As is discussed in Chapter 5, the processing hypothesis only addresses one, albeit important, aspect of reading comprehension—that is, bottom-up processing. It fails to consider the notion that reading (and writing) is an interactive process that requires both bottom-up and top-down (knowledge-based) skills. Thus, the problem is both a processing- and a knowledge-based one; the latter entails a stock of prior experiences and the application of such experiences. In essence, bottom-up skills facilitate top-down skills and vice versa. The knowledge aspect also includes knowledge of *the language in which one is trying to read*. Relative to English, this involves a deep understanding of the alphabetic system on which it is based.

In sum, the notion of a psychology of deafness and language comprehension might pertain to those deaf individuals who have difficulty internalizing a sufficient amount of the essential properties of English. Due to the severity of their hearing impairment, these individuals experience difficulty in using a phonological code in working memory for handling verbosequential stimuli associated with a phonetic language such as English. This difficulty persists despite advances in technology (e.g., amplification systems) and instructional emphasis on utilizing information from other sources such as print (orthography), speech reading, residual hearing, and tactile aspects (e.g., proprioceptive and kinesthetic).

It is important to stress that this difficulty is task-specific; that is, it is related to the requirements of a task relative to the language on which it is based. Thus, we can infer that the short-term working memory of ASL-using students and other deaf students, who have not acquired a high proficiency in English, is not deficient per se, but rather qualitatively different. Of course, the short-term working memory of deaf students who have not acquired any language at as early an age as possible is underdeveloped, at least, and possibly deficient in many respects. A qualitative difference implies a psychology of deafness such that the development of adequate English language and literacy skills might be an unrealistic goal for many students with severe to profound hearing impairment.

FINAL REMARKS

This chapter provided an overview of the interrelationships among cognition, intelligence, and language. Relative to cognition and intelligence, much of the focus was on the Piagetian model and an information-processing model that involves three broad stages. This focus is justified by the amount of research conducted within these models on individuals with severe to profound hearing impairment.

It was argued that a better understanding of the performances of deaf individuals on higher-level Piagetian and other cognitive tasks requires a better understanding of the language proficiency of these students. This argument is supported by the growing evidence of an interactive relationship between thought and language. This interactive relationship is not isomorphic (i.e., one-to-one); rather, it can best be described as reciprocal, especially for higher-level development in both domains.

Assuming an adequate level of language and experiential development between the two groups, future research studies using Piagetian tasks should reveal no significant differences between deaf and hearing individuals. Although translating instructions into a sign language does not address the adequate acquisition of language and accompanying experiences; it does address the reliability and validity of the tasks for some deaf individuals. If deaf children perform inferior to hearing children, and their performance affects academic achievement, then there needs to be a plan to (Paul & Jackson, 1993, p. 265):

1. Improve academic or nonacademic performance, rather than just to label the cognitive/intellectual ability of the individual;
2. Help individuals use their cognitive/intellectual ability more effectively in both academic and nonacademic settings.

In our view, insights into the notion of a psychology of deafness are more likely to emerge from the research conducted within the purview of information-processing. Research on short-term working memory and reading shows that working memory can handle the verbosequential properties of English most efficiently via the use of a phonological-based code. In conjunction with an interactive theoretical view of reading, this paradigm might account for the difficulties that deaf individuals experience in acquiring a spoken language and its printed representation.

Due to the limits of present technology and of compensatory-instructional principles for dealing with verbosequential properties of English, it seems that there is a psychology of deafness and language comprehension for many, if not most, deaf individuals. This does not mean, however, that these students cannot achieve literate thought—that is, the ability to engage in critical and reflective thought. Literate thought depends upon the adequate development of a bona fide language at as early an age as possible. The acquisition of a bona fide linguistic system is the subject of the next chapter.

FURTHER READINGS

Block, N. (Ed.). (1981). *Readings in philosophy of psychology* (Vol. 2). Cambridge, MA: Harvard University Press.

Brainerd, C. (1978). *Piaget's theory of intelligence.* Englewood Cliffs, NJ: Prentice-Hall.

Clark, H., & Clark, E. (1977). *Psychology and language: An introduction to psycholinguistics.* New York: Harcourt Brace Jovanovich.

Garnett, C. (1967). *The world of silence: A new venture in philosophy.* New York: Greenwich Book Publishers.

Martinich, A. (Ed.). (1985). *The philosophy of language.* New York: Oxford University Press.

Penrose, R. (1989). *The emperor's new mind: Concerning computers, minds, and the laws of physics.* New York: Oxford University Press.

C H A P T E R 4

PRIMARY LANGUAGE
DEVELOPMENT

The controversy over the best way to educate deaf children in this country raged from the 18th Century into the 20th. Hundreds of articles appeared in print, salvos of criticism were fired back and forth, and claims and counterclaims were made as each camp tried to win over parents and supporters. While the pure oralist proclaimed that speech was the way, the combinist argued that it was necessary to fit the method to the child, not the child to the method. (Gannon, 1981, p. 361)

Deaf children with ASL are intellectually, emotionally, and linguistically indistinguishable from hearing children with English. (Neisser, 1983, p. 282)

The two passages above set the tone for much of this chapter on the primary language acquisition of deaf individuals. The first passage refers to the ongoing debate between the two prominent communication philosophies: oralism and total communication (i.e., "combinist"). Recent perspectives on this debate can be found in several texts (e.g., Moores, 1987; Paul & Quigley, 1990). With a focus on the development of English literacy, this controversial debate has produced new perspectives on the relationship between the primary and secondary forms of a spoken language (e.g., see Paul & Jackson, 1993; see also Chapter 5 of this text).

The second passage could be considered an impetus or even a justification for the use of American Sign Language (ASL) in infancy and early childhood for all children with severe to profound impairment (e.g., Johnson, Liddell, & Erting, 1989; see also, the discussions in Liddell &

Johnson, 1992; Erting, 1992, and Chapter 6 of this text). Support for the use of ASL can be gleaned from what is considered the "failures" (and oppression, e.g., Reagan, 1990) of both oralism and total communication. These failures are said to be attributed to the fact that neither communication philosophy is readily accessible or a complete representation of English input for most deaf students. It is also possible to find evidence to the contrary, as indicated by the first passage (e.g., see Babb, 1979; Luetke-Stahlman, 1988a, 1988b; Washburn, 1983).

As discussed in Chapter 2, the acquisition of a first language (indeed any language) seems to be "impossible" or "magical." Yet, the comprehension and production of a bona fide language presents little difficulty for most typical hearing children. Hearing children's ability to understand and produce the spoken message is limited primarily by the extent of their linguistic and cognitive development (de Villiers & de Villiers, 1978; Goodluck, 1991; Ingram, 1989).

Despite this seemingly effortless task, there is much controversy surrounding theory and research on the acquisition of language by children. There is disagreement regarding (a) methodologies for gathering data, (b) interpretation or categorization of data within the various linguistic components (e.g., morphology, semantics), and (c) the construction of grammars or theories that achieve explanatory adequacy or that best fit the data (Bohannon & Warren-Leubecker, 1985; Ingram, 1989; Stevenson, 1988). These debates have renewed the long-standing arguments regarding rationalism versus empiricism (e.g., Demopoulos, 1989; Matthews, 1989) and its most recent offspring: learnability versus teachability (e.g., Rice & Schiefelbusch, 1989).

Describing the primary language development of deaf children is a more complicated matter. Such descriptions can include a spoken and/or signed language or some other communication form (e.g., finger spelling, cued speech). The approach taken in this chapter is to describe the language development of deaf children and adolescents relative to the particular type of input to which they are exposed in infancy and early childhood. We chart this development in relation to two broad communication categories, which contain a number of approaches: oral English (OE) and total communication (TC). In addition, we attempt to provide a synthesis of a representative sample of research data on the acquisition of ASL by deaf children.

Based on the description of the primary language development of deaf children via the use of representative research and discussion articles, there is sufficient information to present tentative conclusions for some long-standing controversial questions:

1. How well do deaf children acquire the primary form (speech and/or signs) of English?

2. What is the relationship between the acquisition of a particular primary form and the subsequent development of literacy and academic achievement?
3. Do any of the communication forms provide a representation of English that is as complete as that provide by the spoken form (i.e., speech)?

A further discussion of literacy, and particularly the discussion of question 2 above, is taken up in Chapter 5. In addition, the use of ASL in a bilingual or an English-as-a-second-language program is discussed in detail in Chapter 6. Prior to synthesizing the research on the language development of deaf children, it is important to describe briefly the typical language acquisition of hearing children.

THE DEVELOPMENT OF LANGUAGE

With little difficulty, most hearing children learn the languages of their society, that is, the ones to which they are exposed. This process appears effortless and relatively simple; however, an in-depth analysis reveals its complex and intricate nature. Despite voluminous research, the exact nature of this language learning process is still being debated (e.g., Crystal, 1987; Goodluck, 1991; Ingram, 1989; Stevenson, 1988). Even the manner in which child language development should be studied abounds with controversies.

It is extremely difficult to interpret the language performance of children, especially in the early stages of development. One major controversy is the extent to which nonlinguistic data (e.g., context cues) should be used as an adjunct to linguistic data in descriptions of language development. Another area of difficulty is the relationship between comprehension and production (de Villiers & de Villiers, 1978; Ingram, 1989; Schlesinger, 1982). These controversies, and others, have placed in question the psychological reality of the various linguistic terminologies (e.g., the semantic relation categories) used in describing child language development (e.g., Schlesinger, 1982). Despite these problems, it is possible to provide a general description of child language development within a conceptual framework of two broad time periods, prelinguistic and linguistic, and within the four components (three linguistic, one nonlinguistic) of language: phonology, syntax, semantics, and pragmatics (nonlinguistic).

Prelinguistic Development

Jakobson (1968) remarked that the prelinguistic period, that is, the period prior to the emergence of a child's first words has only recently attracted the attention of linguists. More recently, this period has come within the purview of developmental psychologists and developmental psycholinguists (e.g., Anisfeld, 1984; Crystal, 1987; Ingram, 1989; Stevenson, 1988). In the past, most researchers viewed this era as uninteresting albeit important to the later linguistic development of the child. Several factors contributed to a renewed, intense interest in this area: (a) the emergence of new apparatus for data collection; (b) the notion that later development is dependent on early linguistic and cognitive precursors; and (c) the recent and continuing focus on the functional aspects of language (e.g., pragmatics) as opposed to the structural aspects (e.g., Callanan, 1991; Gleason, 1988; Menyuk, 1977). In addition to the increasing emphasis on the communicative intent of the utterances, there are a few studies regarding the infant's discrimination of speech sound categories. In essence, the major focus of research in the prelinguistic period has been on the descriptions of linguistic and cognitive processes and their importance to the later mature development of both language and cognition.

Precursors of Phonology

Phonologic precursors can be discussed relative to two aspects of speech: segmental and suprasegmental (Cruttenden, 1979; Crystal, 1987). The segmental aspect refers to the sounds of speech (i.e., vowels and consonants), whereas the suprasegmental aspect refers to such factors as intonation, stress, and rhythm. These aspects of speech can be examined in relation to the findings on speech production and perception capabilities of infants during this period. A good review of theories of speech perception, especially in infants can be found in Ingram (1989).

Segmental Aspect: Production

Kaplan and Kaplan (in Quigley & Paul, 1990) delineated four major stages of prelinguistic development. Stage 1 contains crying behaviors; Stage 2 has other vocalization and cooing behaviors; Stage 3 is the babbling period; and Stage 4 is the transitional period between babbling and the emergence of the first words (see also, Petitto & Marientette, 1991 for research on deaf infants). It should be kept in mind that these stages are not distinct or mutually exclusive, but rather are continuous. In addition, not all children proceed through them in a similar manner or at the same time. Nevertheless, there are some general findings associated with Stages 3 and 4.

The beginning of the babbling stage occurs around the third or fourth month (e.g., Cruttenden, 1979; Crystal, 1987; Ingram, 1989). This stage is characterized by two salient events: (1) the emergence of pulmonic-lingual sounds, and (2) the infant's pleasure in producing such sounds. Pulmonic-lingual sounds refer to those sounds produced as air is interrupted when passing through the tongue along with vowel-like, or vocalic sounds.

In general, it seems that the production of consonants moves from the back of the mouth to the front. Another observed pattern concerns the structure of the babbling syllables. That is, vocalic sounds occur initially followed by consonant-vowel (C-V) combinations. Next to occur are the vowel-consonant-vowel (V-C-V) combinations, then the vowel-consonant (V-C) combinations, and finally the reduplication of C-V combinations (Cruttenden, 1979; Crystal, 1987; Goodluck, 1991; Menyuk, 1977). The development and occurrence of these patterns also seems to influence somewhat the teaching of phoneme-grapheme (sound-letter) correspondences in reading texts (see Brady & Shankweiler, 1991; Carnine, Silbert, & Kameenui, 1990; Durkin, 1989; Stanovich, 1988).

During this period, the child realizes that producing sounds is pleasurable. In fact, this activity may occur with or without the presence of an adult/caregiver. In producing the segmental aspect of speech, the child is beginning to coordinate his or her articulators, specifically, the tongue, lips, and teeth.

Segmental Aspect: Perception

There have been a few studies of the infant's discrimination of speech sound categories (see reviews in Crystal, 1987; de Villiers & de Villiers, 1978; Ingram, 1989; Menyuk, 1977). Discrimination is not similar to recognition or comprehension (e.g., see detailed discussion in Bruner & Bruner, 1968). For example, the investigations of Eimas, Siqueland, Jusczyk, and Vigorito (1971) and Morse (1974) have shown that infants as young as 1 month are responsive to speech stimuli and are able to perceive differences between voiceless /p/ and voiced /b/ phonemes produced by an adult. In addition, infants between the ages of 2 and 7 months inclusive have been observed to possess crude localization abilities for sound as evidenced by these infants turning their heads in the direction of a particular sound. It has also been shown that infants, by the age of 3 months, respond differently to their mother's voice compared to those of other adult females. In general, the infant's ability to discriminate between speech contrasts is superior to his or her ability to discriminate between nonspeech contrasts. This finding implies that sensitivity to speech or speech-like sounds may be unique to human infants during this period.

Recent studies on speech perceptions have revolved around two competing theories (universal and attunement; see Eilers, Oller, Bull, & Gavin, 1984; Jusczyk, Shea, & Aslin, 1984). It seems that both theories agree on that fact that infants possess excellent perceptual ability at birth. Attunement theory, however, seems to allow some (i.e., further) development of this ability over a period of time.

Despite these differences and controversies, Ingram (1989) has argued that it is possible to draw some general conclusions about the speech perception abilities of infants:

> The young infant is born with much greater ability than was ever thought just a few years ago. This fact makes the child's rapid linguistic development a year later less difficult to understand (though no less impressive!). It appears that this innate ability combined with a year's listening experience is sufficient for the young child to begin to recognize language-specific words around the end of the first year. Further, it appears that these perceptions are categorical in that the discriminations are more abrupt at specific acoustic parameters than at others. These two findings make the young infant's speech perception much more adult-like than was ever anticipated. (Ingram, 1989, p. 96)

Suprasegmental Aspect: Production and Perception

Intonation patterns have been observed to emerge during Stage 2 of the babbling phase. By Stage 3, these patterns begin to resemble those of adults. Halliday (1975) has reported that a contrast between rising and falling intonation is produced by the 10th or 11th month. He stated, however, that this contrast is not present in adult speech; rather, it is an idiosyncratic system unique to the child. After analyzing several studies, Bloom and Lahey (1978; see also, the discussion in Ingram, 1989) concluded that the rise-fall contour of infant vocalization may be a more important precursor of sentence types, for example, statements, questions, and explanations. Other researchers have suggested that early intonation patterns are precursors of the later process of determining old information from new information (pragmatic function) and to interpreting direct and indirect speech acts (e.g., Lucas, 1980). In sum, a number of researchers have suggested that infants are sensitive to the suprasegmental aspect prior to the segmental aspect of speech (Eimas, 1985; Morse, 1974; see reviews in Crystal, 1987; Goodluck, 1991; Ingram, 1989; Menyuk, 1977).

Relationship Between Perception and Production

The relationship between speech perception and speech production during the early and later stages of the prelinguistic period is often difficult to describe (Cruttenden, 1979; Crystal, 1987; Ingram, 1989; Menyuk, 1977). One major problem is to explain the discrepancy in time between the perception and production of similar sounds. Another problem is to account for the differences in the structure of these early productions from the later ones. For example, a child can perceive a distinction between the presence or absence of vocalic sounds by the age of 4 months. The child's production, however, does not reflect this distinction until sometime during the second year of life. In general, the data on production during this period reveal sounds with unequal frequency distributions, and these data are not congruent with those on perception. In addition, the relationship between babbling and the emergence of intelligible speech is still not well understood. Menyuk (1977) has delineated three issues which have been the focus of ongoing investigations: (1) the uniqueness of speech to the human infant during the prelinguistic period, (2) the existence of a universal developmental sequence in perception and/or production of vocalization, and (3) the relationship of perception and production to each other and to the later development of speech.

Transitional Stage

There is a transitional period between babbling and the emergence of one-word utterances. During this stage (approximately 9 to 13 months), a change occurs in the child's repertoire of sounds, and this is known as the babbling drift (Brown, 1958). The child shifts from the production of four or more syllable utterances to those of one or two syllables. In particular, the structure of these utterances consists predominantly of plosives and nasals sounds (e.g., /b/, /d/, /g/, /m/, /n/) in conjunction with low vowels (e.g., /ae/ as in bat; see discussions in Cruttenden, 1979; Goodluck, 1991; Ingram, 1989). These syllables are of the C-V type described earlier. Several researchers have suggested that the early and late stages of babbling are vocalizations without reference to meaning. In other words, there is no intention to communicate, and babbling merely reflects the feelings of the infant. In this view, the child seems to be playing with speech production by exercising the vocal organs to gain control over their movements. This development may also be influenced by the reactions from the parents/caregivers. It should be pointed out, however, that precursors of meaning and communicative competence are also developing during this period.

Precursors of Semantics-Cognition

A brief overview of semantic-cognitive precursors necessary for the later development of referents is presented here. More detailed descriptions can be found elsewhere (e.g., Anisfeld, 1984; Bloom & Lahey, 1978; Goodluck,

1991; Ingram, 1989; Lucas, 1980). In many ways, semantic development is isomorphic with cognitive development; however, they are not exactly the same. A semantic category, such as a word, may be indicative of a nonlinguistic conceptual category; however, it is not the same as this category (e.g., schema). Nevertheless, it is safe to conclude that semantic development parallels observed patterns of behavior which correspond to different levels of cognitive development. Thus, prior to the emergence of the first words, semantic and cognitive precursors may be essentially the same.

The development of referents as well as communicative competence is dependent on cognitive processes which emerge during the first 2 years, or during one of Piaget's stages called sensorimotor (Piaget, 1952, 1977). Prior to learning about object concepts and relational concepts, a child must develop the ability to organize information. This process is inoperable without certain concepts such as object permanency, that is, a stable world replete with persons, objects, and events (see also Chapter 3 of this text). Prior to the emergence of intentional and meaningful communication, a child explores the environment for about 1 year. With this exploration comes the realization that persons, objects, and events are separate from the self. By acting on these persons, objects, and events, the child discovers object and relational concepts and realizes that she or he can have an effect on them. Further discussion of the importance of cognition to the development of language has been presented in Chapter 3.

Precursors of Pragmatics

Several investigators have suggested that the precursors of speech acts (Dore, 1974, 1975; Searle, 1969), the functions of speech acts (Halliday, 1975), and the overall communicative aspects of language (Bates, 1976; Bruner, 1974–1975) also emerge during the prelinguistic period. Bruner (1974–1975) stated that a child learns about functions, rules, and referential concepts of language while engaging in joint activities with a parent/caregiver. These concepts and rules are also part of the semantic development of the child. Rules of interactions, for example, are learned as the child and parent/caregiver vocalize and respond to each other. The parent/caregiver considers the child's vocalizations a response; this, in turn, prompts a return response from the parent/caregiver. This interaction establishes the roles of speaker and listener which are important to the communicative process.

These intentional and purposive behaviors have been observed as early as 4 months in the motor patterns of the child (Bates, 1976). The child's endeavors to reach for objects while vocalizing simultaneously have been interpreted as a form of communication. In essence, these vocalizations apparently can perform certain functions without conforming to the linguistic structures of the native-speaking adult. In particular, Halliday (1975) delineated several functions in the early linguistic development of his son: (a) instrumental (*I want*); (b) regulatory (*Do as I tell you*); (c) interactional (*me* and *you*); and (d) personal (*Here I come*). The interactional function was observed to emerged at 9 months; however, it has been observed as early as 4 months (Bates, 1976). Also at 9 months, the personal function emerged. It should be remembered that the primary forms of communication during this prelinguistic period are cries, smiles, eye-gazing, and vocalization. All of this implies that the infant uses these behaviors to express his or her needs.

A "snapshot" of some of the major issues of the prelinguistic period regarding the perception and production of infants is presented in Table 4–1.

Linguistic Development

Prelinguistic development does not simply culminate with the emergence of the first words. In fact, the development of the later stages of this period may parallel the beginning stages of linguistic development (Goodluck,

TABLE 4–1. Some Major Aspects of the Prelinguistic Period Regarding Speech Perception and Production

The Prelinguistic Period

- A lengthy period of very sensitive listening precedes the production of speech in infancy; infants appear to be tuned to human voices from just after birth.
- Mutual eye gazing and patterns of inviting and ending eye contact are soon established by infants and carers. These sequences may have significance for the later turn-taking patterns of conversations when eye signals still remain important.
- The very first sounds, cries, and babbles exercise and develop the capacities of the speech organs, and the child's control over them.
- In their first months infants practice and perfect the habitual and significant sounds of the particular languages to which they are exposed.
- In the first months of life infants begin to use their voices to control others and to get them to do things.
- Many infants appear to use a set of personally evolved sounds to express their needs and meanings systematically.

Source: Adapted from Whitehead (1990, pp. 54, 57).

1991; Ingram, 1989). Occasionally, the child may engage in behaviors which emerged earlier in both the prelinguistic and the linguistic periods. This should not be taken to mean that the child is regressing; rather, the child may be increasing his or her understanding of—in Bloom and Lahey's words (1978)—the form, content, and use of language. The stages of linguistic development discussed here are (a) the one-word stage, (b) the two-word stage, and (c) linguistic maturity. An alternative way to view language development, particularly grammatical development, is to use the stages of Brown (1973) based on mean length of utterance. Although this method is not adopted here, it is briefly discussed later to account for the development of inflectional morphemes. As with prelinguistic development, the development of the linguistic stages are continuous; the labels are used for the purpose of studying various parts of the stages (Cairns, 1986; Crystal, 1987).

The child's first words generally mark the beginning of linguistic development. Depending on the nature of the linguistic criteria established, different ages may be reported for the emergence of the first words (as previously discussed). Dale (1976) cited three general requirements which have been reported in the literature: (1) the child must demonstrate an understanding of the word; (2) the child must use the word consistently and spontaneously with reference to an object or event; and (3) the word must be recognized as one from a native-speaking adult's lexicon. It has been remarked:

> Learning a word—its form and meaning—is no small task. It requires that one be able to identify the form of the word, its beginning and end, so that it can be picked out from the stream of speech and produced, eventually, in a form recognizable to others. And it requires that one learn what it means. This includes learning what *parts* of words mean, since knowing this offers children a way of expanding their current vocabulary much as adults do. (Clark, 1991, p. 31)

Analyses of the first words and later development are presented within the conceptual framework of the linguistic components in the ensuing paragraphs. It has been argued that syntactic analyses are not useful for determining the content of the first words (Bloom, 1973; Brown, 1958). More specifically, it has been documented that syntactic precursors do not appear until the end of the one-word stage (Bloom, 1973; Dore, Franklin, Miller, & Ramer, 1976). Syntax, as a linguistic component, does not emerge until sometime during the two-word stage (Bloom & Lahey, 1978; Crystal, 1987; Goodluck, 1991; Ingram, 1989). Thus, descriptions of the child's first words are primarily discussed relative to development of phonology, semantics, and pragmatics.

Phonologic Development: Second Year and Beyond

A review of the literature reveals three general conclusions regarding the description of the phonologic development of young children (Cruttenden, 1979; Eimas, 1985; Ingram, 1989; Morse, 1974). The first conclusion, presented earlier, is that prior to the age of 2 years, the developmental data on perception and production are equivocal and inconclusive. The second conclusion is that there exist at least three units of phonologic analyses: phonemes, syllables, and words—although most recent analyses seem to focus on the two latter types. The third conclusion is that, in general, there are two approaches to analyzing child phonology: (1) the developmental sequence of the child's sound system can be compared with that of the adult model; or (2) this development can be described with reference to the particular child's strategy, and this, in turn, can be compared with that of the adult model.

Unit of Analysis: Phonemes

Prior to the 1970s, most researchers used the phoneme as the unit of analysis, and their approach was to compare the child's development to that of the adult. Jakobson (1968) attempted to chart the order of phonemic acquisition by using his notion of distinctive feature analysis. He proposed several principles to delineate the order of acquisition; only two are presented here: (1) the description of phonologic development should parallel the mastery of distinctive features; and (2) the system of phonemic contrasts of the child may not always be similar to that of adults in distinguishing between words. It should be seen that the second principle is a move away from the dominant approach of this period. In essence, Jakobson argued that the pattern of phonologic development in all children is systematic and universal. The universal sequence proposed by Jakobson is as follows: (1) children initially differentiate vowels from consonants; (2) then, they make a distinction between oral stop and nasal consonants; (3) next, they distinguish between labial (lip) and apical (tip of tongue) stops; and finally, (4) they differentiate the high vowels from the low vowels.

The difficulties in evaluating this theory are discussed in detail elsewhere (e.g., Crystal, 1987; Ingram, 1989). Some evidence for the theory, that is, the reality of distinctive features, has been observed after the age of 2 years (e.g., Menyuk, 1968). It seems that after children have mastered a particular phonemic contrast, they generalize this knowledge to other phonemes with similar distinctive features. In sum, there appears to be a wide variation in the early phonologic development of children. This development, however, may be systematic and probably should be analyzed relative to the child's system of strategies.

Units of Analyses: Syllables and Words

More recent research has moved away from the phoneme as a unit of speech analysis to either syllables or whole words (e.g., Ferguson & Farwell, 1975). These investigations have shown that a child's phonologic development does not proceed one sound as at time or by mastery of successive distinctive features. Instead, they proposed that development occurs according to certain strategies or rules (see, for example, the discussions in Crystal, 1987; de Villiers & de Villiers, 1978; Goodluck, 1991; Ingram, 1989). de Villiers and de Villiers (1978) cited a major shortcoming of the earlier phonemic and distinctive feature analyses, namely, the failure to consider error types and substitutions in the child's production. These researchers argued that such analyses are important for charting the phonologic development of the child with reference to his or her own system. In addition, this approach sheds more light on the perception/production issue (see also, Menyuk, 1977). A few major points are made here:

1. In general, perception precedes production.
2. Sometimes, both perception and production appear to be simultaneous, and occasionally, production precedes perception.
3. As discussed previously, the sequence of phonemic development in perception may not be congruent with that of production.
4. The contribution of additional unrelated factors (e.g., frequency of occurrence) to the process of phonologic development needs to be studied.

To obtain a sense of the syllable as the minimal unit of perception, consider the following example, *dog*. The speaker/listener does not "hear" three distinct phonemes, for example, /d/ /o/ /g/ because of the influence of the vowel on the consonants. This phenomenon is labeled co-articulation. Thus, speech perception seems to be at the syllable level; that is, *dog* is perceived as one syllable, or acoustic unit.

It should be mentioned here that the speech perception of the phoneme is still important, especially for beginning readers. It is critical to recognize that speech can be segmented into phonemes, which are represented by an alphabetic orthography (e.g., see research reviews in Brady & Shankweiler, 1991; Shankweiler & Liberman, 1989; Stanovich, 1988; Templeton & Bear, 1992; see also, Chapter 5 of this text). In other words, in a writing system such as English, the printed symbols are representative of the sounds of speech, albeit, not a direct one-to-one representation.

The beginning reader needs to understand not only that the speech stream can be segmented into words and syllables, but ultimately that even smaller sublexical units (phonemes) are accessible.

It is not the mere associations between letters and sounds that are important; rather, it is the cognitive awareness of the alphabetic principle that is important (e.g., see reviews in Hanson, 1989; Paul & Jackson, 1993). This awareness contributes to the development of rapid, automatic word identification processes. If students do not have knowledge of the alphabetic principle, exposure or experience with print either does not lead to this knowledge or is an inefficient method for developing it.

This discussion of the perception of the "phoneme" provides the background necessary for addressing two of our questions stated earlier regarding the representation of English via the manual mode and the relationship between the primary and secondary forms of the language. These questions are addressed in more detail in Chapter 5.

Mastery of Phonological Rules

Most of the phonologic rules are acquired by around 6 to 8 years of age (Crystal, 1987; Goodluck, 1991; Ingram, 1989). From age 3 onward, the child attempts to acquire the rules associated with the various inflectional endings of nouns and verbs (Brown, 1973). The more general rules of phonology are acquired prior to the acquisition of the specific or less general rules. The early stages of phonologic development cannot be described relative to phonemic contrasts or distinctive features. This development can be charted only after the acquisition of a certain number of words in the child's lexicon. The strategies that a child develops may relate these words to each other or to an adult model. Finally, these strategies may be dependent on the particular first words acquired by the child.

Syntactic Development: The Transitional and the Two-Word Stage

Several investigators have identified syntactic precursors prior to the emergence of the two-word stage (Bloom, 1973; Dore et al., 1976; see also, the discussions in Crystal, 1987; Goodluck, 1991; Ingram, 1989). The notion of syntax, or that word order is meaningful, is marked by the production of successive utterances which do not, at this time, function as connected or cohesive linguistic units. Bloom (1973), for example, reported that a 16-month-old child consistently used one word (i.e., *wide*) with a certain phrase. She maintained that this lexical unit was not interpretable because it referred to *anything* and *everything*. Other notions of syntactic precursors are (a) the use of a nonsense syllable with a certain lexical unit; (b) the reduplicated production of a single lexical unit successively; (c) the production of a single, phonetically, unstable unit prior to a lexical unit; and (d) the production of two words in combination consistently and restrictively (i.e., not with other word combinations).

The beginning of grammar, particularly syntax, commences with the combination of two or more words in sentences (Dale, 1976; de Villers & de Villiers, 1978; Goodluck, 1991; Ingram, 1989). The syntactic activity during this period prepares the child for the later acquisition of the major transformations of the language. An important question in the two-word stage is whether children possess knowledge of subject and predicate and whether this knowledge is similar to that of adults. Several researchers have suggested that knowledge of the basic grammatical relation between subject and predicate is possessed by children. Bloom and Lahey (1978), however, argue that such knowledge is not syntactic only, but rather semantic-syntactic in nature. They described two kinds of relationships: linear syntactic relationship and hierarchical syntactic relationship. In the former, relational words (e.g., *more, away*) are combined with other words, and the meaning of the relational word determines the meaning relation of the two-word combinations. In hierarchical syntactic relations, these combinations involve the form classes of nouns and pronouns in relation to verbs. The meaning of these combinations (i.e., subject-predicate concepts), however, are not the same as the meaning of the individual words. In the latter combinations, children must know both the category of word order relation between words and semantic relation between words. This position is also supported by Bowerman (e.g., 1973, 1988). In addition, both syntactic and semantic complexity have been used as adequate indices in accounting for the acquisition of the inflectional morphemes by Brown (1973). Essentially, Brown maintained that both components overlap making it difficult to distinguish their relative contribution.

Other researchers agreed that knowledge of subject-predicate is present at this stage, but it is better explained by pragmatic terminology (Bates, 1976; Greenfield & Smith, 1976). These investigators assert that the use of word order by children is in accordance with a given-new concept. In the adult use of this concept, given or known information is presented first, followed by new or unknown information. It has been reported that in children the order is reversed. Thus, the first word in the two-word stage is the comment about the topic which occurs as the second word.

In sum, the notion of syntax is present in the two-word stage. This notion, however, may be inextricably related to those of semantics or pragmatics. Although more research is needed in this area, it is safe to conclude that syntactic analyses alone are not sufficient at the level of two words (e.g., Crystal, 1987, Ingram, 1989).

Semantic Development: One-Term and Two-Term Relations

An important aspect in the language growth of a child is the development of semantic, or meaningful referents (Ingram, 1989; Lindfors, 1980; Lucas, 1980; Schlesinger, 1982). These referents reflect the organization of the child's knowledge concerning persons, objects, events, and relations (Bloom, 1970, 1973; Brown, 1973; Crystal, 1987; Ingram, 1989). The meanings of these one-term and two-term semantic relations have caused considerable controversy (Howe, 1981; Schlesinger, 1982). Essentially, it is argued that these early relations must be analyzed relative to surrounding context. de Villiers and de Villiers (1978) have cited several ways in which the meanings of the first words have been described in the literature: (a) categorization of objects and events; (b) categorization of relations between self and other persons, objects, and/or events; and (c) categorization of relations between others and objects and/or events.

The psychological reality of semantic relations have been questioned due to the possibility of categorizing relations in an infinite number of ways (Howe, 1981; Schlesinger, 1982). In addition, the semantic attributes which contribute to the acquisition of the first words produced and comprehended by children are not agreed on yet. These attributes have been termed functional (Nelson, 1973), perceptual (Clark, 1973; see also, the discussion in Clark, 1991), relational-categorical (Bloom, 1973), and relational (Greenfield & Smith, 1976; see also, the discussions in Bloom & Lahey, 1978; Dale, 1976; Menyuk, 1977).

Nelson (1973) investigated the nature of the first 50 words acquired by children. This investigator remarked that two-word combinations emerge after the acquisition of at least 50 words. Nelson reported her findings in six categories. The common category was general nominals, for example, *milk, dog,* which consisted of 51% of the data. Next with 14% of the data each were specific nominals (e.g., *mommy*) and action words (e.g., *give*). Nelson concluded that the words that are learned initially are those which the child can manipulate; that is, these words are functional.

Clark (1973) reported on the phenomenon of overextensions, that is, the use of a word to reflect a broader category than is appropriate. An example is the use of the word *daddy* to refer to all men encountered. Clark argued that overextensions may be based on perceptual attributes which she classified into six categories: shape, sound, size, movement, taste, and texture. Her data revealed that the most common overextensions are concrete nouns occurring between the ages of 12 and 30 months. A more recent rendition of Clark's view of the development of word meanings can be found elsewhere (e.g., Clark, 1991).

Underextensions, as well as overextensions, were reported by Bowerman (1973, 1988; see also, the discussion in Clark, 1991). Underextensions refers to a word representing a narrower category than is appropriate. This phenomenon is difficult to determine because the child is using the label in a correct, albeit restricted, manner. Bowerman asserted that under-extensions, like overextensions, are related to perceptual attributes of objects. It is suggested that underextensions occur prior to overextensions.

Bloom (1970, 1973) argued that the first words are relational-categorical. These relational words (e.g., *this, uh oh, no more*) reflect the behavior of objects and are predominant in the one-word or one-term utterances. Bloom labels the relation of objects to itself as reflexive-object relation. This semantic category consists of four relations: existence, nonexistence, disappearance, and recurrence. At a later period, Bloom states that children produce words reflecting causality-locative relationships which focus on the various aspects of the communicative situation.

In many ways, the two-term stage is a continuation of those semantic relations identified in the one-term stage (Bloom, 1973; Brown, 1973; Cairns, 1986; Greenfield & Smith, 1976; Ingram, 1989). Greenfield and Smith (1976) argued that the semantic relation in this stage consists only of those expressed in the previous stage. In Bloom and Lahey's words (1978), children in this stage use old function (i.e., relations) to gain mastery of new forms.

Semantic relations expressed in the two-word stage have been described extensively in the literature (Bloom, 1973; Bowerman, 1973, 1988; Cairns, 1986; Cruttenden, 1979). Only the most common relations are discussed here. It is possible to group these relations into eight categories: nomination, attribution, recurrence, possession, notice or exclamation, negation, location, and action. Examples of the first five are: nomination—*that car*; attribution—*big car*; recurrence—*more car*; possession—*mommy car*; and notice or exclamation—*hi car*. The categories of negation, location, and action may be subdivided into further categories. For example, negation may reflect nonexistence (*no cookie*) or disappearance (*allgone cookie*). Location may reflect a noun plus noun category, *mommy car*; or verb plus verb, *walk car*; or noun plus prolocative, *car up there*. Action may reflect an agent-action category, *Daddy read*; or agent-object (noun plus noun), *mommy sock*; or agent-object (verb plus noun), *make cookie*. During this stage, the relations which initially occur in large quantities are possession, recurrence, negation, and location.

On the surface level, it appears that some two-term utterances (e.g., *mommy sock*) can be classified in any one of several relation categories. The interpretation of these semantic relations must be based on the child's intent, and this intent is made clearer by the surrounding context. Bloom (1970) reported an example of one utterance (*mommy sock*) which could express two different semantic relationships with respect to two different contexts. In one context, this two-term relation referred to the concept of mommy putting on her own sock whereas, in the other, mommy was put-ting the child's sock on the child.

Pragmatic Development: The Functions
of One- and Two-Word Stages

As discussed in Chapter 1, one view of pragmatic development is that it entails the acquisition of semantic rules which are necessary for engaging in purposive and intentional behaviors (Bates, 1976; Crystal, 1987; Lucas, 1980). The basic unit of analysis of pragmatics is the speech act (Searle, 1969). Speech acts have been investigated in very young children. For example, Dore (1974, 1975) attempted to describe the development stage of language acquisition by employing Searle's (1969) theory of speech acts. Several primitive speech acts were identified: labeling, repeating, answer-ing, requesting an answer, requesting (action), calling, greeting, protesting, and practicing. Dore suggested that the one- and two-term semantic rela-tions of children contain both a function and form and represent the con-tent of the child's social interactions. Others disagree, however, that these early utterances have a form (e.g., Bloom & Lahey, 1978; Halliday, 1975). An interesting finding reported is that some of the primitive speech acts of the child are different from the more mature adult's speech acts. These differences contribute to the difficulty of interpreting the intentions and purposes of the child. Dore maintained, however, that the development of clearer intentions and purposes parallels the acquisition of more advanced linguistic competency. Thus, the child eventually uses speech acts which are in accordance with those of the native-speaking adult.

The basic context for speech acts, or rather communicative compe-tence, is social interactions. During the prelinguistic period, the child ex-presses the beginnings of purposive and intentional behaviors in his or her motor patterns. Typical behaviors include crying, vocalizing, eye-gazing, smiling, and various attempts to reach for objects in conjunction with some of these behaviors. By the second year, due to an increase in mobility and cognitive structures, the communicative gestures consist of showing, giv-ing, and pointing (e.g., Bates, 1976). This phase commences with the child showing an object to an adult. Then, the child engages in such behaviors as giving objects and pointing out objects (i.e., deixis). The major func-tion of these acts is to direct the adult's attention to the object. The atten-tion and acceptance of the adult/caregiver is important for the child. The emergence of the first words coincides with these early communicative behaviors of showing, giving, and pointing. A more detailed description of the substance and function of interaction/deixis can be found elsewhere (e.g., Lindfors, 1980; Lucas, 1980).

The functions of speech acts have also been reported by Halliday (1975). Halliday's Phase I, described earlier, contained four functions. Halliday maintains that during Phase II the child continues to master the functions of language by using utterances which resemble those used by adults. In addition, Halliday reported that a fifth function, heuristic, emerges during this phase around the 13th or 14th month. This function entails the use of vocalization in exploring and learning about the environment. In the earlier heuristic period, a child demands the names of objects, and later on, this behavior evolves into questioning behaviors.

Halliday asserts that it is possible to make a distinction between the *mathetic* and pragmatic functions of language. The mathetic function is the use of language to learn about persons, objects, and events in the environment. The precursors of this function are the personal and heuristic functions. The pragmatic function refers to the regulation of others' behaviors and attempts to satisfy personal needs. The precursors of this function are the instrumental and regulatory functions. The interaction function contributes to the development of both the mathetic and pragmatic functions. In sum, Halliday argues that the functions of language are expressed in isolation prior to the age of 2 years. During the second year, however, a child's utterance contains both mathetic and pragmatic functions.

Comprehension-Production Issue

Central to the analyses of the first words is the comprehension-production issue. This issue was discussed earlier relative to the sounds of speech; it is presented here with respect to the nature of the first words. The productions of children have received more attention than the corresponding comprehension of words. The paucity of research is not due to a lack of interest, but rather to the difficulty of measuring the comprehension of children (see discussions in Bloom & Lahey, 1978; Crystal, 1987; Goodluck, 1991; Ingram, 1989).

It has been suggested that the one-word utterances of children are analogous to the sentences of adults (Ingram, 1989). This phenomenon is termed holophrastic speech, implying that children understand more than they say. Although the word-or-sentence hypothesis has been discussed extensively, most of the evidence seems to support Bloom's (1973) argument that the extent of children's early knowledge is restricted to lexical meanings, not grammatical meaning, that is, syntax or relations between words.

The question of whether comprehension precedes production or vice versa has been investigated. For example, Huttenlocher (cited and discussed in Quigley & Paul, 1990) studied the performance of four 1-year-old children. The researcher devised procedures to assess comprehension by minimizing the influence of contextual cuing. A list of words with precise meanings, that is, those understood by the subjects, was obtained. This is contrary to Clark's (1973) and Bowerman's (e.g., 1973, 1988) contentions that obtaining precise meaning is extremely difficult at this stage. The results of this study also supported Bloom's (1973) arguments. In sum, Huttenlocher concluded that at the one-word stage: (a) the comprehension of children is dependent on contextual cues rather than on verbal comprehension, and (b) there are no instances of overextensions, thus, comprehension of lexical items precedes production.

In another study, Shipley, Smith, and Gleitman (1969) investigated the comprehension issues in two groups of children: one group used single-word utterances and the other used telegraphic two- and three-word sentences. Commands were presented to these children in single words, telegraphic speech, or well-formed sentences. Conflicting results were reported. The single-word group responded best to commands of first words, thus substantiating the claim that comprehension precedes production at this stage. The telegraphic group, however, responded best to well-formed commands. This latter result cannot be interpreted in the same way as the former.

In sum, Bloom and Lahey (1978) and others (e.g., Crystal, 1987; Ingram, 1989) suggest that different kinds of questions should be asked concerning comprehension and production. Instead of investigating which one precedes the other or the relationship between the two, they suggest studying the processes that underlie each and the relationship of the two processes to linguistic and cognitive development. They also suggest that "the developmental gap between comprehension and speaking probably varies among different children and at different times, and that the gap may be more apparent than real" (Bloom & Lahey, 1978, p. 238; see also, the influences of the perspectives on language and thought on this issue in Gelman & Byrnes, 1991).

Linguistic Maturity

As the child proceeds through the three-word stage and beyond, it still is difficult to assess the relative contributions of each linguistic component *in isolation* to this development. For example, it was mentioned earlier that Brown (1973) documented the developmental sequence of the first inflectional morphemes. Although syntactic and semantic complexity were adjudged to be good indices of development, it is difficult to isolate the relative contributions of each component. There are contributions of pragmatics; however, the precise nature of these effects have not been determined (see discussion in Crystal, 1987).

Beyond the three-word stage, the child begins to produce and comprehend linguistic forms and functions of a more complex nature. Now the child is learning the general, adult rules which govern the application of rules for the various linguistic components. The child plays an active role by discovering regularities and formulating hypotheses regarding the application of the rules (Cairns, 1986; de Villiers & de Villiers, 1978; Ingram, 1989; Menyuk, 1977). Through the joint social interaction or deixis, the child acquires semantic referents and functions for persons, objects, and events, in his or her environment. The form of the referents entails the combinations of the arbitrarily defined symbols from phonology, morphology, and syntax. The application of linguistic form, content, and function correspond to a rule system (Bloom & Lahey, 1978; Crystal, 1987; Goodluck, 1991; Ingram, 1989).

The mature linguistic forms are acquired through the processes of modulation and refinement. The basis of these processes is the acquisition of morphemes which alters meaning and form (Brown, 1973). The early syntactic-semantic utterances are modulated and subsequently expanded (or refined) into structures similar to those used by adults. Initially, two operations are in effect: embedding and conjoining (Brown, 1973). An example of embedding is: *no cookie* and *make cookie* becomes *make no cookie*. *No cookie,* which expresses a functional relation, is inserted or embedded into *make cookie* to form a grammatical relation. An example of conjoining is: *mommy make* and *make cookie* becomes *mommy make cookie*. In conjoining, two grammatical relations sharing a common term are conjoined with the redundant term deleted. In sum, an increase in semantic information parallels the increase in structure complexity, and this phenomenon is reflected in the complex utterance produced (Lucas, 1980).

Beyond the three-word stage, the syntactic development of the child consists of "using" the major transformations of the language (Cairns, 1986; Crystal, 1987; de Villiers & de Villiers, 1978; Goodluck, 1991). Initially, the child adheres to a noun-verb-noun or subject-verb-object word order which present problems in some transformations, notably passivization. Nevertheless, the major transformations, for example, question formation (e.g., wh- questions and yes/no questions) and relativization (i.e., use of relative pronouns—*who, whom,* and *that*) are acquired in a systematic manner. Within the question formation category, yes/no questions are acquired before wh- questions and this, in turn, is acquired before tag questions (e.g., *You ate the cookie, didn't you?* or *You didn't eat the cookie, did you?*). There are also smaller acquisition steps within each group of questions. Further discussion of the acquisition process can be found elsewhere (e.g., Cairns, 1986; Crystal, 1987; Dale, 1976; Russell et al., 1976). In general, most children have internalized much of the grammar of the language by the age of 4 or 5 years and have mastered nearly all of the grammar by age 9 or 10.

As stated earlier, semantic development (and pragmatic development) is essentially isomorphic to cognitive development (e.g., Ingram, 1989;

Lucas, 1980). Pragmatics consists of using the rules of semantics. Semantics referents can be categorized as objective and agentive, action, dimensional, and spatial and temporal. The beginning of social interaction or deixis is characterized by the identification of referents with corresponding labels (e.g., Bruner 1974–1975). This process helps the child organize knowledge about persons, objects, and events. The growth in vocabulary and other linguistic variables is hypothesized to be influenced by these interactions (e.g., see discussions in Gelman & Byrnes, 1991; Ingram, 1989; Lucas, 1980). From one perspective, for example, Piaget's model of cognition, most of the semantic referents are acquired by the second stage. This is nearly congruent with syntactic development. By the age of 10, 11, or 12 years, the child has reached linguistic maturity; that is, she or he has mastered most, if not all, of the finite set of the native-speaking adult *rules* regarding the form, content, and function of language.

Some highlights regarding the cognitive and linguistic development of children, particularly during the early phases of this development, are presented in Table 4–2.

TABLE 4-2. Highlights of the Early Cognitive and Linguistic Development of Children

Emergence of the First Words

- First words can only be fully understood within the contexts in which they are uttered. Some of them are not just labels but stand for sentence-like commentaries or instructions.
- Two-word combinations are examples of early grammatical language; the words are put together to express the child's perception of actions and relationships.
- In the years from 2 to 4, children evolve grammatical rules that produce some errors of over-generalization in plurals and tenses. They also invent verbs and nouns by analogy with conventional forms.
- Words refer to actual experiences and things in the world but they also stand for concepts or classifications in the minds of speakers.
- Concepts are generalized categories; they classify similarities, differences and hierarchies (or families) of connected ideas, objects and happenings.
- Concepts are usually thought to have core meanings, perceptual information and linguistic signs. Personal associations also play a part in the complex development of concepts.
- Thinking with concepts develops with language use.

Source: Adapted from Whitehead (1990, pp. 60, 74)

LANGUAGE DEVELOPMENT AND DEAF CHILDREN

Through observations of a young hearing child, say a 5 year old, in the home and school environments, it is possible to describe the nature of the language she or he is using. That is, one can label it as Spanish, French, or English, or even bilingual combinations such as Spanish and English and so on. It is much more difficult, of course, to determine the communicative and grammatical competence of this hypothetical hearing child.

On the other hand, describing the primary language development of a deaf child is much more complicated. It is true that most deaf children in the United States are *exposed* to English in infancy and early childhood (e.g., King, 1981; Moores, 1987; Paul & Quigley, 1990). As emphasized by Quigley and Kretschmer (1982), the description of this "exposure" needs to consider two issues: (1) the nature of the language input; and (2) the nature of the communication mode used, that is, manual or oral.

Relative to these issues, it can be stated that some deaf children are exposed to English (language input) via the use of speech (communication mode—oral). Other deaf children may be exposed to English (language input) via the use of signs (communication mode—manual) or signs and speech (communication modes—manual and oral). Still others may be exposed only to American Sign Language (language input), which only involves the use of signs (communication mode—manual; however, nonmanual cues are important too; see Chapter 1). It could be argued that exposure to English in a signed form also involves some exposure to ASL because of a few overlapping aspects between the signed systems and ASL. Nevertheless, exposure to some aspects of ASL is not commensurate with exposure to ASL as language input in the same way that exposure to or use of a few French words is not commensurate with "knowledge" of the French language.

In light of the discussion above, it should not be surprising that there have been very few research studies that attempted to determine the communicative and grammatical assessment of deaf children, especially with respect to the use of English via the various signed systems. Some of the research, cited in this chapter, involved retrospective studies employing secondary language assessments, that is, reading and writing, in evaluating the efficiency of language/communication approaches in developing a primary language. There are a few studies, however, which are developmental, that is, these studies attempted to chart some aspect of primary language development.

The goal of this section is to describe the language development of deaf children relative to three broad categories: oral English (OE), manually coded English, and ASL. Oral English approaches have been motivated by the oralist philosophy and manually coded English approaches by the total communication (TC) philosophy. Although the use of ASL is philosophically feasible within the TC philosophy, its impetus has come from two broad movements: the legitimacy of ASL as a language and the "depathologizing" of deafness. As much as possible, research findings are reported in this section within each of these categories with reference to the various components of language described previously, for example, syntax and semantics.

Descriptions of the major communication and language categories and some specific approaches used within the categories have been provided in Chapter 1. It is important to emphasize repeatedly that the descriptions and categories may be idealized versions of what usually occurs in practice. This is due mainly to the inconsistent and unsystematic use and application of the rules for the systems by many, but not all, practitioners (e.g., see reviews in Paul & Quigley, 1990; Quigley & Kretschmer, 1982). From another perspective, the type of signing that occurs in the use of some signed systems resembles that which can be labeled as "foreign talk" (discussed in Luetke-Stahlman & Luckner, 1991). This includes the use of short sentences, the paraphrasing of certain sentence constructions or lexical items (words), reductions or omissions of certain grammatical elements such as inflections (e.g., -ly, -ed) and certain function words (e.g., the, of). An example has been provided by Luetke-Stahlman and Luckner (1991, p. 9), the following sample:

> of Signed English (was) taken from teachers' spontaneous language . . . (under-
> lined words were signed as well as spoken):
> OK—*any* other *word?*
> *Yea,* I *would* not *like to go there,* too.
> You do not *want* to *walk through* that *water,* right?
> You don't *scream* out . . .
> . . . like a *pig's room—alright* . . . OK

It is helpful to remember the somewhat arbitrary and idealized nature of the descriptions and categories to consider the various language and communication approaches on a continuum ranging from least representative to most representative of the grammar of standard English. The relationship of the various approaches to standard English is depicted in Figure 4–1. ASL is not included in Figure 4–1 because it is a language with a grammar different from that of English. The manner in which each of the signed codes represents a written English word determines its placement on the continuum. For example, the English word, *beautifully,* can be represented by one manual marker [sign] as in English-based signing; two manual markers, one for *beautiful* and one for *-ly* as in SEE II (signing exact English); or one manual marker for each letter as in finger spelling (specifically, the Rochester method). With this line of reasoning,

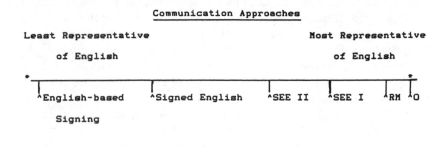

Note: SEE I = seeing essential English

        SEE II = signing exact English

        RM = Rochester method

        O = oral approaches including cued speech

FIGURE 4-1. Relationships of Communication Approaches to the Written Structure of Standard English.

finger spelling (Rochester method) would be considered the most representative of the structure of English (i.e., written English), followed by SEE I (seeing essential English), SEE II, signed English, and English-based (or English-like) signing. Because all OE approaches, including cued speech, use standard English, these are considered most representative of the structure of English, particularly, *spoken* English. This concept of a continuum allows for the various gradations in the communication and language approaches that are likely to occur in actual practice.

The relative merits of the various communication approaches used in developing language in deaf children are shrouded in controversy. Most of the arguments, however, are polemic rather than data based. The controversy which still exists after more than 200 years (e.g., McAnally et al., 1987, in press; Moores, 1987) is indicative of the notion that none of these approaches has proven adequate for *all* deaf children. In fact, it is possible that a universal approach does not exist (Moores, 1987; Paul & Quigley, 1990; Quigley & Kretschmer, 1982).

It will be obvious that much of the research on this issue is descriptive in nature. That is, there have been few attempts to work toward an "explanatory adequacy" as espoused by Chomsky (1975; see also Chapter addition, not enough attention has been paid to the nature of the systems relative to the representation of English. Finally, there needs to be additional discussion on the notion that *a* language should be developed at as early an age as possible.

Oral English

Research on oral English (OE) is presented relative to cued speech and traditional oral-English methods (e.g., unisensory and multisensory approaches). In general, students who are exposed to these methods are those with severe to profound hearing impairments. The most promising effects of oral-education programs have been observed for a small select group of students (i.e., high socioeconomic status [SES]) in incontestably, intensive oral programs such as Central Institute for the Deaf (CID) and St. Joseph Institute for the Deaf in St. Louis, Missouri (Connor, 1986; cf., Geers & Moog, 1989; Luetke-Stahlman, 1988a). Nevertheless, it is still true that there is a need for "well documented research, demonstrating the value and need for oral methods" (Lane, 1976, p. 137).

Cued Speech

Most of the research on cued speech (CS) has been conducted on students in countries other than the United States; however, the use of cued speech in the United States seems to be increasing (e.g., Quenin & Blood, 1989). Examples of early research are the works of Ling and Clarke (1975) and Clarke and Ling (1976), who analyzed the receptive abilities of students who had been exposed to CS for 2 years. The test stimuli consisted of cued and noncued words, phrases, and sentences. Results indicated that students understood cued stimuli significantly better than noncued stimuli. Cued words were easier than cued phrases which were easier than cued sentences. The investigators also reported that the students' phonetic (i.e., pronunciation) errors can be grouped into patterns that can be addressed in a systematic remedial speech and language program.

Nicholls and Ling (1982) analyzed the speech reception abilities of Australian students with hearing impairments exposed to cued speech for 4 years. Test stimuli were presented under seven conditions that resulted from all possible permutations of three variables: audition, cues, and speech reading. The scores of the students for two conditions, speech reading plus cues, and audition, speech reading, and cues were significantly higher than those for all other conditions. In addition, the use of cues did not negatively affect the students' abilities to speech read or to use their residual hearing. The researchers concluded that CS might be a viable option for students with severe to profound hearing impairment who cannot progress adequately in conventional oral-education programs.

Mohay (1983) studied the effects of cued speech on the English language development of three children—two had a profound hearing impairment and one child had a severe hearing impairment. The children started their education in a traditional oral program and then transferred to a CS program. The researcher observed that the children's use of word combinations (i.e., two- or three-words) increased after exposure to cued speech. It was suggested, however, that certain factors such as growth in cognitive ability might have been responsible for the increase in production rather than the use of CS.

More recent studies on hearing adults (Abraham & Stoker, 1984; Chilson, 1985) and adults with hearing impairment (Gregory, 1987) have provided additional support for the positive effects of cued speech on speech reading skills. In general, the adults obtained significantly higher speech reading scores on speech stimuli presented with cues. Thus, many of these studies seem to confirm the results of a survey by Quenin and Blood (1989): "Cued Speech is viewed as a vehicle for conveying spoken language and as a tool in speech development" (p. 288).

The assumption that the use of cued speech has a positive effect on the development of a language, particularly reading skills, is the subject of several articles in a recent publication (*Cued Speech Journal, 1990*). From another perspective, Liedel and Paul (1991) have argued that cued speech may play a critical role in the development of rapid word identification skills (i.e., bottom-up skills) for reading. The development of rapid word identification skills in English is dependent, in part, on the cognitive representation of the phonological and morphological properties of English (see Chapter 5). Liedel and Paul have developed a model in which cued speech is part of an interactive-interaction bilingual-bicultural program for ASL-using deaf students. This model is based on a social-cognitive interactive view of reading. In addition, this model is another example of a recent survey finding: "Cued Speech may be a component of both oral and total communication approaches to teaching hearing-impaired students" (Quenin & Blood, 1989, p. 288).

Cornett (1991) has also recognized the role of cued speech in the development of reading via the development of phonological awareness. This recognition is based on some research evidence and on the fact that Cornett designed the CS system to reflect the phonological aspect of any spoken language (see Chapter 1). In emphasizing the importance of cued speech for reading, Cornett quoted the concluding paragraph of a study by Alegria, DeJean, Capouillez and Leybaert:

To come back to our initial point, the present work strongly suggests that the lexicon developed by the deaf with Cued Speech has properties that are *equivalent* to the phonology of the hearing subjects. In both cases the internal representations of the words are compatible with their orthographic representation. This allows the use of phonological coding to identify unfamiliar words and, as said before, can prime the whole process of reading acquisition. (Cornett, 1991, p. 36)

Traditional Oral Programs

The benefits of unisensory methods, especially the acoupedics approach, have been reported in several case studies (Pollack, 1984). Long, Fitzgerald, Sutton, and Rollins (1983), for example, documented the achievement of a $4\frac{1}{2}$-year-old girl. The language development of the girl was proceeding at a rate similar to her hearing counterparts. A description of the essential components of this approach (also known as auditory-verbal), specifically the training aspects for clinicians, can been found in a recent article (Caleffe-Schenck, 1992).

Some of the most impressive results of traditional oral methods can be found in studies on students enrolled in indisputably, comprehensive programs. Lane and Baker (1974) compared the reading grade level scores of former students at CID to students with hearing impairment in other investigations. The reading achievement growth of the former CID students was 2.5 grades for a 4-year education period. This growth rate is much greater than that observed in national surveys (Allen, 1986; CADS, 1991; Trybus & Karchmer, 1977).

In a later study, Doehring, Bonnycastle, and Ling (1978) examined the language comprehension abilities of CID students, some of whom were integrated in regular-education programs. The results indicated that the students performed at or above grade level on reading tasks. It was concluded that the performances of the CID students were influenced by their intensive auditory-oral training.

The success of orally trained students has been documented in more recent studies and reviews (Geers & Moog, 1989; Luetke-Stahlman, 1988a; Paul & Quigley, 1990; Quigley & Paul, 1986). Students in intensive, comprehensive oral-education programs are more likely to develop better language, reading, and academic skills than are students in other educational programs and those exposed to approaches that do not completely represent the grammar of English (e.g., see Figure 4–1, presented previously).

Luetke-Stahlman (1988a) examined the performances of hearing-impaired students who were between the ages of 5 to 12 years old and exposed to two groups of approaches. One group of approaches consisted of oral English and other forms representing either a language (e.g., ASL) or a fairly complete representation of a language (e.g., SEE I, SEE II, cued speech). The other group consist of approaches that are not considered to be a complete representation of a language (e.g., SE [including manual English] and PSE [i.e., English-based signing]). The researcher controlled several variables statistically, for example, age and aided and unaided hearing acuity. The literacy battery consisted of tests involving portions of *Woodcock-Johnson Psychoeducational Battery, The Johns Sight Word List for Third-Graders,* and the *Northwestern Syntax Screening Test* (Lee, 1969). A speech intelligibility measure was also included.

The results indicated that the students exposed to OE and other systems in this group of approaches performed significantly better than students in the other group on six of the seven measures used. Luetke-Stahlman (1988a) concluded that it was important to be exposed to instructional approaches that are either a bona fide language or a complete representation of a language. This study is considered again later in the discussion of the signed systems.

It can be inferred from the Luetke-Stahlman's study that deaf students with a working knowledge of the primary form of English may acquire adequate English literacy skills. This issue has been investigated extensively in a recent study by Geers and Moog (1989), who argued that the primary oral form of English is indispensable. Geers and Moog studied 100 oral students with profound hearing impairment enrolled in programs in the United States and Canada. The overwhelming majority of these students (80%) were mainstreamed for all or most of the school day. The researcher proffered several statements to explain the well-developed language and cognitive skills of many of the students. For example, they concluded that:

(a) It is possible for profoundly hearing-impaired children, by the time they are 16 years of age, to achieve reading skills commensurate with those of normal-hearing students.

(b) Children with profound hearing impairment who have a combination of favorable factors—including at least average nonverbal intellectual ability, early oral education management and auditory stimulation, and middle-class family environment with strong family support—have a potential for developing much higher reading, writing, and spoken language skills than in reported for hearing-impaired people in general.

(c) *The primary factors associated with the development of literacy in this orally educated sample are good use of residual hearing, early amplification, and educational management, and—above all—oral English language ability, including vocabulary, syntax, and discourse skills.* (Geers & Moog, 1989, p. 84, emphasis added)

It is interesting to note that some of these "primary factors" have been noted for deaf students in total communication programs to be discussed later (e.g., Delaney, Stuckless, & Walter, 1984; Moores & Sweet, 1990). It might not be obvious that most of the primary factors listed above document the very strong relationship between the primary (especially, oral) and secondary forms of a language such as English.

Additional insights into the success of orally trained students have been reported in two survey studies (McCartney, 1986; Ogden, 1979). In one study, it was remarked that "this group is atypical in comparison to the national population and the national hearing-impaired population," that is, they "have better than average education, careers, and annual salaries" (McCartney, 1986, p. 135). The students in both surveys attributed their success to the factors mentioned previously, namely, early education, early amplification, parental involvement, and oral-communication skills. They also felt that it was important to have the desire to be integrated into regular-education programs and the mainstream of society.

Despite the differences in the various oral approaches, success has been observed for students with severe to profound hearing impairment. This success seems to be based on the common features across most programs, for example, early identification of hearing impairment, involved parents/caregivers, and the development of oral-communication skills via the areas of speech, speech reading, and residual hearing (e.g., see discussions in Levitt, 1989; Ling, 1990; Ross, 1990; Silverman & Kricos, 1990.

Total Communication

Many TC signed systems have been in use for about 20 or more years. Not surprisingly, the little research evidence that exist does not indicate a particular approach as being superior to all others for all or even most deaf students. Although it has been reported that certain aspects of the English grammar can be taught, for example, morphology and vocabulary, the rate of acquisition for deaf students seems to become slower, compared to hearing students. Nevertheless, there is some evidence to indicate that one of the most important variables is how well a particular system represents the structure of English. For most students to benefit from these specific systems, however, practitioners (parents and teachers) need to improve their use of them. We synthesize a representative sample of studies in the various categories mentioned previously: Rochester method, seeing essential English, signing exact English, and English-based signing (previously known as Pidgin Sign English).

Rochester Method

Quigley (1969) examined language, reading, and academic achievement of students in nine residential schools. He reported that students exposed to the Rochester method (RM) performed significantly better than those students who were exposed to simultaneous communication. The average 18-year-old student exposed to RM was reading at about the fifth-grade level.

Stuckless and Pollard (1977) examined the ability of college-age deaf students to process both print and finger spelling. It should be recalled that finger spelling entails the use of hand shapes to represent letters of the English alphabet. Stuckless and Pollard reported that the processing ability of the students was strongly related to their level of English competence. In addition, it was noted that print was easier to process than finger spelling. This finding, and other similar findings, have been confirmed in additional studies. It seems that information presented in print is easier to process than that presented in any of the language/communication approaches (see reviews in Moores, 1987; Paul & Quigley, 1990; Quigley & Kretschmer, 1982).

Looney and Rose (1979) showed that finger spelling can be used as an effective aid in teaching certain English morphemes such as -ed and -er. Twenty-four prelingually deaf students, age 8 to 15 years, participated as subjects. After demonstrating the ability to express through writing and finger spelling a few basic English kernel patterns, these subjects were randomly assigned to three groups. Group 1 was exposed to the Rochester method, Group 2 to print, and Group 3 was the control group. The two treatment groups were exposed to a systematic, 4-week instruction of selected morphological rules, that is, those involving past tense inflectional suffixes. The researchers administered pre- and posttests to assess their ability to recognize, select, determine grammaticality, and to produce the appropriate past tense morphemes.

The results indicated that both treatment groups made significant gains whereas the control group failed to demonstrate such a trend. In addition, no significant differences were reported between the two treatment groups. This led the researchers to conclude that finger spelling, as well as print, is useful in representing inflectional suffixes when taught in a systematic manner. It was also noted that maximum benefits result when students have some understanding of basic English sentence patterns such as *The boy is happy*. Finally, it is important to provide systematic and consistent instruction over a period of time.

Very few programs use the Rochester method as the sole approach (Moores, 1987; Paul & Quigley, 1990). Many programs may use this approach in a few classes, especially with junior and senior high students with hearing impairment (Baker & Cokely, 1980). An in-depth discussion of how finger spelling, one aspect of the RM, is perceived and produced can be found elsewhere (e.g., Akamatsu, 1982; Padden & Le Master, 1985; see also, Wilbur, 1987).

In a recent study, Akamatsu and Stewart (1989) investigated the use of finger spelling by five trained teachers of deaf students. They found that these teachers did not frequently employed finger spelling. In general, when finger spelling was used, it was primarily for the purpose of conveying a specific English word. The clarity of finger spelling use varied with the intent of finger spelling, that is, to use or teach an English word. Nevertheless, the data on clarity motivated the answer to one of their most important question:

> What are deaf children expected to do with the fingerspelled words of their teachers? They are expected to learn English words and their spellings, to recognize the words in print, and to write them correctly. How they can learn all this in the relative absence of clear and accurate fingerspelling models is still an open question. (Akamatsu & Stewart, 1989, p. 369)

In essence, the role and importance of finger spelling for the development of rapid word identification skills needs further study. For example, it has been reported that good deaf readers use both finger spelling and a phonological code (see Chapters 3 and 5) for the temporary retention of linguistic stimuli in short-term memory (e.g., Hanson, Liberman, & Shankweiler, 1984; see also, the reviews in Hanson, 1989; Paul & Jackson, 1993). Poor readers do not predominantly used either finger spelling or a phonological code.

Although finger spelling, specifically as it is used in the Rochester method, is theoretically most representative of the structure of written English, the empirical data have not been convincing enough to consider this approach a panacea either now or when it was a prevalent method during the 1960s (Quigley, 1969).

Seeing Essential English

Schlesinger and Meadow (1972) described the primary language acquisition of four deaf children (see also, the discussion in Chapter 6 on the use of ASL). Three of their subjects were exposed to at least some SEE I signs. The beginning of these subjects' exposure to SEE I ranged from 15 months to 3 years of age. Fairly substantial development was observed in both syntax and vocabulary, and some support was found for Bloom's (1970) two-word syntactic-semantic relations. The data on one subject were analyzed with respect to the pivot-grammar proposed by Braine (1963a, 1963b), the counterfindings on pivot-grammar argued by Brown (1973), and the relations proposed by Bloom (1970). It was reported that the bulk of the data supported Brown's arguments against pivot-grammar. In addition, the use of two-word/sign utterances by this subject seemed to support Bloom's contention that such utterances tend to expose a variety of structural meanings in relation to the surrounding context cues. For example, this subject signed/spoke: *Daddy shoe.* This is an example of the agent-object relation in which the subject is attempting to tell her father to remove his shoes and get into the sandbox with her.

The data on another subject focus on the acquisition of some English morphological rules. It was found that this subject, exposed to SEE I markers at age 3, began to use the markers by age 4. In sum, on the basis of spontaneous language samples and tests of grammatical competence (Menyuk, 1963), it was concluded that these deaf children were acquiring grammatical competence in the same sequence as hearing children; however, the rate of development was slower.

Raffin and his associates (Gilman, Davis, & Raffin, 1980; Raffin, 1976; Raffin, Davis, & Gilman, 1978) focused on the use of SEE I markers by students, especially sign-markers representing some of the most common English morphemes such as -*s* (plurality and third-person singular), -*ly* (adverb), -*er* (comparison), and -*ed* (past tense). The findings indicated that the order of acquisition of the markers of students with hearing impairment was qualitatively similar to that of hearing students (Brown, 1973). In other words, students with hearing impairment proceed through developmental stages at a slower rate than and produce errors similar to those of younger hearing students. It was also observed that acquisition and use of the SEE I markers were influenced pervasively by teachers' use of the markers. That is, the more systematic and consistent teachers are in using the sign markers, the more likely students are to acquire and use them.

In a more recent investigation, Washburn (1983) discussed the educational achievement results of students in three public school districts who had been exposed to seeing essential English. Based on an analysis of scores from 1977 to 1981, the researcher stated that the average reading grade levels of SEE I students were from one to two grades higher than those of other students with hearing impairment in other programs. In addition, the SEE I students in grades 11 and 12 of one program scored in the top 20% of all *hearing* high-school students taking the reading comprehension subset of the *Stanford Achievement Test.* The mean reading level of the top group was slightly above the seventh grade. Experimental research, however, is needed to determine if the use of SEE I *caused* the differences in scores between students exposed to this method.

We have already discussed the work of Luetke-Stahlman (1988a) previously. It should be recalled that students exposed to SEE I were considered to be in a group that had been exposed to a system which was a fairly complete representation of the structure of English. This type of exposure was deemed to be responsible for their performance on the battery of tests in this study.

The results of the Luetke-Stahlman's study confirmed the findings of an earlier study by Deal and Thornton (1985); however, Deal and Thornton argued that much more research is needed on the assumptions of the so-called "more complete signed systems." These researchers investigated the comprehension levels of deaf students who were exposed to stories via the use of SEE I and sign English (a synonym for English-based or English-like signing). Although the results indicated that the SEE I trained students outperformed the sign English trained students, "the overall comprehension scores for both groups was less than or equal to 50%" (p. 275).

Signing Exact English

No signed system is widely implemented in its entirety; however, many of the signs used in the education of students with hearing impairment come from signing exact English (SEE II; Jordan, Gustason, & Rosen, 1979; Jordan & Karchmer, 1986). The creators of SEE II have developed educational materials to aid in the using of the system (Gustason, 1983).

Babb (1979) investigated the language and academic performances of students with profound hearing impairment exposed to SEE II for about a decade. Half of the students were exposed to SEE II in the home (i.e., via parents/caregivers) and at school. The other half were exposed to the system at school only. Results indicated that the group exposed to SEE II in the home and at school performed significantly better than the group exposed to SEE II at school only on all measurements. The median grade achievement of the home-plus-school group was slightly above the seventh-grade level. Students in both the Babb (1979) and Washburn (1983) studies had higher achievement levels than those reported in every national survey conducted by the Center for Assessment and Demographic Studies at Gallaudet University (Allen, 1986; CADS, 1991). Impressive results of students exposed to SEE II have also been reported in the study by Luetke-Stahlman (1988a), discussed previously.

Signed English

Bornstein, Saulnier, and Hamilton (1980) and Bornstein and Saulnier (1981) followed 18 students with severe to profound hearing impairment enrolled in residential and day schools for 5 years. The researchers reported that the receptive vocabulary and syntactic development of the students were qualitatively similar, albeit quantitatively reduced, when compared to that of hearing counterparts. Analyzing the students' use of the SE markers over the 5-year period, the researchers found that very few students were using the markers consistently. In fact, the oldest students, who were about 10 years old, were using only one half of the 14 inflectional sign-markers.

In a more recent study, Gardner and Zorfass (1983) examined the oral language development of a 3-year-old child with a severe impairment. The child was exposed to SE from the age of 13 months. As the oral development (i.e., speech) of the child increase, the use of signs or sign-markers decrease. The child was severely hearing impaired *and* benefitted enormously from the use of amplification. This indicated that audition was the primary mode of receiving communication, rather than vision, which is the case for most students with severe to profound hearing losses. The results of this case study provide further support for the importance of audition in the development of spoken language skills such as speech and speech reading.

There is some evidence that the placement of SE signs above words impacts positively the reading comprehension scores of deaf students (e.g., Robbins, 1983; see also, the discussion in King & Quigley, 1985). Other research has shown that this technique can be used to improve deaf students' word identification skills (e.g., Stoefen-Fisher & Lee, 1989). These positive results should be interpreted with caution because SE does not deal with "complex" English words, that is, words that involve markers not included in the system (i.e., more than the 14 SE markers). The limitations of the system, relative to advanced literacy skills, has been demonstrated by the work of Luetke-Stahlman (1988a). Finally, there are problems in using signs in the printed form, especially for the purpose of reading. It has been remarked:

> One problem the authors have struggled with is that they can follow the left-to-right convention for writing words in sequence but cannot use that convention for sequencing of sign actions within words; e.g., a right-handed sign that moves from the mouth to the ear moves backward and slightly to the right; the reverse image illustrated (as one would see the signer) shows the sign moving to the signer's right, which means it moves to the reader's left. This right-to-left movement disrupts the left-to-right sequence of standard print. Such backtracking could lead to omission of the final parts of signs or to the reversal of two parts. (Maxwell, 1987, pp. 345–346)

Finally, it should be noted that the overall results of the use of the SE system have not met the expectations of its creator (e.g., see Bornstein, 1982). This has led to a modification of the theory of using SE (Bornstein, 1982); that is, it is debatable that the structure of English needs to be "completely" represented all or even most of the time. In addition, the completeness of this representation becomes less critical as the deaf individual becomes older. Theoretical debates aside, there is no compelling evidence that deaf individuals have acquired a high level of competency in either the primary or secondary mode of English via the use of SE.

English-based Signing

Much of the signing that occurs in total-communication classrooms resembles some form of Pidgin Sign English (PSE). Strictly speaking, PSE might be better labeled as English-based or English-like signing in which few sign-markers are used (Paul & Quigley, 1990; cf., Luetke-Stahlman & Luckner, 1991). This description is still applicable to deaf individuals who attempt to sign to hearing persons who do not know ASL. As with the signing of hearing persons, there are variations in the signing of deaf persons. However, it is likely that the signing of deaf individuals, especially those with a limited knowledge of English, contains a good deal of ASL-like grammatical aspects. The signing of both hearing and deaf individuals in English/ASL contact situations needs to be researched further.

There is another framework for describing "English-based" or "English-like" signing. For example, many teachers and other practitioners have difficulty using the more complex signed systems such as SEE I and SEE II in a consistent, systematic manner (Kluwin, 1981; Marmor & Petitto, 1979; Mitchell, 1982; Strong & Charlson, 1987; cf., Luetke-Stahlman, 1988b). In addition, they *borrow* signs from several systems to suit their communication needs. These reduced and inconsistent variations of signing combine some grammatical aspects of ASL with those of the various signed systems within an English word order.

With the above caveats in mind, it is possible to describe the "achievement" of students exposed to this form of communication in early childhood, including in school settings. Because of the dearth of "experimental" research, it is difficult to conclude that the use of this particular form of signing "causes" the achievement. This difficulty is compounded by the variability across signers in using English-based signing.

The first study examined is one which described the communication approach used in school and at home as total communication. Griswold and Cummings (1974) investigated the expressive vocabulary of 19 preschool deaf children, ages 2 to about 5 years old. Results indicated that a composite vocabulary list of 493 words and expressions were used by two or more students. However, the size of the vocabulary was smaller than that reported for hearing children of comparable ages. In spite of this, the composition of the vocabulary of the deaf children was similar to that of hearing children regarding (a) the proportion of nouns and verbs, (b) the number and usage of specific prepositions, (c) the usage of numbers (words), and (d) the usage of specific question words. The deaf children, however, differed from the hearing children in that they rarely used connectives, articles, and auxiliary/modal verbs. These investigators concluded that a correlation existed between the size of the vocabulary and two other variables: the length of time spent in a preschool program and the amount of exposure to total communication in the home environment.

In another study, Crandall (1978) studied the developmental order of manual English morphemes. The subjects used a communication approach labeled as manual English. Manual English entailed the use of signs from an ASL lexicon and sign markers representing morphemes (e.g., *-ed, -ly*), demonstratives (e.g., *this, that*), and articles (e.g., *a, an, the*) from SEE II and from a basic text on manual communication (O'Rourke, 1973). Twenty pairs of hearing mothers and their young deaf children served as subjects. In particular, Crandall was interested in ascertaining whether the developmental order of the morphemes used by the deaf children was (a) related to age, (b) similar to that of hearing children of comparable age, and (c) related to their mother's use.

In general, all three hypotheses were supported. Mixed results, however, were obtained for the first hypothesis. It was reported that the deaf children's production of the inflectional morphemes did not increase significantly with age. The mean number of morphemes per utterance, however, did show an increase with age. Relative to developmental order, it was found that the first six morphemes used by the deaf children were similar to those documented for hearing children (Brown, 1973). This finding is consistent with those obtained in other studies (Raffin, 1976; Raffin et al., 1978; Schlesinger & Meadow, 1972). Finally, Crandall remarked that the mother's use of the morphemes influenced the child's use of these same morphemes. This last finding is typical of others in that it reveals the importance of the home environment.

Layton, Holmes, and Bradley (1979) examined the emergence of semantic relations in deaf children in a "PSE-using" environment. Three children, ages $5\frac{1}{2}$, $6\frac{1}{2}$, and 7 years, 7 months, served as subjects. They had been exposed to sign language 9 to 15 months prior to the inception of the study. Sign language is taken to mean a total communication system in which speech is simultaneously combined with manual signs, predominantly selected from an ASL lexicon. The signs needed for inflections and articles were selected from SEE II (Gustason, Pfetzing, & Zawolkow, 1975). The subjects were exposed to signed/spoken utterances that were one-word/one-sign in advance of their productions. For example, a subject at the one-word/one-sign stage was exposed to two-word/two-sign sequences.

The findings indicated that the semantic-syntactic categories of the deaf subjects were proportionately different from those reported for younger hearing children at less developed and equivalent linguistic levels (Bloom, Lightbown, & Hood, 1975). For example, hearing children produced more recurrence utterances (*more*), whereas the deaf subjects produced more state, negation, and attribution utterances (for examples and detailed explanations, see Bloom & Lahey, 1978). It was noted that these latter types of utterances did not emerge until a later stage of hearing children's development. The investigators attempted to account for these differences by suggesting that (a) deaf children were exposed to advanced categories prior to their understanding of the basic concepts; and (b) the differences may be due to a difference in age, that is, the older deaf subjects processed at a more sophisticated cognitive level than that of the younger hearing subjects in the study by Bloom et al. (1975). Finally, the researchers argued that instructors of hearing-impaired children should be aware of the "normal" developmental patterns of hearing children.

The studies presented thus far seem to indicate that the use of English-based signing is effective for primary language development if it is used in the home and its practitioners use structures that follow the developmental patterns of hearing children. The work of Brasel and Quigley (1977) is representative of what is known about the effects of English-based signing (in this case, manual English or PSE) on English literacy skills. The research design permitted the investigation of the effects of type of communication (oral and manual), type of language (ASL and English), and intensity of early language input. Eighteen deaf students between 10 and 19 years of age were located in each of four language groups: manual English (termed PSE), average manual (considered ASL), intensive oral (IO), and average oral (AO). The intensive oral group represented those students who received intensive oral training involving both the school and the parents. The parents of the average oral group left the education of their children to the schools. The parents of the manual English and average manual groups were deaf parents whereas those of the two oral groups had normal hearing.

The results indicated that the manual English group significantly outperformed both oral groups in five of the six major syntactic structures as measured by the *Test of Syntactic Abilities* (Quigley, Power, Steinkamp, & Jones, 1978). In addition, the manual English group significantly outperformed all other groups on all subtests of the *Stanford Achievement Test* (SAT). On the Paragraph Meaning subtest, the manual English group's mean score was 7.24 years which was nearly 2 years better than the nearest group, intensive oral. The overall mean score of the manual English group on the SAT was 5.25 years.

The findings of the Brasel and Quigley study were interpreted as indicating that both type of communication and type of language input are essential variables in the language development of deaf children and that manual English might be a superior system for teaching deaf students. Nevertheless, it is still not clear how English should be represented manually. The manual English group in the Brasel and Quigley study read as

well as both the SEE II (home-plus-school) group in the Babb (1979) study
and the high-school SEE I group in the Washburn (1983) investigation.

Delaney et al. (1984) suggested that exposure to manual communication is not sufficient by itself for developing English literacy skills. The
achievement levels of three groups of students with profound hearing impairment were compared in a school that changed from oral education to
total-communication education. The results showed that the TC students
had higher achievement levels than both the transitional students (i.e.,
exposed to oral and TC methods) and the oral students (i.e., exposed to
oral methods prior to the change). The achievement level of the TC students was similar to that of the best group in the Brasel and Quigley
(1977), Babb (1979), and Washburn (1983) studies. Delaney et al. stated
that several other factors were probably responsible for the students'
achievement level, for example, involvement of parents and school personnel, well-established curricula, and the presence of some oral-communication skills.

As discussed previously, the results of Luetke-Stahlman (1988a) do
not support the findings of Brasel and Quigley (1977). In conjunction with
the findings of the study by Deal and Thornton (1985), it is clear that no
signed system (or even English-based signing) is superior for all or even
most deaf students. Nevertheless, some guidelines for selecting and using
a signed system in the education of deaf students need to be developed.
Some of the major highlights of the various studies within each signed
system are listed in Table 4–3.

American Sign Language

Traditionally, the study of spoken languages has contributed to much
of the prevailing linguistic thinking. The study of sign languages, however,
has only recently attracted the attention of linguists and psycholinguistics.
There is general agreement that ASL is a bona fide language (Klima &
Bellugi, 1979; Lane & Grosjean, 1980; Liddell, 1980; Wilbur, 1987), although there seems to some disagreement on how ASL is used or should
be described (e.g., see the special issue of *Deaf American,* 1990). Some
recent research focuses on comparing the processing of sign languages with
that of spoken languages (e.g., see discussions in Bellugi, 1988; Petitto,
1988). There seem to be similarities in stages and processes, for example,
the reduction or deletions of morphemes (e.g., Newport & Meier, 1985),
overgeneralizations of rules, and the influence of markedness on hand
shapes (e.g., McIntire, 1977). More research is needed on how skills can
be transferred from a sign language to a spoken language (Paul & Quigley,

TABLE 4–3. Summary of Findings of Studies Within the Signed Systems

Rochester Method	
Quigley (1969)	The average 18-year-old student exposed to RM was reading at about the fifth-grade level.
Stuckless & Pollard (1977)	The processing ability of deaf students was strongly related to their level of English competence.
Looney & Rose (1979)	Finger spelling can be used as an effective aid in teaching certain English morphemes such as -ed and -er.
Akamatsu & Stewart (1989)	The clarity of finger spelling use varied with the intent of finger spelling, that is, to use or teach an English word.

Seeing Essential English	
Schlesinger & Meadow (1972)	It was concluded that deaf children were acquiring English grammatical competence in the same sequence as hearing children; however, the rate of development was slower.
Gilman, Davis, & Raffin, 1980; Raffin, 1976; Raffin, Davis, & Gilman, 1978)	The acquisition and use of the SEE I markers were influenced pervasively by teachers' use of the markers. The more systematic and consistent teachers are in using the sign markers, the more likely students are to acquire and use them.
Washburn (1983)	SEE I students in grades 11 and 12 of one program scored in the top 20 percent of all hearing high-school students taking a reading comprehension subtest of the *Stanford Achievement Test.*

(continued)

TABLE 4-3. *(continued)*

Deal & Thornton (1985)	The results indicated that the SEE I trained students outperformed the sign English trained students; however, the overall comprehension scores of both groups were less than or equal to 50 percent.

Signing Exact English

Babb (1979)	Results indicated that the group exposed to SEE II in home and at school performed significantly better than the group exposed to SEE II at school only.

Signed English

Bornstein, Saulnier, & Hamilton, 1980; Bornstein & Saulnier, 1981)	Analyzing the students' use of the SE markers over a five-year period, it was found that very few students were using the markers consistently.
Bornstein (1982)	The completeness of representing English structure becomes less critical as the deaf individual becomes older.
Gardner & Zorfass (1983)	Results of this case study provide further support for the importance of audition in the development of spoken language skills such as speech and speech reading.
Robbins (1983)	Placement of SE signs above words positively impacted reading comprehension of deaf students.

English-based Signing

Griswold & Cummings (1974)	It was concluded that a correlation existed between the size of vocabulary and two other vari-

TABLE 4-3. *(continued)*

	ables: the length of time spent in a preschool program and the amount of exposure to total communication in the home environment.
Brasel & Quigley (1977)	Findings were interpreted as indicating that both type of communication and type of language input are essential variables in the language development of deaf children and that manual English might be a superior system for teaching deaf students.
Crandall (1978)	In general, the developmental order of the morphemes used by deaf children was similar to that of hearing children of comparable age and related to their mother's use of the morphemes.
Layton, Holmes, & Bradley (1979)	Findings indicated that the semantic-syntactic categories of deaf subjects were proportionately different from those reported for younger hearing children at less developed and equivalent linguistic levels.
Delaney, Stuckless, & Walter (1984)	Findings indicated that exposure to manual communication is not sufficient by itself for developing English literacy skills. Several other factors were probably responsible for the students' achievement levels, for example, involvement of parents and school personnel, well-established curricula, and the presence of some oral-communication skills.

1987a, 1987b, in press; Quigley & Paul, in press) or on important differences between ASL and English that pose problems for late second-language learners (e.g., Brown, Fischer, & Janis, 1993). This last issue is of importance for teaching deaf students whose first language is ASL to read and write standard English (see Chapter 6 of this text).

Descriptions of ASL grammar abound in controversy similar to any other new field of scientific inquiry (e.g., attempting to establish new terminology or directions for research). This situation, in turn, makes it extremely difficult to describe the acquisition of ASL grammar by deaf children and adolescents. For example, the feasibility of applying spoken language analyses (e.g., mean length of utterance, one-word stage) to a sign language is not always acceptable (e.g., Wilbur, 1987). The meaning of a sign needs to incorporate its accompanying nonmanual cues (Baker & Cokely, 1980; Liddell, 1980; Wilbur, 1987). As another example, there are disagreements among ASL linguists on how to transcribe or represent simple S-V-O sentences such as *The boy hit the girl* (e.g., Gee & Kegl, 1982; see also, the discussion in Gee & Goodhart, 1988).

In spite of these problems, it is still possible to state that the language development of deaf children learning ASL is comparable to that of their hearing peers. It has even been argued that ASL should be the first language for most deaf children because of its accessibility and the fact that it might be easier to learn than any form of English (e.g., see Johnson et al., 1989; Liddell & Johnson, 1992; see also Chapter 6). In the ensuing paragraphs, we present a sample of the findings regarding the development of ASL. This is intended to provide the reader with a brief overview, not an exhaustive treatment. A more detailed treatment of these issues can be found elsewhere (e.g., Bellugi, 1988; Bellugi & Klima, 1985; Klima & Bellugi, 1979; Liddell, 1980; Lane & Grosjean, 1980; Lucas, 1990; Newport & Meier, 1985; Petitto, 1988; Wilbur, 1987).

Phonological "Parameters" and the First Signs

Systematic research on the structure of ASL signs began with the work of Stokoe (1960). He studied the formation of signs (*cherology*), and treated it as analogous to the phonological system of spoken languages. Just as spoken words can be divided into phonemic elements, signs can be divided into smaller "cheremic" (hand) elements. Stokoe described three elements of a sign: (1) the handshape, (2) the location of the hand with reference to the body, and (3) the movement of the hand. These he labeled *dez, tab,* and *sig* (see Chapter 1). Battison (1974) argued for a fourth element, called orientation, which refers to the orientation of the palm (e.g., to differentiate between the sign for SHORT and that for TRAIN; see Figure 4–2). The distinctive features in spoken language are combined from vowels and

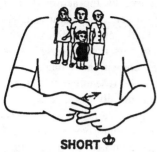

SHORT ♛
Side of right H rubs back and forth
on side of left H-hand

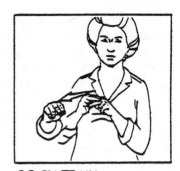

GO-BY-TRAIN

Noun: TRAIN

FIGURE 4-2. Signs for SHORT and TRAIN. SHORT—From *Signing Exact English,* Gustason, G., Pfetzing, D., & Zawolkow, E. (1980), published by Modern Signs Press, Inc., Los Alamitos, CA. Reprinted by permission of the publisher. TRAIN—*A Basic Course in American Sign Language* by Humphries, T., Padden, C., & O'Rourke, T. J. (1980), (p. 94). T. J. Publishers, Inc., Silver Spring, MD. Reprinted by permission of the publisher.

consonants. In a similar manner, the four elements described here are combined to produce a sign. As mentioned later, the phonology of signs has evolved into a complex, dynamic system of analysis (e.g., Stokoe, 1990; Wilbur, 1987).

One of the most interesting studies of the prelinguistic period has been the work of Petitto and Marentette (1991). Based on their observational study, these researchers have argued that there is a form of babbling, manual babbling, that is unique to deaf infants of deaf parents. This finding seems to support the assertion that speech is not critical for the babbling stage. By focusing on similarities between manual and vocal babbling, Petitto and Marentette (1991) remarked "that there is a unitary language capacity that underlies human signed and spoken language acquisition" (p. 1495). It should be mentioned also that some research has shown that deaf infants engage in vocal babbling. This has been interpreted to mean that babbling is "innate" because the deaf infants did not have adequate access to the sound system of their hearing parents (e.g., see discussions in Crystal, 1987; Ingram, 1989).

The first words of hearing children have been reported to emerge between the ages of 10 to 13 months (Dale, 1976; de Villers & de Villers, 1978). Because of the use of gestures, there is some debate as to when the first "linguistic signs" emerge (as opposed to prelinguistic gestures; see, e.g., Petitto, 1986, 1988). In any case, the age range of the first "signs" of deaf children has been reported to be from 7 or 8 months to about 13 months (Hoffmeister & Wilbur, 1980; Schlesinger & Meadow, 1972).

One area of phonological research has focused on the acquisition of handshapes (e.g., Hoffmeister & Wilbur, 1980). In general, similar to hearing children, deaf children acquire easier (unmarked) elements prior to more difficult (marked) elements. A good example of this type of research is the work of McIntire (1977), who studied the acquisition of handshapes in one deaf child at ages 13, 15, and 21 months. The researcher found that pointing and grasping handshapes were acquired initially (e.g., A, S, L, 5, C, and "baby O"). The acquisition of more complex handshapes (e.g., H, W, 8, X) occurred with the increasing maturity of cognitive and physical abilities. In addition, substitutions produced by the subject involved similar phonological elements, for example, using the 5 handshape instead of the F handshape to sign CAT. This phenomenon parallels substitution of phonemic elements in hearing children. Thus, the phonological development of deaf children appears to be similar to the phonological development of hearing children. That is, both proceed from easier, less marked elements to more difficult, more marked elements and both substitute easier, similar elements for more difficult ones.

Stokoe (1990) discussed several stages in research on sign language. He remarked that the "deep interest" in sign language phonology is characteristic of a real breakthrough in research on ASL. As Stokoe stated:

> In this stage, linguistics of sign language comes of age; instead of working to "break the code," researchers are engaged in finding the latest way to microanalyze its smaller and smaller fractions. . . . How many parameters of a sign are there, and which of various counts is correct? Do signs have parameters in the strict sense of that term at all? Are signs to be considered the result of rules operating on bundles of simultaneous features contained in HOLD and MOVE segments . . . ? Are signs, rather, composed in syllabic form with morae of movement and position . . . ? Is there something called "autosegmentation" going on in tiers . . . ? Are facial expressions and other nonmanual actions part of sign phonology . . . ? More generally, is a sign language like ASL more interesting because of its similarity to spoken languages or because of its differences? (Stokoe, 1990, p. 5)

Morphological and Syntactic Development

As remarked by Siple (1978): "It is easy to say that the grammar of ASL is uniquely its own; but it is more difficult to identify and describe the actual syntactic devices used" (p. 10). This statement has been echoed more or less since that time (e.g., see discussion in Gee and Goodhart, 1988). Part of the problem is with the ASL/English contact situations, which lend support for a sociolinguistic perspective of the grammar and use of ASL, rather than a "pure" linguistic perspective (e.g., see Bochner & Albertini,

1988; *Deaf American,* 1990). As discussed in Chapter 2, the particular perspective, linguistic, sociolinguistic, or some other one, depends on the metatheoretical views of the theorists and researchers. Another issue is the use of linguistic terms that are relevant to the use of space and motion as in sign languages: reduplication, verb directionality, and systematic non-manual cues (for a discussion of these terms see Baker & Cokely, 1980; Liddell, 1980; Wilbur, 1987).

The few studies on morphological and syntactic development discussed briefly here are concerned with some major linguistic structures: negation, the pronominal reference system, and classifiers. Only a few studies are discussed, including some of the earlier ones, that set the stage for further research. For example, Hoffmeister and Wilbur (1980) reviewed a number of studies on the beginning stages of the acquisition of negation. They found that, in the earlier stage, the use of the sign for *no* is present as well as the more frequent negative headshake. The later stage is characterized by the emergence of two signs *not* and *can't*. Similar to hearing children learning a spoken language, the notion of *can't* is acquired prior to that of *can*. It was concluded that these developmental stages appear to parallel those reported for hearing children learning English (Brown, 1973).

Hoffmeister and Wilbur (1980, citing Hoffmeister's dissertation work) described a study on the acquisition of the pronominal reference system of ASL. A deaf child of deaf parents served as a subject. Results are presented in five stages. In Stage 1, for example, it was reported that pointing behaviors refer to objects that are visible in the immediate environment such as the signer or objects. The subject indicated a possessor-possessed relationship by initially pointing to an object and then pointing to the self. Analogously, Nelson (1973) and Bates (1976) also found similar deictic (pointing) gestures which preceded the spoken language development in young hearing children. These pointing behaviors of the deaf child were also the precursors to other pronominal concepts, for example, plurality, the use of *that* and *all,* which are later executed by formal adult signs.

Near the end of Stage 2 and the beginning of Stage 3, the previously learned operations began to refer to events and objects not in the immediate environment. By Stage 4 (age 4 years, 2 months), reflexivization (e.g., use of self signs, myself, yourself, etc.). Finally, it was concluded that this deaf subject had mastered the ASL referential system by Stage 5 (4 years, 5 months of age; for another discussion of personal pronouns, see Petitto, 1988).

Bellugi and Klima (1985) provided in-depth analyses of three morphological subsystems of ASL: formal distinction between nouns and verbs, spatial marking for verb agreement, and the transition of pronouns from gesture to sign. The latter system is of interest here because it seem to reflect a transition from a prelinguistic period to a linguistic one. As about age 10 months, the deaf child uses the pointing gesture (i.e., index finger) to refer to personal pronouns, for example, first and second. The pointing gesture is also used for other functions such as indicating objects. The *transition* stage begins during the second year of life. For example, the child starts to use "name signs" (i.e., proper) instead of first and second person pronouns. Around the 21st month, the pointing gesture reemerges; however, it is a pronominal sign which is part of a linguistic system. The use of this sign is similar to the behavior of hearing children who reverse (i.e., misplaces) the words *I* and *you*. The deaf child discontinues the reversal of these pronouns until about age 2 years, 3 months. At this point, the child's pronoun system is similar to that of the adult language in this area. It was noted that both deaf and hearing children's development and use of the pronoun system followed similar stages.

The presence of classifiers in American Sign Language was indicated in the seminal work of Frishberg (1975). Several studies have been conducted in this area (e.g., Gee & Kegl, 1982; Kantor, 1980; Liddell, 1980; Luetke-Stahlman, 1984; Wilbur, Bernstein, & Kantor, 1985). For example, Kantor (1980) studied the acquisition of ASL classifiers by deaf children. Similar to classifiers in spoken languages, ASL classifiers appear as part of syntactic forms (e.g., the verb or the noun) and reflect certain semantic properties of their noun referents. Nine deaf children, ages 3 to 11 years, of deaf parents served as subjects. Like other studies on the acquisition of ASL, these findings indicated a developmental sequence similar to those that have been identified for hearing children learning a spoken language (de Villiers & de Villiers, 1979; Menyuk, 1977). In particular, it was reported that classifiers emerged around age 3 and were mastered by 8 or 9 years of age. It was concluded that classifiers are not acquired as lexical items, but rather as a complex syntactic process. The researcher concluded that rule acquisition in both ASL and spoken language is affected by similar phonological and syntactical environments.

Luetke-Stahlman (1984) studied the recognition of classifiers by hearing-impaired students in both residential and public-school settings. The 22 residential students were between the ages of 5 to 16 years whereas the 17 public-school students were from 4 to 15 years old. Results indicated that residential students had higher recognition scores than the public-school students. The older residential students (i.e., 10 to 16 years old) had higher scores than both the younger residential students (i.e., 5 to 9 years old) and the older public-school students. No differences were found between younger residential students and younger public-school students (5 to 9 years old). Because knowledge of classifier constructions is a fairly good index of knowledge of the grammar of ASL, Luetke-Stahlman concluded that residential hearing-impaired students are more proficient in ASL than their public-school hearing-impaired counterparts.

Semantic-Pragmatic Development

The few studies cited here illustrate the attempt to discuss semantic-pragmatic development in American Sign Language. For example, Newport and Ashbrook (1977) conducted a study to compare the emergence of semantic relations in deaf children learning ASL as a first language to that of hearing children learning English as a first language (Bloom et al., 1975). Five young deaf children served as subjects. In general, the findings indicated that the *existence* relation emerged prior to *action* relations which preceded *state_*relations. In addition, *nonlocatives* emerged prior to *locatives*. A detailed description of these relations can be found in Bloom and Lahey (1978) and Lucas (1980). It was concluded that the sequence of the acquisition of semantic relations by deaf children was similar to that reported for hearing children despite the differences in modality and syntax.

Kantor (1982) conducted phonologic, syntactic, semantic, and pragmatic analyses of data obtained from interactions of two deaf mothers with their deaf children. This researcher was interested in describing the modifications of deaf mothers in communicating with their children and in describing the developmental sequence of deictic (pointing) behaviors and modulated verbs in deaf children exposed to ASL. In general, the researcher reported that the deaf mothers, similar to hearing-speaking mothers, modified their language to fit the child's, that is, they used more simple and direct structures. The developmental sequence of the pointing behavior and verb modulations were essentially similar to those reported early in this section by Hoffmeister and Wilbur (1980). Kantor remarked that pointing, in the early stage, indicated a few semantic relations, for example, the use of demonstratives (i.e., *this, that,* etc.). Additional semantic and pragmatic functions emerged at a later stage with the occurrence of locatives, pronominals, and indexing referents present in the context.

FINAL REMARKS

In this chapter, we attempted to present some major highlights regarding the development of language in both hearing and deaf children. The main focus was on the language development of deaf children via the use of three broad approaches: oral English, total communication, and American Sign Language. Relative to the TC approaches, we synthesized a sample of research data on some of the major signed systems with students with severe to profound hearing impairment.

There is evidence that some deaf students can acquire a high level of competence in English as a first language. However, most students with severe to profound hearing impairment do not, suggesting that there is no superiority of either oral English or TC approaches for all deaf children and adolescents. Relative to the TC approaches, there seems to be several reasons for this lack of success, for example, the inconsistent and unsystematic use of the signed systems by practitioners, how well and how much of the English structure that the various systems represent, and whether this representation is similar to that of spoken English. Although oral English approaches may be theoretically complete representations of standard English, deaf student have difficulty developing English via these approaches due to their dysfunctional auditory system.

As discussed in Chapter 5, this difficulty in acquiring the English language and its accompanying culture, including the academic culture, has a pervasive influence on deaf students' acquisition of literacy skills. Even more important, this situation questions whether English should be a first language for all or even most deaf students. Indirect support for this assertion has come from the research on American Sign Language. Not only is ASL a bona fide linguistic system, but also, the development of ASL in deaf children seems to parallel the development of hearing children in a spoken language, such as English.

Whether the acquisition of English is or should be easier for ASL-using deaf students is the topic of Chapter 6. However, there seems to be sufficient evidence to argue that, under comparable conditions, ASL may be essentially easier and faster for many deaf students to acquire at a competent level than the manually coded English systems. We are not implying that ASL is or should be the first language for most students with severe to profound hearing impairment. The crux of our argument is that researchers and scholars still need to resolve the issue of acquiring a *first language at as early an age as possible for most deaf students*. This issue is the major focus of our Conclusion chapter (Chapter 9).

FURTHER READINGS

Baker, C., & Padden, C. (1978). *American Sign Language: A look at its history, structure, and community.* Silver Spring, MD: T.J. Publishers.

Berwick, R. (1986). *The acquisition of syntactic knowledge.* Cambridge, MA: MIT Press.

Goldin-Meadow, S., & Mylander, C. (1984). Gestural communication in deaf children: The effects and non-effects of parental input on early language development. *Monographs of the Society for Research in Child Development, 49,* nos. 3–4.

Jackendoff, R. (1983). *Semantics and cognition.* Cambridge, MA: MIT Press.

Markowicz, H. (1977). *American Sign Language: Fact and fancy.* Washington, DC: Gallaudet University Press.

Pollack, D. (Ed.). (1980). *Amplification for the hearing impaired* (2nd ed.). New York: Grune & Stratton.

C H A P T E R 5

READING AND WRITING

To completely analyze what we do when we read would almost be the acme of a psychologist's dream for it would be to describe very many of the most intricate workings of the human mind, as well as to unravel the tangled story of the most remarkable specific performance that civilization has learned in all its history. (Huey, 1908/1968, p. 8)

What drives reading and writing is this desire to make sense of what is happening—to make things cohere. A writer achieves that fit by deciding what information to include and what to withhold. The reader accomplishes that fit by filling in gaps . . . or making uncued connections. All readers, like all writers, ought to strive for this fit between the whole and the parts and among the parts. (Tierney & Pearson, 1983, p. 572)

It can be inferred from the passages above that reading and writing are extremely complex skills and that they are interrelated, that is, they share similar underlying processes. The similarity between reading and writing, often termed the reading-writing connection, has been motivated by both theories of the writing process (e.g., see discussions in Rubin & Hansen, 1986; Tierney & Leys, 1984) and reading comprehension, particularly interactive theories of reading (see Rumelhart, 1985; Samuels & Kamil, 1984). However, as discussed in this chapter, there are some differences between reading and writing. To simplify, this can be seen in the following statement: Good writers are almost always good readers; good readers have the potential to become good writers. Although reading is the process of understanding written language, there is a strong, reciprocal relationship between reading and writing which has important implications for instruction.

There is also a complex, intricate relationship between "conversational" language (i.e., speech) and the language of print (e.g., Shankweiler & Liberman, 1989; Sticht & James, 1984; Taylor & Taylor, 1983). This relationship can be gleaned from a careful study of models of reading comprehension, especially interactive models. Both reading and writing build on the knowledge base and the grammatical base of a spoken language. In addition, there is a strong connection between listening skills and reading skills. Although it is possible to learn some aspects of language via the use of literacy skills, it is much more efficient to possess a working knowledge of all components of the language, for example, phonology, morphology, syntax, and semantics, prior to beginning reading (e.g., Shankweiler & Liberman, 1989).

The strong interrelations among language, reading, and writing aspects relative to the English language account for much of the difficulty of deaf students in obtaining high-level literacy skills. As is discussed in this chapter, the nature of these relationships explains in part why deaf students with good oral-aural skills are often better readers than other deaf students—including those who know ASL—who do not possess these skills (see Chapter 4 of this text; see also Quigley & Paul, 1989). This seems to support the notion that the sign-print connection is not commensurate with or not similar to the speech-print connection. In essence, the cross-modal properties of speech and print are different from those of sign and print.

It should be emphasized that literacy is not simply speech written down. It is true that reading is the process of comprehending written language which requires knowledge of print factors such as orthography, words, grammar, convention of discourse, anaphoric reference rules, and linguistic redundancies (e.g., Dechant, 1991; Just & Carpenter, 1987; Nickerson, 1986). However, knowledge of the language of print—albeit, extremely important—is not sufficient for attaining adequate literacy skills. As stated by Nickerson (1986) and others (e.g., Adams, 1990; Anderson, Hiebert, Scott, & Wilkerson, 1985), good readers have knowledge of the following: (1) how the world works; (2) social situations; (3) goals, purposes, intentions, and plans; (4) ethics and human nature; (5) logical inference rules; and (6) topics in which one is reading.

The two groups of factors listed above are reflective of one of the major themes of this chapter: Literacy is an interactive process in which readers and writers attempt to construct or compose a working model of meaning. The construction or composition of meaning requires the coordination of both bottom-up and top-down skills. An overreliance on top-down comprehension skills in reading leads to a misinterpretation of the meaning of the passage. The absence of bottom-up, lower-level skills during writing impedes the use of higher-level skills of intent and organization and makes it difficult for other readers to understand the printed representation of the writer's message.

In this chapter, we illustrate the impact of deafness on the development of reading and writing skills. Two groups of reading models are discussed: reading-comprehension theories and literary critical theories. The focus is on reading comprehension theories because we are interested in the acquisition of reading skills. We present and discuss the reading achievement levels of deaf students in reference to interactive theories.

The background information on reading processes and achievement is necessary for the section of the chapter dealing with the writing process. After discussing the current understanding of writing, we provide information on the written language levels of deaf students. For both reading and writing, we argue for a closer interrelationship among theory, assessment, curriculum, and instruction. Finally, we present our reflections on further research and instructional efforts.

THEORETICAL MODELS OF READING

There are two groups of theoretical models that are concerned with the condition of reading and, in some cases, writing: reading-comprehension and literary critical or reading and literacy (Lemley, 1993; Wagner, 1986). Although there are some overlapping features, there are also paradigmatic differences between the two groups. The concept, paradigm, is often used as a research tool to understand extant theory within a scientific field (e.g., Ritzer, 1991). The use of the word paradigm here is similar to that described by Ritzer:

> A paradigm is a fundamental image of the subject matter within a science. It serves to define what should be studied, what questions should be asked, how they should be asked, and what rules should be followed in interpreting the answer obtained. A paradigm is the broadest unit of consensus within a science and serves to differentiate one scientific community (or subcommunity) from another. It subsumes, defines, and interrelates the exemplars, theories, and methods and instruments that exist within it. (Ritzer, 1991, p. 120)

With the conceptual framework above in mind, research on reading has been concerned with the decoding and comprehension of the written language of English. Theorists and researchers focus on the acquisition of reading skills that are critical for high reading achievement levels, typically within either cognitive or social-cognitive purviews (Bernhardt, 1991; Samuels & Kamil, 1984). Descriptions of the reading process attempt to explain how and why some children acquire these skills and why others have great difficulty. Instructional implications include the use of techniques to improve the development and application of successful reading skills. It is also possible to label this as a "deficit" view of reading development (Lemley, 1993); however, this is a metatheoretical position (see discussion in Paul & Jackson, 1993).

Literary critical, or literacy, theorists and researchers are primarily interested in the *context* of the application of skills associated with literacy (Lemley, 1993; Wagner, 1986). This context contains several dimensions, for example, literary works (i.e., literature), history, socioculture, and sociolinguistics (e.g., Wagner, 1986). Within this perspective, reading and writing skills are subsumed under the broad notion of literacy. For example, in some societies, being literate may include the ability to read or write in the context of literate thought, that is, the ability to engage in reflective or critical thought (Olson, 1989; Wagner, 1986). In addition to the array of skills and functions associated with these skills, literacy also encompasses the views and beliefs of particular societies toward these functions and skills. This broad perspective makes it difficult to come to a theoretical understanding of literacy because of the variety of views that exist across societies.

As mentioned previously, there is some overlap between the two broad groups of theories, particularly with the focus on the skills of reading and writing. Despite paradigmatic differences, both groups have important implications for developing literacy skills in deaf children and adolescents (Lemley, 1993). Within a technological, information-intensive society such as the United States, the ability to read and write is extremely important (e.g., Adams, 1990; Anderson et al., 1985), even for individuals with hearing impairment (e.g., King & Quigley, 1985; Paul, 1993).

The major goal of literacy instruction should be literate thought. If reading and writing skills—albeit important—are difficult to develop in deaf students, then other viable means of developing literate thought should be explored. In any case, the major focus of this chapter is on the development of reading and writing skills. Thus, much of the information presented draws from the theories and research within the paradigm of reading comprehension theories with some information from literary critical theories.

Reading-Comprehension Theories

A vast amount of theoretically based and empirical research information has been accumulated on reading since the classic book by Huey (1908/ 1968) from which one of the passages at the beginning of this chapter is taken. Many issues raised in Huey's work continue to be refined—for example, the extent to which word recognition involves serial versus parallel processing of component letters; direct versus phonologically mediated lexical access; and bottom-up (sequential/hierarchical) versus top-down (context-driven), and/or interactive processing of printed information (Dechant, 1991; Samuels & Kamil, 1984; Vellutino, 1982).

These issues are present in the major principles of the three broad groups of reading comprehension theories: bottom-up, top-down, and interactive. The following descriptions of the models should be considered prototypes, not representative of a model or theory associated with a specific person. For example, at least five interactive models have been identified (Grabe, 1988, 1991); our goal is to present characteristics that are common across these models, rather than an in-depth discussion of one specific interactive model.

Bottom-up Models

Bottom-up, or text-based, models place a great deal of emphasis on the recognition (identification) of letters and words. The process is referred to as bottom-up because it begins with the perception of letters and words on the page, proceeds through the analyses at several successive levels involving larger units (e.g., phrases, sentences), and culminates with the construction of meaning at the top, that is, in the readers' minds. This type of processing is linear and hierarchical. Thus, readers need to be successful with the processing of the smallest units (letters, words) before they can proceed to the next level of analysis. The total information from these levels of analyses leads or adds up to "meaning"

Relative to the processing of words, two types are often debated in the literature, the processing of the word as a whole unit as in whole word or look-say methods or the processing of letters or strings of letters such as letter clusters (*bl, ch, str*) as in phonics methods (Adams, 1990; Chall, 1983). The issue of the place and form of decoding in beginning reading in bottom-up models has been at the heart of a long-standing controversy in reading instruction. There are many variations of phonics programs; however, one of the major goals should be the use of a system that teaches students about the nature of the alphabetic principle, the system on which English written language is based (Adams, 1990; Shankweiler & Liberman, 1989).

Knowledge of the alphabet system does entail a working knowledge of letter-sound correspondences. The importance of this knowledge has been described:

> Research indicates that the most critical factor beneath fluent word reading is the
> ability to recognize letters, spelling patterns, and whole words, effortlessly, auto-

matically, and visually. Moreover, the goal of all reading instruction—comprehension—depends critically on this ability. (Adams, 1990, p. 14)

As discussed later, reading comprehension also depends on other important skills; nevertheless, lack of adequate bottom-up processing can interfere and possibly prevent the development of higher-level reading skills.

Bottom-up models assert that meaning resides in the text. It is the reader's task to "extract" that meaning from the page or the whole passage. Despite the shortcomings and criticisms of these models (Grabe, 1988, 1991; Samuels & Kamil, 1984), they have demonstrated the importance of knowledge of the alphabet system. In addition, it has been shown that the use of context clues—albeit important in resolving misunderstandings—actually plays a minor role in lexical access in highly literate readers. Finally, another issue that is gaining wide acceptance is the fact that beginning readers and skilled readers who encounter difficult passages engage in phonological coding, that is, the conversion of printed symbols on the page to their phonological equivalents (e.g., Rayner & Pollatsek, 1989; Samuels & Kamil, 1984). As discussed previously (see Chapter 3), the notion of phonological coding is also important for deaf readers.

Top-Down Models

Top-down theorists assert that the only purpose of reading is comprehension, and this should be emphasized from the beginning. Reading is said to begin with the information that is in the readers' heads, not with what is on the printed page. Examples of top-down models can be seen in the works of Goodman (1976, 1985) and Smith (1975, 1978). Both of these scholars reject what they term the emphasis on reading as a precise process which involves exact, detailed, sequential perception and identification of letters, words, spelling patterns, and larger units.

Goodman (1976, 1985) asserted that reading acquisition is similar to language acquisition. He labeled reading as a psycholinguistic guessing game in which readers make more accurate guesses about meaning based on a sample of the text. The more linguistic and nonlinguistic (i.e., world) knowledge that readers have in their heads, the less time they will spend on lower-level text-related variables. This in turn leads to the development of rapid, advanced skills in reading.

Relative to Goodman's model, Samuels and Kamil (1984) remarked that this view "always prefers the cognitive economy of reliance on well-developed linguistic (syntactic and semantic) rather than graphic information" (p. 187). In addition, Goodman's model has had the greatest impact on views of reading instruction, particularly early reading instruction. It is not uncommon to hear about "THE psycholinguistic approach to reading or THE whole language approach to reading" (Samuels & Kamil, 1984, p. 187).

The views of Smith (1975, 1978) have also been somewhat influential, and similar to those of Goodman's. Smith stated that the primary process is that of "prediction." He presented four main arguments for the primary role of prior knowledge, context, and prediction in reading and against the precise sequential/hierarchical view of reading. First, individual words are often polysemous (have multiple meanings) and their intended meanings can only be obtained from context aided by prior knowledge. Second, there are more than 300 "spelling-to-sound correspondences rules" of English, and there is no precise way of knowing when any of the rules must apply or when an exception to the rules is being encountered. Third, the amount of visual information from print that the mind can process at any given moment in reading is limited to four or five letters or other units. And finally, short-term working memory is limited; only a small number of items can be stored at any time, and increased input leads to displacement of items already in storage. For children to use prediction in learning to read, Smith asserted that the reading material must be meaningful to children and that they must feel free to use their prediction skills even though this will result initially in errors rather than precise reading.

Similar to bottom-up models, top-down models are also considered to be linear. Despite the shortcomings of top-down models, they have shown that reading is a predictive process and that an adequate knowledge of the culture and, specifically, the language in which one is trying to read are important. These skills, in conjunction with the automatic word identification skills associated with bottom-up processing, form the basis for the group of models labeled interactive.

Interactive Models

Because of the criticisms and research data against the linear bottom-up and top-down models (e.g., Grabe, 1988, 1991; Lipson & Wixson, 1991; Samuels & Kamil, 1984), several interactive models have emerged in recent years—for example, Rumelhart's schema-interactive, Stanovich's interactive compensatory, and Perfetti's verbal efficiency models (Grabe, 1988). Interactive models emphasize the reader as an active information processor whose goal is to construct a model of what the text means. Two aspects of the models are of primary importance: (1) the central role of background knowledge in constructing meaning from texts, and (2) a number of dynamic processing strategies ranging from the specific aspects of decoding print to the metacognitive strategies of consciously monitoring one's processing of information. Comprehension is driven by preexisting concepts in the readers' heads as well as by the information from the text.

Thus, the construction of meaning requires the development and coordination of both bottom-up and top-down skills and occurs at many different levels of analysis such as lexical, syntactic, schematic, planning, and interpretative.

Most of the interactive models include notions of rapid and accurate letter and word recognition, that is, automatic processing "that does not depend on active attentional context for primary recognition of linguistic units" (Grabe, 1988, p. 59). For example, Perfetti's model (1985) places a great deal of emphasis on word recognition. There are sufficient data to argue that good readers recognize lexical forms at a processing rate that is faster than the time it takes to use context and predicting cues (Rayner & Pollatsek, 1989). Rapid, automatic word identification skills permit the use of higher-level comprehension skills.

Some interactive models, for example, Rumelhart's schema-interactive model (1980), emphasize the organization of knowledge in long-term memory (see discussion of memory in Chapter 3). Schema has been described as:

> an abstract knowledge structure. A schema is abstract in the sense that it summarizes what is known about a variety of cases that differ in many particulars. . . . A schema is structured in the sense that it represents the relationships among its component parts. (Anderson & Pearson, 1984, p. 259)

The schema concept provides a powerful tool for organizing knowledge into meaningful units which aids in acquisition, storage, and retrieval. The effect of meaning on memory functioning is well documented; words are easier to recall than unrelated letters, sentences easier than unrelated words, and so forth. In fact, any body of semantically related data is easier to retrieve from memory than any comparable body of semantically unrelated data. Schemata are the devices by which knowledge is organized into meaningful units and incoming data (such as from a text) are incorporated into the existing schemata, modify such schemata, or help form new schemata. Finally, schemata, at various levels, are combined with related schemata into higher order, and usually with more general schemata.

The following text with interpretations illustrates the interactive process of reading.

> He plunked down $5 at the window. She tried to give him $2.50, but he refused to take it. So when they got inside she bought him a large bag of popcorn. (Collins, Brown, & Larkin, 1980, p. 387)

After reading the first sentence, the good reader might hypothesize that this scenario takes place at either a racetrack, a movie theatre, or a bank. This hypothesis is the result of both bottom-up and top-down processing (Mason & CSR, 1984). With bottom-up processing, the reader might remark that "plunking down of $5" means the same as "buying." The word, window, can be interpreted to be that which exists at a house, bank, or ticket office. Relative to top-down processing, the reader has other interpretations which are competing for attention. The reader might decide that individuals do not plunk down money at a house window. It is possible to give money at either a bank window, a ticket window at a movie theatre, or a ticket window at a racetrack. These hypotheses compete with others until the situation become clear to the reader, possibly after reading the next two sentences (Mason & CSR, 1984).

Despite the influence of interactive views of reading, there are still strong proponents for the other two views. In essence, very few theorists espouse a "pure" bottom-up or top-down processing. For example, Rayner and Pollatsek (1989) remarked that their model of reading is basically bottom-up with some top-down processing. It should be obvious that interactive models are not above criticism (e.g., Carnine et al., 1990). In spite of the purported importance of prior knowledge, specific knowledge needs to be learned in school because of the nature of academic subjects such as science and social studies and because everyday knowledge might not be sufficient for reading these subjects. Such knowledge is part of classroom instruction.

A summary of the major points of the three groups of reading comprehension theories is provided in Table 5–1.

Factors Associated with the Reading Process

One of the biggest contributions of interactive theories is the notion of interaction among groups of factors associated with the reading process. The three groups of factors that have been delineated and discussed in several texts on the teaching of reading are text-based, reader-based, and context-(or task-) based (e.g., Lipson & Wixson, 1991). Some important text-based factors are vocabulary (word knowledge), grammar (i.e., phonology, morphology and syntax) of the language, orthography, and other features associated with the text (e.g., headings, boldface entries, parentheses, and so forth). For example, there seems to be a strong relationship between knowledge of word meanings and reading comprehension (e.g., Anderson & Freebody, 1979; Nagy & Herman, 1987; Paul & O'Rourke, 1988); however, this relationship is still poorly understood. Knowledge of the language of print is an important factor for both first-language and second-language readers (Bernhardt, 1991; Grabe, 1988, 1991; Paul, Bernhardt, & Gramly, 1992).

Reader-based factors include prior knowledge, metacognitive skills, and motivation and interests (see discussions in Dechant, 1991; Lipson & Wixson, 1991; Mason & Au, 1986). It should be clear that prior knowl-

TABLE 5-1. Major Points of the Three Groups of Reading Theories

Bottom-up Models

- There is a great deal of emphasis on the recognition (identification) of letters and words.
- The process begins with the perception of letters and words on the page, proceeds through the analyses at several successive levels involving larger units such as phrases and sentences, and culminates with the construction of meaning at the top, that is, in the readers' minds.
- The models have demonstrated the importance of knowledge of the alphabet system.
- The use of context clues actually plays a minor role in lexical access in highly literate readers.

Top-Down Models

- The only purpose of reading is comprehension, and this should be emphasized from the beginning.
- Reading is said to begin with the information that is in the readers' heads, not with what is on the printed page.
- In one top-down model, reading acquisition is similar to language acquisition.
- Models have shown that reading is a predictive process and that an adequate knowledge of the culture and, specifically, the language in which one is trying to read are important.

Interactive Models

- These models emphasize the reader as an active information processor whose goal is to construct a model of what the text means.
- Comprehension is driven by preexisting concepts in the readers' heads as well as by the information from the text.
- The construction of meaning requires the development and coordination of both bottom-up and top-down skills and occurs at many different levels of analysis such as lexical, syntactic, schematic, planning, and interpretative.

Source: Adapted from Bernhardt (1991), Grabe (1988), and Samuels & Kamil (1984).

edge entails knowledge of text-based factors and that associated with the immediate and larger culture and the topics in which one is trying to read.

Context (or task) factors refer to the purposes of reading, the setting in which reading is accomplished, and instructional factors. There is evidence that reading comprehension varies according to the purposes and task requirements. For example, readers perform better when they have a clear idea of what is required of them after reading a passage (see discussions in Dechant, 1991; Lipson & Wixson, 1991; Mason & Au, 1986). Relative to setting, the meaning of a passage depends on the broader context in which it is read. For example, reading about a scientific discovery in a science text will have a different effect than reading the same discovery in *The National Enquirer* or *Readers' Digest*. Finally, both the content of instruction and the methods of instruction have effects on the reader's comprehension of passages.

In discussing and synthesizing the research on reading and deafness, we relate the findings of a sample of investigations to the three broad categories above, that is, text-based, reader-based, and context-based, when applicable. More detailed descriptions and summaries of reading research on both hearing (e.g., Barr, Kamil, Mosenthal, & Pearson, 1991; Pearson, Barr, Kamil, & Mosenthal, 1984) and deaf children (e.g., King & Quigley, 1985; Quigley & Paul, 1989) can be found elsewhere. Prior to discussing this research, it is important to provide a historical synthesis on the reading achievement level of students with severe to profound hearing impairment (see also, Quigley & Paul, 1986, 1989).

READING ACHIEVEMENT AND DEAFNESS

Descriptions of the reading achievement of deaf students are based on the results of their performances on standardized tests, both of general achievement and reading. The following discussion is presented relative to three areas: (1) performance on tests other than the *Stanford Achievement Test* (SAT); (2) performance on the SAT, including the normed versions; and (3) performance of select subgroups not included in the SAT sample. Despite improvements in the construction of the tests and the implementation of early intervention, there are two general themes that can be gleaned from the findings. One, the overwhelming majority of 18- to 19-year-old deaf students do not read above a fourth-grade level. Two, this "plateau" has been in existence since the beginning of the formal testing movement (Quigley & Paul, 1986).

Performance on Tests Other than
the Stanford Achievement Test

The work of Wrightstone, Aronow, and Moskowitz (1963) is illustrative of this area. These researchers conducted a national study to develop special reading norms for deaf students. Using the Elementary Reading Test of the Metropolitan Achievement Test, they assessed the reading ability of

5,307 deaf students between the ages of $10\frac{1}{2}$ to $16\frac{1}{2}$ years old. The students were selected from 73 special schools (and classes) in the United States and Canada. More than half of the sample had a hearing impairment greater than 85 dB in the better unaided ear.

Furth (1966b) reanalyzed the data from the Wrightstone et al. study and compared them to the grade norms for hearing children. Using a fourth-grade reading level as the criterion for functional literacy, Furth concluded that most deaf students are functionally illiterate. In fact, he reported that less than 25% of the deaf students between the ages of $14\frac{1}{2}$ and $16\frac{1}{2}$ years reached about the fifth-grade reading level. In addition, Furth noted that the mean reading grade level increased about one grade *during a 5-year period.*

Performance on the SAT

A number of studies reported the performance of deaf students on the SAT, normed on hearing students. For example, Babbini and Quigley (1970) studied the performance of deaf students on several mathematics, language, and reading variables over a 5-year period. The students were selected from six residential schools. Relative to reading achievement, Babbini and Quigley reported findings similar to those of the Wrightstone et al. (1963) study. It was found that there was an improvement of one-third grade per year for reading. The mean reading grade (i.e., Combined Reading on the SAT) for this sample was 4.6. One of the most significant observations made by the researchers was the high intercorrelations among all the subtests. Babbini and Quigley argued that the SAT was primarily assessing the language abilities of the deaf students, rather than their educational achievement. They argued further for the development of an achievement test normed on deaf students.

The Center for Assessment and Demographic Studies has conducted a series of national investigations on the educational achievement of deaf students. The results of two early studies (DiFrancesca, 1972; Gentile & DiFrancesca, 1969) were used to develop a version of the SAT that had norms for students with hearing impairment. We are interested in the findings of the normed versions for 1974 (Trybus & Karchmer, 1977), 1983 (Allen, 1986), and 1991 (CADS, 1991).

Despite the special adaptations, Trybus and Karchmer (1977) reported a median grade level of 4.5 for deaf students at 20 years of age. They noted that only 10% of the best reading group was reading at or above the eighth-grade level. Allen (1986) noted that the median reading level for the 1983 sample was still below the fourth grade. In the most recent report (CADS, 1991), the average reading level of the 18-year-old deaf student in special-education programs is below 3.5 grades.

A summary of the language and reading performances of deaf students across several exemplary studies is depicted in Table 5–2.

Select Subgroups

The findings of the national surveys should be interpreted with caution because they tend to obscure the performances of students in individual programs, in special programs, or in mainstreamed or integrated classrooms (Paul & Quigley, 1987a, 1990; Quigley & Paul, 1986). For example, some students in total communication programs perform better than the national norms (e.g., Delaney et al., 1984; Luetke-Stahlman, 1988a). In addition, these surveys do not include students with severe to profound hearing impairment in special, comprehensive oral programs such as the Central Institute for the Deaf (Lane & Baker, 1974) or students in integrated classrooms (e.g., Geers & Moog, 1989; Messerly & Aram, 1980). Several students in these latter groups are reading on a par with or better than their *hearing* counterparts.

What differentiates these deaf students from others with low-reading achievement? The work of Luetke-Stahlman (1988a, 1988b) suggested that it is important for deaf students to be exposed to either languages or manual systems that completely encode spoken English (e.g., cued speech, seeing essential English, signing exact English. Delaney et al. (1984) argued that academic achievement, particularly reading achievement, is not dependent solely on type of instructional input. Other important factors include the skills and knowledge of the teacher, design of the curricula, involvement of parents/caregivers, and the development of oral-communication skills.

A number of the factors mentioned above were reiterated by the research of Geers and Moog (1989), which was discussed in detail in Chapter 4. In essence, Geers and Moog (1989) emphasized the reciprocal relationship between the oral and written forms of a language (see also, Shankweiler & Liberman, 1989; Vygotsky, 1962). As discussed in Chapter 3, one important manifestation of this relationship is the use of a phonological-based code in short-term working for the comprehension of syntactic structures. It is also important to have knowledge of the alphabetic principle, the system on which the English written language is based.

A Perspective on the Reading Process of Deaf Students

Despite the low levels of reading achievement described above for most students with severe to profound hearing impairment, it has been argued that the reading process of deaf students is qualitatively similar to that of

TABLE 5-2. Summary of the Reading Performance of Deaf Students: Center on Assessment and Demographic Studies (CADS)

· CADS Surveys	
Gentile & DiFrancesca (1969)	The investigators reported the results of the Stanford Achievement Tests administered to about 12,000 students ages 7 to 19 years in special-education programs. Eighty-two percent of all students were reading at a mid-fourth grade level and lower. The mean grade levels for both the 15- and 16-year-old were 4.4 for Paragraph Meaning (Reading).
DiFrancesca (1971)	The SAT was administered to about 17,000 students between the ages of 6 and 21 years old. The highest mean grade level on the Paragraph Meaning subtest (Reading) was 4.3 for the 19-year-old students. The average reading grade-level growth was 0.2 grade levels per year.
Trybus & Karchmer (1977)	The reading achievement growth was reported for a 3-year period (1971–1974). The median reading grade level for 20-year-old deaf students was about 4.5. The overall growth in reading achievement was 0.8 grade level, or slightly less than 0.3 grade level per year.
Allen (1986)	The researcher reported that the median reading grade level of the 1983 sample was below the 4th grade. It was suggested that the plateau effect might be due to a high proportion of students with additional disabilities at the upper age levels.
CADS (1991)	The average reading level of 18-year-old deaf students has been reported to be below 3.5 grades.

hearing students, including second-language learners (e.g., Hanson, 1989; Hayes & Arnold, 1992; Paul, 1993). Relative to the reading-comprehension theories discussed previously, it seems that many reading instructional programs for deaf students have been influenced by top-down models, particularly the whole language approach (see Abrams, 1991; Dolman, 1992) influenced by Goodman (1976, 1985). Much of the impetus for this approach seems to come from the work of Ewoldt (1981), based on four deaf students. Ewoldt was a colleague of Goodman.

Given the importance of both bottom-up and top-down skills in reading, we feel that research and instructional practice for students with severe to profound hearing impairment should adhere to the basic tenets of interactive theories of reading (see also, Dolman, 1992; Kelly, 1993). This view has been termed a 'deficit' model (see discussion in Lemley, 1993); however, this is a metatheoretical perspective that cannot be resolved by the scientific method (Paul & Jackson, 1993). As we have indicated previously:

> The poor reading performance of most deaf students may be viewed within an interactive theoretical framework in which the reader uses specific skills (e.g., decoding and inference) to hypothesize at various linguistic levels (e.g., lexical, syntactic, semantic, textual) about the information contained in the text . . . In relation to this, the reading difficulties of deaf students may be attributed to deficits in experiential (e.g. world knowledge), cognitive (e.g., inferencing), and linguistic (e.g., word knowledge) variables. Other variables of equal importance are educational and socioeconomic in nature. (Quigley & Paul, 1989, p. 5)

Research on Selected Text-based Factors and Deafness

Much of the reading research on deaf children and adolescents has been conducted on text-based factors such as vocabulary, syntax, and figurative language (King & Quigley, 1985; Moores, 1987; Paul, 1993; Paul & Quigley, 1990). There is some research on the use of finger spelling to increase deaf students' understanding of the orthographic structure of print, specifically for word identification purposes (e.g., Hirsh-Pasek, 1987). Research on the importance of using a phonologic code during reading was presented in Chapter 3. If fluent word reading is deemed critical for and is influenced by comprehension skills, there needs to be a greater focus on the development and use of bottom-up skills (e.g., see discussion in Paul, 1993).

Words and Word Meanings

There have been extensive studies on deaf children's knowledge of words and word meanings (e.g., Fusaro & Slike, 1979; Hatcher & Robbins, 1978;

LaSasso & Davey, 1987; Paul, 1984; Paul & Gustafson, 1991; Schulze, 1965; Silverman-Dresner & Guilfoyle, 1972; and various surveys by the Center for Assessment and Demographic Studies). In our view, the most extensive investigation of deaf children's reading vocabulary knowledge was conducted by Silverman-Dresner and Guilfoyle (1972). The researchers constructed definitions for a final list of 7,300 words taken from two sources: the *Dale-Chall List* of 3000 familiar words (Dale & Chall, 1948) and from the *Children's Knowledge of Words* (Dale & Eicholtz, 1960). The major purpose of the study was to develop a set of age-graded vocabulary lists which reflected the actual reading vocabulary levels of deaf students from age 7 to 17 years. It was reported that deaf girls knew more words than deaf boys and that older deaf children knew more words than the younger ones.

Other studies compared the lexical knowledge of deaf children with that of hearing counterparts. In general, the results revealed that the vocabulary knowledge of deaf children is quantitatively reduced when compared to hearing peers. In addition, if deaf students have problems with other language variables, notably, syntax and orthographic knowledge, this tends to make it difficult for them to "infer" the meaning of the word via the use of adequate context clues (e.g., see discussion in Paul & O'Rourke, 1988).

That knowledge of words is important for deaf students has been documented in the few studies that examined the relationship between lexical knowledge and reading comprehension. For example, LaSasso and Davey (1987) analyzed the performance of 50 prelingually, profoundly hearing-impaired students, whose ages ranged from 10 to 18 years. Their findings indicated that vocabulary knowledge is an effective predictor of reading comprehension performance. Their results were confirmed in a later study by Paul and Gustafson (1991) who studied the relationship between knowledge of multimeaning words and reading comprehension. These researchers noted that there is a strong correlation between knowledge of two meanings of words and reading achievement scores.

To understand better the relationship between knowledge of words and reading comprehension, several researchers have attempted to study factors that contribute to the difficulty of a word (e.g., MacGinitie, 1969; Paul, 1984; Paul & Gustafson, 1991; Walter, 1978). Word difficulty is influenced by numerous factors, for example, prior knowledge, conceptual load, ability to use context clues, pronunciation, context surrounding the word, letter frequency, word frequency, and multiplicity of meanings (Anderson & Freebody, 1985; Nagy & Herman, 1987; O'Rourke, 1974; Paul & O'Rourke, 1988). In addition to the text-based and reader-based factors listed above, word difficulty might also be influenced by task-based factors, specifically those due to construction of vocabulary tests such as test format (e.g., multiple-choice, free response) and difficulty of the items themselves (see discussion of item difficulty and vocabulary tests in Curtis, 1987).

In an early study, MacGinitie (1969) examined the effects of context and multiplicity of meanings on both hearing and hearing-impaired subjects. The researcher developed a test which contained the target word, the correct word meaning, and three single-word distractors. The following illustrates four test items:

1. BEAR	forest	wild	paw	animal
2. BEAR	forest	wild	paw	carry
3. BEAR	burden	weight	land	carry
4. BEAR	burden	weight	land	animal

The ages of the hearing-impaired subjects ranged from 9 to 20 years. Their scores were compared with a group of hearing subjects in grades four and eight.

Results revealed that the scores of the hearing subjects were depressed by misleading contexts. Contrariwise, the scores of the hearing-impaired subjects were not affected by the contexts. As expected, the hearing subjects knew more words and more meaning of words than the hearing-impaired subjects.

Walter (1978) compared the lexical knowledge of deaf and hearing children. Subjects were 199 profoundly, hearing-impaired subjects whose ages ranged from 10 to 14 years old. Their performance was compared to 277 hearing age-peers. As expected, the youngest hearing age-subgroup performed better than the oldest deaf age-subgroup. It was also reported that the gap between the two overall groups (hearing and deaf) increased as the frequency of the words decreased. In light of these findings, Walter argued that previous estimates of the vocabulary knowledge of deaf students were spuriously high. That is, there was an overestimation of the word knowledge of deaf students, particularly on general achievement tests.

In addition to examining the relationship between vocabulary knowledge and reading comprehension, Paul and his collaborators (Paul, 1984; Paul & Gustafson, 1991; Paul, Stallman, & O'Rourke, 1990) assessed the comprehension of high-frequency words by both hearing and hearing-impaired subjects. For example, Paul and Gustafson (1991) were interested in answering the following questions:

1. Are there differences between deaf and hearing subjects on knowing either one meaning or two meanings of the same multimeaning words?
2. Does lexical knowledge improve with the age of the subjects?
3. Is comprehension of two meanings of words more difficult than comprehension of one meaning of the same words?

Forty-two deaf students and 42 hearing students served as subjects. The ages of the deaf subjects ranged from 10 to 18 years and the ages of the hearing subjects ranged from 8 to 11 years.

As expected, the hearing subjects had significantly higher scores than the deaf subjects relative to selecting both single meanings and two meanings of the same words. Surprisingly, no significant effects of age on selecting two meanings of words were observed for either group of subjects. It was also found that selecting two meanings of words was significantly more difficult than selecting one meanings of words for both groups.

Paul and Gustafson (1991) argued that knowledge of multimeanings of words is important for reading comprehension. For example, approximately two thirds of the words that appear in the spoken and written language contexts in the primary grades are multimeaning words (e.g., Johnson, Moe, & Baumann, 1983; Searls & Klesius, 1984). Comprehension difficulties might surface if students are not aware of the secondary or other meanings of words which appear in print. There is still a need to determine which particular meanings or the number of meanings of words that are used in reading materials for hearing and deaf students.

The research cited above on multimeaning words has important implications for instructional practices and curricular materials. These implications have also been stated by Conway in his study of the semantic relationships in the word meanings of students with hearing impairment:

> Traditional programs of learning definitions for lists of words should give way to learning words in semantically rich contexts. The contexts can serve as bridges to old information and as foundations for developing further conceptual interrelationships. . . . Such rich contexts should also include use of semantic mapping . . . and adaptations of networking strategies. (Conway, 1990, p. 346)

Another area for further research is to examine the issue of acquiring word meanings from context (i.e., during reading). There are numerous factors which impact this issue—text-based (e.g., difficulty of words and syntactic structures, and the contexts surrounding the words); reader-based (e.g., knowledge of language variables, and the amount and variety of reading experiences); and task-based factors (e.g., the type of assessment used). Because of these factors, it is not clear if deaf readers, especially poor readers, can acquire or derive many word meanings during the act of reading (e.g., see the various viewpoints and discussions in Davey & King, 1990; deVilliers & Pomerantz, 1992; Paul & O'Rourke, 1988).

Syntax

The research on syntax has focused on several general issues, three of which are: (1) comprehension of the structures and the frequency of structures in reading materials, (2) the effects of factors such as instructional methods and context of passages, and (3) the effects of short-term working memory on the comprehension of syntax. The more recent studies have attempted to "explain" deaf students' "difficulty" of certain syntactic structures within the framework of Chomsky's Universal Grammar (e.g., Lillo-Martin, Hanson, & Smith, 1991, 1992) and other "language" hypotheses (e.g., Wilbur, Goodhart, & Fuller, 1989). The selection of the studies discussed in this section is representative of much of the research on syntax and deaf individuals.

The work of Quigley and his associates (e.g., Quigley, Power, & Steinkamp, 1977; Quigley, Smith, & Wilbur, 1974; Quigley, Wilbur, & Montanelli, 1974, 1976; see also, the review in Russell et al., 1976) detailed the performance of a national stratified, random sample of deaf students between the ages of 10 and 19 years old on tests of comprehension of various syntactic structures presented singly in sentences. Table 5–3 depicts summary information on (1) the order of difficulty of various syntactic structures for both deaf and hearing students, and (2) the frequency of occurrence of each structure in reading series from Houghton-Mifflin (McKee, Harrison, McCowen, Lehr, & Durr, 1966).

Inspection of Table 5–3 reveals that the average 8-year-old hearing student scored higher on the various tasks than the average 18-year-old deaf student. In addition, there exists a huge gap between the age when deaf students comprehend various syntactic structures in single sentences and the typical age level when the same structures appear in a typical reading series. Given the fact that reading series might also present problems for deaf students relative to vocabulary and other text features, the use of present, unadapted materials might be inappropriate for most deaf students.

Despite the quantitative delays in syntax, Quigley and his associates also demonstrated that deaf students were acquiring syntactic structures in the same manner (i.e., qualitatively similar) as younger hearing students. That is, the deaf students proceed through stages, made errors, and use some strategies that were similar to those of hearing students. This qualitative similarity can also be seen in the written language productions of deaf students discussed later.

Since the extensive studies by Quigley and his collaborators, there have been several studies that focused on specific syntactic structures, for example, anaphoric relationships within conjoined sentences, indefinite pronouns (e.g., Wilbur & Goodhart, 1985), modals (e.g., Wilbur et al., 1989), and relative clauses (e.g., Lillo-Martin et al., 1992). For example, Wilbur et al. (1989) examined hearing-impaired students ability to comprehend English modals (e.g., *will, won't, would, can, could, shall*, etc.). One-hundred eighty seven subjects, between the ages of 7 and 23 years, participated in the study. These students met the same criteria as those in the Quigley's studies that were summarized above.

TABLE 5-3. Summary of Performance on Syntactic Structures and Their Frequency of Occurrence per 100 Sentences in the *Reading for Meaning* series.

Structure	Deaf Students Average Across Ages %	Age 10 %	Age 18 %	Increase %	Hearing Students Average Across Ages %
Negation					
be	79	60	86	26	92
do	71	53	82	28	92
have	74	57	78	21	86
Modals	78	58	87	29	90
Means	76	57	83	26	90
Conjunction					
Conjunction	72	56	86	30	92
Deletion	74	59	86	27	94
Means	73	57	86	29	92
Question Formation					
Wh- Questions					
Comprehension	66	44	80	36	98
Yes/No Questions					
Comprehension	74	48	90	42	99
Tag Questions	57	46	63	17	98
Means	66	46	78	32	98
Pronominalization					
Personal					
Pronouns	67	51	88	37	78
Backward					
Pronominalization	70	49	85	36	94
Possessive					
Adjectives	65	42	82	40	98
Possessive					
Pronouns	48	34	64	30	99
Reflexivization	50	21	73	52	80
Means	60	39	78	39	90
Verbs					
Auxiliaries	54	52	71	19	81
Tense					

TABLE 5-3. *(continued)*

Structure	Deaf Students Average Across Ages %	Age 10 %	Age 18 %	Increase %	Hearing Students Average Across Ages %
Sequencing	63	54	72	18	78
Means	58	53	71	18	79
Complementation Infinitives and Gerunds	55	50	63	13	88
Relativization Processing	68	59	76	17	78
Embedding	53	51	59	8	84
Relative Pronoun Referents	42	27	56	29	82
Means	54	46	63	18	82
Disjunction & *Alternation*	36	22	59	37	84

Structure	Level at Which Structure First Appeared	Frequency in 6th Grade Text
Negation be	1st Primer—13	9
Conjunction Conjunction	1st Primer—11	36
Question Formation Wh- Questions Comprehension	2nd Primer—5	6
Yes/No Questions Comprehension	1st Primer—5	3
Pronominalization Backward Pronominalization	4th grade—1	0 (4 per 1,000)

(continued)

TABLE 5–3. *(continued)*

	Frequency of Occurrence	
Structure	Level at Which Structure First Appeared	Frequency in 6th Grade Text
Possessive Adjectives	1st grade—4	27
Possessive Pronouns	3rd Primer—1	0 (3 per 1,000)
Reflexivization	2nd grade—1	2
Verbs Auxiliaries	1st grade—1	18
Complementation Infinitives and gerunds	2nd Primer—4	32
Relativization Processing	3rd Primer—2	12
Disjunction and Alternation	1st grade-1	7

Source: Adapted from Quigley, Wilbur, Power, Montanelli, & Steinkamp (1976).

Wilbur et al. (1989) reported that the students' comprehension of English modals was related to the level of reading achievement. In addition, the researchers analyzed their data with respect to an order of acquisition. They discussed this order of acquisition relative to the predictions of three hypotheses: developmental, theoretical, and syntactic (e.g., use of syntactic transformations). The researchers concluded that the acquisition of English modals requires more than just a knowledge of transformational rules—there is a need to consider semantic and pragmatic aspects (e.g., as in the theoretical position). As stated by these researchers:

> To approach an adequate account of the English modals, much more than transformational rules are needed. In the last decade, the case has been made for the importance of including proper pragmatics and semantic considerations, both in the classroom and in testing situations. (Wilbur et al., 1989, p. 16)

Several other researchers have argued that a better understanding of deaf readers' knowledge of English syntax requires an analysis that goes beyond the sentence level (e.g., Ewoldt, 1981; McGill-Franzen & Gormley, 1980, Nolen & Wilbur, 1985). For example, McGill-Franzen and Gormley (1980) examined deaf children's comprehension of truncated passive sentences (e.g., *The window was broken*) presented in context and in isolation. Results indicated that the subjects understood the structure better in context than in isolation.

In another study, Ewoldt (1981) argued that deaf students could actually bypass the specific English syntactic structure and proceed directly to meaning. Her results are based on the performances of four deaf students between the ages of 6 years, 11 months to 16 years, 11 months. The researcher claimed that deaf students did not "overrely" on text information; in fact, the researcher argued for a top-down approach to reading instruction. The whole language approach has been derived from top-down models (e.g., Goodman, 1976, 1985) and is a widely used approach in the education of deaf children (e.g., see discussion in Dolman, 1992).

Taken together, there seems to be some evidence that deaf students can understand syntactic structures better in context than in isolation. However, there are still several issues that need to be resolved by further research. Similar to the research on context and vocabulary knowledge, the use of context to comprehend syntax is indicative of the students' ability to *derive* the meaning of the structure. Deriving the meaning of structure—like deriving word meaning—might be more indicative of reading skill. This skill, however, is also influenced by the "type" of context clues that exist in the passage. For example, it is possible to describe the context (typically, a phrase or sentence) that surrounds a word as misdirective, directive, and nondirective (see reviews of research in Davey & King, 1990; Paul & O'Rourke, 1988). There needs to be further research on descriptions of context (perhaps, two sentences or a paragraph) that surround a particular syntactic structure. This research is necessary in order to understand the effects of context on deaf students' comprehension of syntax.

As discussed previously, there is substantial evidence that the ability (especially, the speed) to recognize (or comprehend) words in isolation is indicative of reading ability. Of course, it is also important for readers to derive the meanings of words from context, especially if there is a breakdown in comprehension. However, it is critical that readers do not have to spend too much time on deriving words or word meanings.

The intent of this discussion is to show that the same logic might apply to syntax. There is ample evidence that knowledge of syntax in isolation is important for reading comprehension, as discussed previously in the work of Quigley and his collaborators. Additional support has been provided by Negin (1987), who reported that syntactic segmentation significantly affects hearing-impaired students' ability to comprehend narrative and expository reading materials. It is important for readers to be able to derive the meanings of certain structures during reading, particularly if there is a breakdown in comprehension. However, good readers do not have to spend a preponderant amount of time figuring out the meaning of a specific structure.

We have discussed the work of Lillo-Martin et al. (1991, 1992) in Chapter 3. Recall that these researchers argued that deaf students' difficulty with reading is not due to specific syntactic comprehension problems. Rather, it is due to an underlying processing deficit—that is, lower-level phonological processing. This is a strict bottom-up perspective which may not be complete within the framework of interactive theories of reading, discussed in this chapter. In all fairness, Lillo-Martin et al. remarked that their findings should not be interpreted to mean that poor deaf readers never have "structural" problems. Rather, researchers and educators should be open to the possibility that some syntactic problems may be related to a processing deficit.

Figurative Language

It is not immediately obvious that the English language contains a significant number of idiomatic and other figurative expressions. The most obvious examples are figures of speech such as simile (*Running around like a chicken without a head*) and metaphor (*The night was a blanket*). Examples of idiomatic expressions include *It's raining cats and dogs* and She's *out of her mind*.

The bulk of figurative expressions take the form of verb-particle phrases and multimeaning words (Paul, 1984; Payne, 1982). Examples of verb-particle phrases include *look up*, *ran into*, and *rip off*. Common examples at the word level are *head* of the class, *hands* of the clock, and *eye* of the needle. It has been argued that one of the fastest-growing groups of figurative expressions is the verb-particle phrases (Payne, 1982).

Research on the comprehension of figurative language is difficult to conduct because of the interactions and influence of other language variables such as vocabulary and syntax. Nevertheless, the reader, even the beginning reader, will encounter numerous instances in print (e.g., Dixon, Pearson, & Ortony, 1980). There is research showing that both deaf and hearing readers, especially second-language readers, have difficulty with figurative language (e.g., see discussions in Grabe, 1988, 1991; King & Quigley, 1985). In addition to vocabulary and syntax, the use of figurative expressions is another language variables that is often controlled for in the development of special reading series (e.g., Quigley & King, 1981–1984; Quigley, Paul, McAnally, Rose, & Payne, 1990, 1991).

Many students with severe to profound hearing impairment have difficulty comprehending figurative expressions in printed materials (e.g., Conley, 1976; Giorcelli, 1982; Payne & Quigley, 1987). For example, Giorcelli (1982) constructed a test of figurative expressions that entailed the following areas: analogical and syllogistical reasoning, associative fluency, linguistic problem solving, interpretation of anomaly, and discrimination between paraphrases of novel and idiomatic metaphors. Two groups of subjects, hearing and deaf, served as participants. The ages of the 25 hearing students ranged from 8 years to 9 years, 4 months. The ages of the 75 deaf subjects ranged from 9 years, 9 months to 19 years. Giorcelli reported that the hearing subjects performed significantly better than the deaf subjects on the total test and on 7 of the 10 subtests. Similar to the research of Quigley and his associates on syntax reported previously, the researcher found that the 18-year-old deaf students did not perform as well as the 9-year-old hearing students. In fact, there was little improvement in the performance of deaf students beyond 13 to 14 years of age.

Payne and Quigley (1987) assessed both deaf and hearing students' comprehension of the verb-particle figurative expressions. The ages of the 45 deaf subjects ranged from 10 to 19 years whereas the ages of the 45 hearing subjects ranged from 8 to 12 years. The researcher developed a test with 64 items using verb-particles at three levels of semantic diffi-culty (literal, e.g, *walks out*, semi-idiomatic, e.g., *washes up*, and idiom-atic, e.g, *gives up*) and in five syntactic patterns (SVA—subject, verb, adverb; SVAO—subject, verb, adverb, object; SVOA—subject, verb, object, adverb; SVPO—subject, verb, preposition, object; and SVAPO—subject, verb, adverb, preposition, object). Similar to Giorcelli's findings, the researchers reported that the hearing subjects performed significantly better than the deaf subjects on all levels of semantic difficulty and for all syntactic structures.

Some researchers have documented that deaf students can understand metaphorical expressions if the vocabulary and syntax are controlled (e.g., Iran-Nejad, Ortony, & Rittenhouse, 1981) or if there is sufficient context to disambiguate the meaning of the expressions (e.g, Houck, 1982; Page, 1981). It has also been suggested that deaf students may learn the expres-sions as a whole and that vocabulary and syntax do not present problems (e.g., Wilbur, Fraser, & Fruchter, 1981). Nevertheless, there is research showing that knowledge and explanation of figurative expressions (e.g., simile, metaphors, idioms, and proverbs) are related to the reading com-prehension levels of deaf students (Fruchter, Wilbur, & Fraser, 1984; Orlando & Shulman, 1989).

In essence, similar to the research on vocabulary (e.g., Paul, 1984; Paul & Gustafson, 1991), it is difficult for many deaf readers to "derive" the meaning of figurative expressions from context. This is due to two major difficulties: (1) Deaf students may not have the level of reading competence to use context clues, and (2) the context of the reading mate-rial typically does not "reveal" the meaning of the expression.

Research on Selected Reader-based and Other Factors and Deafness

The research on the effects of reader-based and other factors (e.g., task-based) on deaf students' reading ability has not been as systematic and extensive as the research on the effects of selected text-based factors (see discussions in King & Quigley, 1985; Paul, 1993). We have discussed at least two well-documented reader-based factors, degree of hearing impairment and internal mediating system, and one other well-documented factor, parental hearing status elsewhere in this text (see Chapters 4 and 6). Although there are other factors, for example, cognitive style, content of tests and texts, instructional practices, and test-taking strategies, our focus in this section is on three of the most critical—and highly related—reader-based factors: prior knowledge, inferencing, and metacognition (an in-depth discussion of other reader-based and other variables can be found in King & Quigley, 1985; see also the discussion in Limbrick, McNaughton, & Clay, 1992).

The work of Wilson (1979) is representative of the research on deaf students and inferencing. Based on his analysis of previous studies, this researcher hypothesized that one of the major reasons for deaf students' difficulty with reading materials beyond the third grade was their difficulty in making inferences. The task of making inferences is predominant for the higher reading levels due to the abstract and implicit nature of the information. The researcher documented deaf students' problems with inferences in a series of short passages in which inferencing was studied in various syntactic environments and with vocabulary controlled.

The ability to make inferences in, for example, answering questions is highly related to the prior knowledge and metacognitive abilities of the students (for hearing students, see, e.g., Baker & Brown, 1984; Fincher-Kiefer, 1992). There is some research showing that students with severe to profound hearing impairment have the ability to use their prior knowledge to comprehend aspects of the text (e.g., Kluwin, Getson, & Kluwin, 1980) or to organize information for retelling a story (i.e., story grammar; e.g., Griffith & Ripich, 1988). As discussed previously, the research on deriving word meanings and syntax can be interpreted as deaf students' having the skill to apply prior knowledge and metacognitive aspects. However, it should be clear from several studies that deaf students either do not have adequate prior knowledge or metacognitive skills or do not apply these skills during reading tasks (e.g., see discussions in King & Quigley, 1985; Strassman, Kretschmer, & Bilsky, 1987).

The notion that reading is thinking, reasoning, or essentially a higher-level cognitive activity and that instruction should be based on this principle can be found in several reviews and analyses of the research literature (e.g., Erickson, 1987; Martin, 1993; Paul, 1993). Because of the similarity between cognition and reading, some researchers have argued that an improvement in the cognitive thinking skills of students will lead to a subsequent improvement in their reading skills (e.g., Martin, 1993; Naglieri & Das, 1988). Reading beyond the literal stage (i.e., reading for meaning) has been described as follows:

The evaluative, inferential reading comprehension act, among other things, is a culturally-loaded, linguistic, metacognitive response to the printed word. . . . the deaf . . . [should] . . . be exposed to advanced comprehension tasks commensurate with the maturity of their thinking abilities. Inferential and critical reading should be taught as natural extensions of the thinking process. (Erickson, 1987, p. 293)

Two recent studies are discussed as examples of the research on two important reader-based variables, prior knowledge and metacognition. The purpose of one study, Strassman (1992), can be stated as a question: "What metacognitive knowledge do deaf students have about school-related reading" (p. 327)? Twenty-nine students with severe to profound, prelingual hearing impairment and between the ages of 14 years, 7 months to 19 years, 5 months participated in the study. The examiner conducted and videotaped interviews with the students on an individual basis, using the *Reading Comprehension Interview* (Wixson, Bosky, Yochum, & Alvermann, 1984).

The researcher interpreted the results as showing that many deaf students can be classified as passive readers. It was stated that:

It is not clear that these adolescents had metacognitive knowledge about why they did what they did in school-related reading or what the long-term goal of reading in school was. Rather, they seemed to mechanically employ the techniques that they had been taught. (Strassman, 1992, p. 328)

In another study (Yamashita, 1992), the purpose was to determine the relationships among prior knowledge, metacognition, and reading comprehension for students with hearing impairment. Sixty-one students with a degree of hearing impairment ranging from 36 dB to 120 dB participated in the study. The students attended either oral or total communication day classes at the middle and high school levels. Results indicated that both prior knowledge and metacognition are significantly related to reading comprehension. Further regression analyses revealed that metacognition has the strongest effect for all measures of reading comprehension, which was described as answering different levels of questions (e.g., see Booth, 1985; Raphael & McKinney, 1983).

DEVELOPMENT OF WRITING

Theories and research on writing have been influenced by theories and research on reading. The development of writing has also been affected by the recent thinking on models of instruction—that is, whether writing can be or should be taught to students. In addition, research on writing has been discussed relative to the type of research inquiry, namely, the use of quantitative or qualitative methods. Implicit in all theories of both reading and writing is the notion that children are active "little scientists." That is, they construct hypotheses about how the language works in both the oral and written mode (e.g., see discussion in Ruddell & Haggard, 1985).

Perhaps the best way to discuss writing is to divide perspectives into two broad categories: product and process (e.g., Czerniewska, 1992; Laine & Schultz, 1985; Paul & Quigley, 1990). Traditional research and instruction on writing has focused on the products whereas the more recent research emphasis is on the process of writing (Bereiter & Scardamalia, 1983; Hillocks, 1986). As is discussed later, this should not be construed as an *either-or* situation. The process of writing does involve knowledge of the product.

The Product View of Writing

The products of writing refer to items such as spelling, punctuation, capitalization, grammar, and legibility (e.g., Czerniewska, 1992; Laine & Schultz, 1985). Relative to bottom-up theories of reading, proponents of this view maintain that written English literacy is dependent on knowledge of the alphabet system, or the relationship between sounds (phonemes) and their letter representations (graphemes) (e.g., see discussions in Brady & Shankweiler, 1991; Templeton & Bear, 1992). Similar to bottom-up skills of reading, the acquisition and development of writing is hindered if the student does not possess automatic lower-level skills such as the mechanics mentioned previously.

There have been a number of studies that demonstrated that poor readers are also poor writers (e.g., see research review in Chall, Jacobs, & Baldwin, 1990). This has also been reported for many students with severe to profound hearing impairment (Moores, 1987; Paul & Quigley, 1990). One assumption is that to be a good writer, one must be *at least* a good reader. Another assumption is that writing skills, similar to reading skills, must be taught (see discussions in Chall et al., 1990; Czerniewska, 1992).

Despite the linearity of the product, or bottom-up, view of writing, it is important for the writer to possess fluent lower-level skills in mechanics. However, lower-level skills are not sufficient. It has been shown that a number of good readers do not become good writers (e.g., see discussions in Bereiter & Scardamalia, 1983; Czerniewska, 1992). These findings have led some scholars to call for a "paradigm" shift in the view of the development of writing.

The Process of Writing

One predominant recent view is that writing is a *social process* (e.g., Czerniewska, 1992; Laine & Schultz, 1985). The underpinnings of this viewpoint can be found in the work of Vygotsky (1962), whose views have also influenced social-interactionist theories of language development (see Chapter 2 of this text). Support for the social view of writing can be found also in the current literary critical theories mentioned previously (e.g., see Lemley, 1993).

Because writing is an aspect of language, it is a social process whose meaning, role, and value vary across contexts or communities. Within this framework, writing is not merely or only a representation of an individual's thoughts. Similar to the use of language, a person writes to "generate" or "create" meaning. In other words, written language is not an attempt to represent or reflect "reality"; it is the writer's creation or construction of "reality."

The social process of writing emphasizes what can be called higher-level cognitive aspects, for example, organization, purpose, and audience. The lower-level skills such as legibility and grammar are dealt with afterwards as needed. That is, after producing or completing a draft, students might receive assistance with grammar and mechanics from other student-writers or teachers.

One popular model of writing development contains the stages of planning (topic generation and organization), composing (the first draft), and revising (editing, rewriting) (e.g., see discussions in Laine & Schultz, 1985; Whitt, Paul, & Reynolds, 1988). These stages are not always mutually exclusive. For example, a writer might choose to compose and revise at the same time. During the composing stage, the writer might decide to reorganize the manuscript.

The social process of writing seems to be a predominant top-down approach. In our view, this approach is linear and has shortcomings similar to the product, or bottom-up, approach. It is most beneficial to view writing as an interactive social-cognitive process that is similar to the process of reading (e.g., Rubin & Hansen, 1986; Tierney & Leys, 1984; Tierney & Pearson, 1983).

The notion of similar underlying processes imply that both reading and writing involve the construction of meaning. In addition, writing, like reading, entails the interaction between the individual and the text that the individual is attempting to compose. There is a reciprocal relationship between the top-down (e.g., organization and intent) and bottom-up aspects (e.g., spelling, grammar) of writing. In essence, writing develops as a result of and in conjunction with reading (Adams, 1990; Anderson et al., 1985).

To understand and research the process of writing, some scholars have argued for the use of "holistic" methodology (e.g., see discussions in Bereiter & Scardamalia, 1983, 1987; Czerniewska, 1992) and natural instructional approaches (e.g., see discussion in Laine & Schultz, 1985). As remarked by Bereiter and Scardamalia (1983), holistic approaches "insist on viewing natural behavior in its full context and . . . seek to break down the rigid division between observer and observed" (p. 21). Nevertheless, there is no superiority or "God's eye view" associated with any particular type of methodology. Consequently, a better understanding of writing, and any other phenomenon, as both a cognitive and social process entails the use of both quantitative and qualitative methodologies (e.g., Bereiter & Scardamalia, 1983, 1987).

In tandem with the naturalistic research methodology, there has been a push for natural instructional approaches, especially in the areas of reading and writing (e.g., Czerniewska, 1992; Laine & Schultz, 1985). Relative to writing, the natural approaches assert that writing is not "something" that can be taught in a linear fashion—that is, the imparting of knowledge from teachers to students. It has been stated that:

> The emphasis of these and other contemporary approaches to writing is on generating meaning (rather than correctly recording or transmitting what already exists). . . . Teachers are doing more writing themselves and learning to discuss their own composing processes. They write in class with their students, share drafts of their own writing, and ask students to comment and make suggestions. Students see that writing isn't difficult only for kids and magic for teachers. (Laine & Schultz, 1985, p. 16)

RESEARCH ON WRITTEN LANGUAGE

In this section, three issues are discussed: (1) the use of written language productions; (2) research on written language and hearing children, with an emphasis on the relationship between oral and written language development; and (3) research on written language and deaf children. In conjunction with the information on STM and reading achievement (see Chapter 3), our discussion of the issues above should highlight the major reasons for the great difficulty that many students with severe to profound impairment have with the development of both reading and writing skills.

Use of Written Language Productions

Until the recent great upsurge of interest in American Sign Language and manually coded English (see Chapter 4), much of the research on the language of deaf children was conducted on written language productions. This is in distinct contrast to hearing children where primary spoken language is usually the focus of interest. The major reason for this situation was that the spoken language of many deaf children and adolescents is extremely limited and often unintelligible and therefore not readily available for inspection and analysis.

There is some research showing that written language productions are not completely reflective of what deaf students can do in the primary mode, that is, via the use of English-based signed systems or the use of sign communication in general (e.g., see discussion in and the research of Everhart & Marschark, 1988). For example, Everhart and Marschark (1988) interpreted their results as indicating that "literalness evidenced in written English need not be indicative of the more general cognitive literalness assumed from such results by previous researchers" (p. 191).

From another perspective, spontaneous written language productions are generally considered to be among the best indicators of a deaf child's level of mastery of English. However, there are a number of problems associated with the use of written language productions. These problems are discussed in the ensuing paragraphs.

1. Typically, some external stimulus is used to elicit a written sample— a picture, picture sequence, short film, request to write a story or letter, and so forth. The validity and reliability of these techniques often are unknown. If it is found that certain vocabulary items, morphological structures, syntactic structures, or other linguistic units of interest do not appear in the writing samples elicited, it is difficult to determine whether this is due to the deaf child's inability to produce such structures, or whether it is merely that the stimulus used did not elicit them.

2. Some linguistic units (e.g., infinitival complements—Mary wanted *to make a million dollars*) might appear in the written productions, but in insufficient numbers or variety to allow for study and analysis.

3. Some constructions (e.g., some types of relative clauses) appear in linguistic environments such that it is difficult to understand them and their role in a sentence.

4. As probably every teacher of deaf children knows, the written language productions of many deaf children are often as unintelligible as their spoken language.

Despite these problems of eliciting and analyzing written language productions, such productions are valuable indicators of deaf children's understanding of English and of the internalized language structure with which the child is working. Researchers have employed two broad methods for eliciting written productions: *free response* and *controlled response* (see also, the discussion in Chapter 8). Free-response methods refer to the spontaneous, freely produced samples of writing. Controlled-response methods entail the use of techniques to control or manipulate the behavior of a subject or informant by holding certain linguistic variables constant (e.g., see discussion in Cooper & Rosenstein, 1966). The linguistic method of presenting pairs of sentences which differ on only one structure and asking subjects for judgments of the sentences' grammaticality is one example.

With a focus on the products of writing, analyses of the written language productions of deaf students have been influenced by the prevailing linguistic theories, typically, structural linguistics or Chomsky's transformational generative grammar. Although dividing lines between free response and controlled response studies and traditional and generative frameworks are not always sharp, the categories serve adequately for grouping the data on the written productions of deaf students. We also discuss research on the written language of deaf students which has been influenced by the emerging paradigm of the process of writing, particularly the interpretation of the writings of deaf students beyond the sentence level, that is, at the multi-sentence level.

Research on Written Language and Hearing Children

A number of studies have explored the developmental stages of writing in the written language productions of elementary-age hearing children (e.g., see reviews in Chall et al., 1990; Czerniewska, 1992; Hillocks, 1986; Ruddell & Haggard, 1985). In general, there is a strong relationship between the early written productions of children and their oral language development. For example, there is a progression from multiple conjoined sentences (e.g., use of conjunctions such as *and*) to embedded sentences (e.g., relative clauses—*The boy who kissed the girl ran away*). This progression exemplifies the increase in the complexities of the writings throughout the elementary grades.

There are several examples of this continual increase in complexity in both oral and written language. Research on hearing children between the ages of 9 to 15 years showed increases in certain language variables such as clauses, particularly subordinate clauses and adverbial clauses, except those of time and cause. It should be noted that these clauses appear more often in the written language productions. In fact, examining the increase relative to age revealed a larger increase for written language than for oral language. By the intermediate grades, for example, grades 6 and 7, the written language productions of children were considerably more complex than their oral language productions.

Several researchers/scholars have interpreted these results as demonstrating the strong early relationship between 'oral' (i.e., speech) and written language productions (e.g., Chall et al., 1990; Ruddell & Haggard, 1985). This reciprocal relationship is deemed important for the later development of advanced reading and writing skills (e.g., see also, Brady & Shankweiler, 1991; Templeton & Bear, 1992). For example, written language influences the organization of the mental lexicon, fostering a deeper appreciation of the phonological and morphological aspects of words. In addition, this deeper understanding of the alphabet system facilitates the further development of both reading and writing.

Other scholars have interpreted the findings as indicative of stages of written language development. For example, Danielewicz (in Ruddell & Haggard, 1985) delineated four major activities of these stages in which children:

1. *unify* spoken and written language, making few distinctions between the two;
2. *distinguish* between spoken and written language by reducing coordinating conjunctions;
3. *strip* features of spoken language from written production; and
4. features typically associated with written language. (p. 68)

es Danielewicz's study and others support the strong early etween oral and written language, they also showed that there progression . . . in differentiation among spoken and written language, spelling, and syntactic complexity" (Ruddell & Haggard, 1985, p. 68).

Research on Written Language and Deafness

The research on the written language of deaf students is discussed relative to two broad areas: the sentence level and multisentence level. At the sentence level, we present data from both free-response and controlled-response studies, influenced by both traditional/structural and generative theories. The more recent studies, focusing on the multisentence level, view writing as a process.

Sentence Level—Free Response: Traditional Framework

The two predominant findings of the early traditional free-response studies were: (1) Deaf students had lower performances on written language than younger hearing children, and (2) the writings of deaf students varied greatly from standard English (e.g., Heider & Heider, 1940; Stuckless & Marks, 1966; Templin, 1950). For example, Heider and Heider (1940) analyzed the written language productions of deaf students, ranging in age from 11 to 17 years, and those of hearing students, ranging in age from 8 to 14 years. Results revealed that deaf subjects used fewer words and clauses (e.g., shorter sentences) than did hearing subjects. Deaf subjects did not attain the average sentence length of 8-year-old hearing children until they were 17 years old (see also Myklebust, 1964). Relative to the notion of complexity, Heider and Heider reported that hearing subjects produced more complex sentences than did deaf subjects. They found that the deaf subjects were typically 17 years old before they used the same proportion of compound and complex sentences in their compositions as did 10-year-old hearing subjects (see also Taylor, 1969).

Although the written language development of deaf students showed improvement with the advancement of age, it seemed to plateau at about the level of the 9- or 10-year-old hearing student. There was the emerging view that deaf students did not have a command of the grammar of English, particularly in the areas of vocabulary and syntax (e.g., see Templin, 1950 for an historical precursor to later studies). This inadequate command of standard English was deemed to be the "global" reason for the written language performance of deaf students. This resulted in the prevalent use of, for example, stereotypic phrases. In addition, it was found that deaf children use more determiners, nouns, and verbs than did hearing children and fewer adverbs, auxiliaries, and conjunctions.

With the above view in mind, several researchers described the errors and rigid writings of deaf students. For example, it was noted that deaf students produce errors of *addition* (adding unnecessary words), *omission* (of words needed to make the sentence correct in standard English), *substitution* (of wrong words), and *order* (word order departing from that of standard English) (e.g., the work of Myklebust, 1964). Myklebust (1964) and Simmons (1963) also documented a number of "carrier phrases," which were found to appear more often in the rigid writings of deaf students than in the writings of hearing students. Examples include: *I see a* _____ , *There is a* _____ , and *They had an idea.* It has been argued that the presence of stereotypical phrases might be either an artifact of the test instrument used or of the "structural" approach to teaching language to deaf students (e.g., see van Uden, 1977; Wilbur, 1977).

Some prominent reading researchers, concerned mainly with hearing children, have attempted to provide a global interpretation of these early studies on deafness. For example, it has been remarked that:

> Both the Heider and Heider and the Templin studies point to a significant relationship between oral and written language development. The opportunity for oral language experience through hearing would appear to exert direct influence on performance in written language. (Ruddell & Haggard, 1985, p. 68)

It should be emphasized that these studies were descriptive in nature. This information is important; however, a better understanding of free-response data emerged with the generative grammar theories (e.g., Chomsky, 1957, 1965), which focused on explanatory adequacy. That is, these theories attempted to explicate the *rules* that children use to produce sentences at various developmental levels. As discussed in Chapter 2, the idea of language being "generative" refers to the fact that there is a limited number of highly abstract mechanisms used (at a subconscious level) for the processing (comprehension and production) of a theoretically infinite number of sentences. These abstract mechanisms are often described in terms of "rules" for sentence processing (production or interpretation).

Sentence Level—Free Response: Generative Grammar

The grammatical data in this section are presented relative to four categories: phrase structure rules, the lexicon, morphological rules, and transformational rules (Russell et al., 1976). The work of Taylor (1969) is used to illustrate these aspects because this researcher pioneered a kind of analysis new for deaf children's written language—a transformational-generative analysis. In addition, many of Taylor's findings have been confirmed by other researchers.

In Taylor's study, subjects were 35 deaf children at each of four grade levels. The subjects were required to write written compositions in response to their viewing of a movie called "The Ant and the Dove" (i.e., one of Aesop's Fables). Some of the major findings of this study are discussed in the ensuing paragraphs.

Relative to phrase structure rules, Taylor found four types of omissions: prepositions (e.g., *The ant slept the bed)*, determiners (e.g., *The ant saw grasshopper)*, direct objects (e.g., *A girl threw in the water)*, and verbs, particularly copulas (e.g., *The bird away)*. Determiner omissions were the most frequent at all age levels, followed by prepositions, direct objects, and verbs. However, at age 10, verbs were the second most frequent omission, and by age 12, verbs had become the least frequent omission. These findings led Taylor to conclude that one of the earliest standard English rules mastered by young deaf children is that the predicate of a sentence must contain a verb. That is, a sentence must contain a noun phrase and a verb phrase.

It was reported that the major type of redundancy occurred with prepositions, for example, *The ant walked to home* and *He thanked to the dove*. The frequency of occurrence of this type of redundancy did not decrease much over the age range of the subjects in Taylor's study. In comparing the occurrence of omissions and redundant use of prepositions, the researcher established a pattern of development that has been shown to be typical of language acquisition in younger hearing children. The pattern is as follows: (1) the failure to apply a rule until it is learned, (2) the gradual acquisition of the rule and its increasingly correct use, (3) the subsequent "overgeneralization" of that rule to environments where it should not be applied, and (4) predominant correct use of the rule.

Relative to the lexicon category, Taylor experienced difficulty in interpreting data revealing deaf children's violations of selectional restrictions. Errors that could confidently be attributed to violation of selectional restrictions were very infrequent. The only two categories that appeared to be clear were "combinations of determiners and nouns which were mutually incompatible with respect to the feature count (e.g., *a water and the few grass*) or with respect to the feature plural (e.g., *a scissors and a pliers*)" (Taylor, 1969, p. 124). No discernible improvement in deaf children's performance in this area could be detected within the 10- to 16-year age range of the subjects.

Finally, deaf subjects made few substitutions of one major category of English for another. Nevertheless, they did not noticeably improve their performance in this area across the age range studied by Taylor. The researcher remarked that sentences containing such phenomena were not grossly variant, and could be readily interpreted by readers. Taylor hypothesized that variant structures such as *Mother table the food* are related to such functional shift use of nouns as verbs in such expression as *table the motion.*

Relative to the morphology category, it was observed that the performances of deaf students improved with the advancement of age. Most of the difficulties occurred in the area of verb inflections, followed by singular-plural inflections (e.g., *The sheeps*, and *Six boy*) and possessive inflections (use of *'s* and *s'*). It should be emphasized that the errors that deaf students produced were similar to those made by younger hearing children. For example, in verb inflection, the most frequent errors were omissions of inflectional endings—for example, *So she fly and get a leaf.* The next type of common error was overgeneralization of the correct form—*The dove was scared and flied away*, followed by the incorrect application of the correct rule as in *The circle broked.* The least frequent of verb morphological variances occurred as incorrect tense marking in sentences such as *Dove saw ant can't swim.*

Taylor (1969) also examined deaf children's use of three major types of transformational rules in her study: conjunction, nominalization, and relative clauses (see the discussion of research on syntax by Quigley and associates in the section on reading presented previously). Compared with some other categories, there were relatively few transformational variances. However, the researcher concluded that this was not because deaf children performed well in this area. It was because the children rarely attempted to use complex transformations. The students did not show a significant decline in the number of nonstandard transformational structures they produced with age. Nevertheless, Taylor felt that they showed some increased mastery of transformational rules because whereas the number of variances did not decrease, the number of transformations attempted did increase significantly with age. The types of transformational errors are illustrated in Table 5–4.

The results of Taylor's research indicated that deaf children's written language productions still vary considerably from standard English usage. In general, the 16-year-old students have achieved mastery over many aspects of the production of simple active declarative sentences, particularly of the subject-verb-object order. Nevertheless, even at this age, deaf students still have problems with morphology, especially in areas of noun and verb inflections. In addition, they have difficulties with the determiner and auxiliary systems of English. Students make relatively few mistakes in producing complex transformations; however, they rarely write these constructions. In essence, deaf students know little about complex transformations such as relativization and nominalization. When they attempt to write such transformations, the students produce numerous variant structures. It can be concluded that these deaf children were not just making "errors" in producing English sentences; rather, they were producing "correct" (for them) sentences from rules which were not based on those of standard English.

Besides examining the comprehension of specific syntactic structures by the use of specific tasks discussed previously, Quigley et al. (1976) obtained written language samples from their stratified random national sample of deaf students. Similar to Taylor's findings, only limited instances of the structures studied by the TSA were found in the freely produced written samples. In addition, there seems to be a correlation between the limited productions and the comprehension (i.e., order of difficulty) of these structures.

Sentence Level—Controlled Response: Generative Grammar

Based on transformational generative grammar, a substantial body of research exists which used controlled presentation of stimuli. The use of controlled-response tasks provides additional information on the grammatical competence of deaf students. For convenience, our discussion of these studies is organized around the framework used previously: phrase structure rules, the lexicon, and tranformational rules.

In a study of the use of phrase structure rules, O'Neill (1973) developed a *Test of Receptive Language Competence* in which deaf and hearing subjects were required to judge whether simple sentences generated by

TABLE 5-4. Types of Transformational Errors in Taylor's (1969) Study.

Structure	Error	Sentence
Conjunction	Omission	• A ant see a tree a bird. • Ant walk found animals.
	Misplacement	• The dove got out of the tree and took a leaf threw it down. • The ant ran to its home and get the scissors and hit a man's leg.
	Deletion	• The tool hurt the hunter and yelled. • The hunter scared the dove and flew away. • The ant threw a ball on the ground and put in his room.
	Tense sequencing	• The ant went off and ride the dragonfly.
Nominalization Gerunds and Infinitives		• The ant like to played with insects. • The man began screamed. • He cannot know how to swimming. • The hunter missed to shoot the dove. • The ant saw him what he was doing.
Relative Clauses	Nonuse of pronouns	• The ant held the thing look like circle.
	Copying	• There was a little hole underground which a smart ant lived in it.

Source: Adapted from Taylor (1969).

correct and incorrect rules were "right" or "wrong." In the *omission* section, her deaf subjects (ages 9 to 17 years) made correct judgments on 75% (versus 84% for hearing children) of the items and showed significant improvement with age. In general, the deaf subjects did as well as hearing subjects in selecting the "right" sentences as "right," but they had a tendency to label "wrong" sentences as "right" much more often than did the hearing children. Specifically, the deaf subjects were more likely to accept incorrect sentences in which function words such as determiners, prepositions, and verb particles had been omitted than sentences in which nouns, verbs, and adjectives (content words) had been incorrectly omitted. These findings are in close agreement with those reported by Taylor (1969) for free written production discussed previously.

The *redundancy* category was observed to be slightly more difficult than *omission* for O'Neill's deaf subjects (73% correct overall, versus 85% for hearing subjects). O'Neill found a pattern of results similar to that reported for the *omission* category previously. That is, sentences containing redundant determiners, prepositions, and verb particles were more difficult for deaf subjects to judge than those containing redundant content words. It was also noted that the deaf subjects tended to accept sentences which contained a redundant verb—for example, *The children went walked to the park*.

Relative to the lexicon, O'Neill (1973) developed a selectional restriction subtest, which was the most difficult test for both deaf (69% correct) and hearing (82% correct) subjects. Subjects accepted as correct a wide range of sentences which violated selectional restrictions on nouns and pronouns. Examples include *The desk serenaded Matilda* and *Milk are good for you*.

Relative to morphology, Cooper (1967) found deaf children's knowledge of inflectional morphemes to be superior to their knowledge of derivational markers. This is consistent with the difficulty deaf children have with derived nominals of various types. Cooper's data generally confirm and extend those found by Taylor (1969) in her free data-gathering situation.

Focusing on the negative transformational rule, Schmitt (1969) administered comprehension and production tasks involving the selection of one of four pictures to match correctly a given sentence. He found that most of his deaf subjects (ages 8 to 17 years) understood the meaning of the negative marker *not* in English sentences. However, there was a number of the 8-year-old subjects who failed consistently on this task. Schmitt hypothesized that they were operating with what he called the *no negative rule*, "which specifies the ignoring of the marker 'not' and the treatment of negative sentences as equivalent to affirmative sentences" (p. 124). It might be that such a response is even more typical of the performance of deaf children younger than those Schmitt tested.

Relative to passive transformational rules, Schmitt (1969) had deaf children select the one of four pictures which correctly illustrated the action of reversible passive sentences. Subjects were also required to "fill-the-gap" in sentences to produce passive sentences to describe pictures correctly. The researcher found that few of the deaf children below age 14 could pass his tests, and that even at 17 years of age, many children still could not comprehend the meaning of passive sentences or produce them correctly.

Schmitt's work was extended by Power and Quigley (1973) who used three tasks to investigate the acquisition of the passive voice. In the comprehension task, deaf children were required to move toys to show the action of the passive sentence. Three types of passive sentences were used—full reversible, full nonreversible, and agent deleted (which can be reversible or nonreversible). With the agent-deleted sentences, a forced choice of one of two pictures which represented the action of the sentence was used instead of the toy-movement task. The production task was the same as used by Schmitt (1969). The researchers concluded that even at age 17–18 years the majority of deaf children have a defective rule for the processing of passive sentences. This rule can be stated as "passive reversal of subject-object order to process meaning of such sentences is signaled only by by; tense markers are free to vary" (Power & Quigley, 1973, p. 76). It seems that many deaf students, including the older ones, persisted in interpreting all sentences in terms of the standard subject-verb-object order of the English simple sentence.

Recent Research on the Process of Writing

The studies in this section are a representative sample of the recent research on the process of writing with deaf individuals. Some of the early work in this area was conducted by Gormley and Sarachan-Deily (Gormley & Sarachan-Deily, 1987; Sarachan-Deily, 1982, 1985). Gormley and Sarachan-Deily (1987) analyzed the writing samples of 20 high-school-age students with severe to profound hearing losses. The focus of the study was to examine the similarities and differences between "good" and "poor" writers. The assignment of a writer to a good or poor category was based on the judgments of teachers and the investigators.

The students' written language samples were analyzed relative to three categories: content (e.g., suggestions, reasons, and conclusions), linguistic aspects (e.g., organization and cohesion), and surface mechanics (e.g., spelling, punctuation, and capitalization). Results revealed no significant differences between the two groups on the surface mechanics and most of the linguistic aspects. It should be noted that both groups made a number of errors in these two categories. However, the major difference between good and poor writers was in the area of content. That is, the compositions of good writers were more developed, cohesive, and readable. In short, the major difference was with the use of higher-level writing skills. Although the researchers argued that writing instruction should focus mainly on higher-level skills, they suggested there is also a need to encourage hearing-impaired writers to reread and revise their manuscripts. These activities should help students to reduce their errors in surface mechanics and many linguistic aspects.

Description of the revision strategies of deaf student writers was the major focus of a more recent study (Livingston, 1989). Either the deaf writers, themselves, or their teachers made suggestions for revising the manuscript. The researcher was also interested in whether the revisions actually resulted in an improved final draft.

Twenty-two high-school seniors, between the ages of 16 to 21 years old, participated in the study. The students wrote a story a month for three months. After completing a first draft, each student consulted individually with the teacher. At these conferences, teachers were instructed to provide ideas and suggestions for the purpose of clarification, not for remedying grammatical errors. Students then prepared a second draft of their topics which were read by their peers.

The researcher analyzed the "changes" from the first to the second drafts and the interactions that occurred in the conferences. The "changes" were categorized according to the frameworks developed by Bridwell (1980) and Sommers (1980)—for example, deletion, substitution, addition, and rendering—and according to syntactic level. Results indicated that most of the revisions were initiated by the students themselves, rather than by their teachers at about a 6-to-1 ratio. The most frequent changes were additions and substitutions. Compared to the research on hearing writers, it was found that deaf writers tended to make more additions whereas hearing students tended to make more deletions. However, both groups were similar in their revisions on the syntactic level.

Even more interesting was the observation that the questions/suggestions of teachers of hearing-impaired students were "sentence-specific instead of discourse-based" (Livingston, 1989, p. 25). That is, teachers tended to focus on specific sentences in the story rather than on higher-level skills such as organization and purpose, even for stories that seem to have, for example, no clear purpose. In addition, it was observed that some teachers prefer to comment on the first draft of the student without holding conferences. This procedure tended to result in students' misunderstandings of the written comments of the teacher. Some teachers even attempted to correct directly the grammatical errors in the first drafts of students. Relative to this activity, the researcher reported that:

Most often, students mimicked the correction onto subsequent drafts, but in many instances, the error was carried over. . . . Essentially, the attempt at correction on the part of the teachers was not understood by the students and therefore ignored. (Livingston, 1989, p. 25)

In a recent study, Klecan-Aker and Blondeau (1990) analyzed the written stories of eight students who were severely to profoundly hearing impaired and whose ages ranged from 10 years, 10 months to 18 years, 1 month. The students received speech and language services in an oral/aural program in public schools. Using an elicitation procedure (i.e., simply asking the subjects to write a story), the students wrote stories during their speech and language sessions. No time limits were imposed, and the subjects received the following instructions: "I want you to write a story. Remember, as you write, that stories have a beginning, middle, and end" (p. 277).

The written stories of the subjects were analyzed relative to intra-sentential and intersentential elements: T units (Hunt, 1970), story grammar components (Stein & Glenn, 1979), cohesion, and developmental level relative to the age of the student (Klecan-Aker, 1988). The data on T units in this study were compared to the hearing subjects in an earlier study (Klecan-Aker & Hedrick, 1985). Using descriptive statistics, it was found that the hearing-impaired subjects used fewer clauses and words per T unit than did their hearing peers. In addition, of the various story grammar components—setting, initiating event, attempt, internal response, consequence, and ending—hearing-impaired subjects only had difficulty with one component, internal response. Relative to cohesion, only one structure was examined—conjunctions. Results revealed that the subjects produced more coordinating conjunctions (*and, and so, and then*) than subordinating conjunctions (*because, that, when*). Finally, there was no strong relationship between the developmental level of the stories and the ages of the students. Some of the results, particularly those on T units and conjunctions, supported the early research on the writing of deaf students discussed previously. It should be remembered that the sample size in the current study was small and that subjects were oral deaf students (see Chapter 4 for a discussion of the language development of oral deaf students).

Within the framework of writing as a process approach, a number of recent studies have emphasized strongly that there should be a continual focus on higher-level skills such as organization, intent, and authorship, and that teachers should encourage writers to engage in thinking, planning, and evaluating activities. This focus can be seen in studies that examined the free writing of deaf children in kindergarten (e.g., Andrews & Gonzales, 1991) to students in elementary and secondary grades (e.g., Kluwin & Kelly, 1991) to students in a postsecondary program (e.g., Brown & Long,

1992). The researchers reported that the quality of deaf students' written productions improved over time and there were noticeable changes in content and syntactic complexity.

The emphasis on the process approach does not mean that it is not important to attend to lower-level skills. Some researchers have provided guidelines for teachers to work on skills such as fluency, syntax, and vocabulary (e.g., Luckner & Isaacson, 1990; Paul & Quigley, 1990). In one sense, focusing on the product of writing only (particularly, lower-level skills) is similar to a bottom-up approach in reading whereas focusing on the higher-level skills only (as in a process approach) is a strict top-down model. Given our earlier discussion that reading and writing are related, that is, both lower-level and higher-level skills are important, it seems that viewing writing as a social-cognitive interactive process might yield the most productive research and instructional effects for deaf children and adolescents. In essence, the reading-writing connection, including the impact of the language-thought relationship, has been discussed relative to deaf students (e.g., Kretschmer, 1989; Yoshinaga-Itano & Downey, 1992). It has been stated that:

> A review of the literature substantiates . . . that the ability to produce well-formed narratives may have a significant relationship to reading comprehension and semantic language characteristics. (Yoshinaga-Itano & Downey, 1992, p. 131)

FINAL REMARKS

In this chapter, we described the impact of deafness on the development of reading and writing skills. Relative to reading, the focus was on one group of reading-comprehension theories—interactive theories. It was argued that the reading difficulties of deaf students should be discussed and can be ameliorated within the framework of social-cognitive interactive theories.

The background information on reading processes was necessary to understand extant theory and research on the development of writing. In essence, literacy is an interactive process in which readers and writers attempt to construct a working model of meaning. It is clear that the construction of meaning requires the coordination of both bottom-up and top-down skills.

It is not surprising that our increased understanding of the processes of reading and writing has not altered substantially the low-literacy achievement of students with severe to profound hearing impairment. Perhaps, there needs to be a more concerted effort to ensure the interrelationships of theory, research, assessment, curriculum, and instruction. In addition, there needs to be more research on reading factors that have not been extensively investigated, for example, reader-based factors such as prior knowledge, inferencing, and metacognition.

These suggestions for further research might lead to an improvement—albeit in small increments—of the literacy skills of deaf students. On the other hand, literacy might not be a realistic goal for many students with prelingual severe to profound hearing impairment. This assertion is based not only on the discussion in this chapter, but also on the discussions relative to the relationship of short-term memory and reading comprehension in Chapter 3 and the acquisition of the English language in Chapter 4. Although English literacy development requires much more than the knowledge of the English language, one of the major problems for deaf students is the acquisition of the primary form of English at as early an age as possible.

For many deaf students, it might be more beneficial for educators to concentrate on the development of literate thought—that is, the ability to think critically and reflectively. The impetus for this line of thinking has come from another group of models labeled literary critical theory, which will probably receive an increasing amount of theoretical and research attention. Some of the influences of literary critical theory can be seen in the growing movement for the establishment of bilingual and second-language programs for deaf students. This is the main focus of the next chapter.

FURTHER READINGS

Balmuth, M. (1982). *The roots of phonics: A historical introduction.* New York: Teachers College Press.

Gelb, I. (1963). *A study of writing* (Rev. ed.). Chicago, IL: University of Chicago Press.

Hoffman, J. (Ed.). (1986). *Effective teaching of reading: Research and practice.* Newark, DE: International Reading Association.

Mathews, M. (1966). *Teaching to read: Historically considered.* Chicago, IL: University of Chicago Press.

Thaiss, C., & Suhor, C. (1984). *Speaking and writing, K–12: Classroom strategies and the new research.* Urbana, IL: National Council of Teachers of English.

Zakaluk, B., & Samuels, S.J. (Eds.). (1988). *Readability: Its past, present, and future.* Newark, DE: International Reading Association.

CHAPTER 6

BILINGUALISM AND SECOND-LANGUAGE LEARNING

What is the difference between first and second language learning? It cannot be the case that a language is "learnable" as a first language, but less so as a second language. Is the predisposition to acquire whatever language one is exposed to good for a one-time use only? Does this ability self-destruct after one use, or does the presence of a first language alter the conditions for language learning? Can an explanation of the variability in second language learning tell us anything about language learning in general? (Wong Fillmore, 1989, p. 313)

Because of deaf students' difficulty with English, some educators and researchers have become interested in the nature of second-language learning, specifically the second-language learning of English. This interest has engendered arguments for the establishment of bilingual programs involving the use of American Sign Language (ASL) and English (e.g., Luetke-Stahlman, 1983; Paul, 1990; Paul et al., 1992; Quigley & Paul, 1984; Reagan, 1985; Strong, 1988b). Although there is no consensus on what type of bilingual or second-language learning education program should be established, several models have been described (e.g., see Johnson et al., 1989; Paul et al., 1992; Paul & Quigley, in press; Strong, 1988b). For example, it has been proposed that deaf children be exposed to ASL and English concurrently in infancy and early childhood or that ASL be developed first in a normal interactive manner and English developed later (second-language learning).

A brief survey of the literature on bilingualism and English-as-a-second-language (ESL) reveals that these fields have as many and as deep differences in theory, research, and practice as does the education of deaf students (Bernhardt, 1991; McLaughlin, 1987). This survey is important because there is very little research information available on bilingualism, ESL, and deafness. In light of our conclusions regarding language and literacy development of deaf students as discussed in Chapters 4 and 5, much of the information on hearing bilingual and second-language learners is applicable to deaf students (see also the discussion in Paul & Quigley, 1987b, in press).

The plan for the chapter is as follows. First, we provide some background on bilingualism and second-language learning with hearing students. This entails a discussion of definitions, theories, and a synthesis of a representative sample of research studies. In addition, we address a number of other issues relevant to deafness such as (1) similarities and differences between first- and second-language acquisition, (2) the nature of second-language literacy, particularly reading, and (3) research on bilingualism and second-language learning. Subsequently, we synthesize the research on bilingual educational models for hearing minority students. Based on this synthesis, we describe the basic tenets of our bilingual educational model (see Paul, 1990, 1991; Paul & Quigley, in press; for a detailed description). Our final remarks center on the future of bilingual education and deafness.

DEFINITIONS

It is unsurprising that there is disagreement about what constitutes bilingualism and second-language learning (e.g., Cook, 1991; Crystal, 1987; McLaughlin, 1984, 1987). Bilingualism implies the use of two languages; however, this seemingly simple notion has produced a great deal of confusion in the theoretical and research literature. Factors which contribute to the lack of consensus include the notion of language, language competency, language proficiency, and the time frame in which languages are learned.

One major problem is to decide whether a particular code or symbol system is, in fact, a language. The defining criteria for identifying a distinct language are not unequivocal. For example, some German universities have separate departments for the English (British) and American languages. Norwegians do not always agree on whether they have one language or two (Haugen, 1956).

Relative to deaf students, the notion of a language is a major longstanding, controversial issue. As discussed previously in this text, ASL is a bona fide language which is different in grammar а English and the English-based signed systems. It is clear th. second language for deaf students who come to school knowiₙg ᴀᴏʟ or some other minority language such as Spanish or German. For example, a bilingual situation for some deaf students can consist of exposure to ASL and one of the English-based signed systems or ASL and oral English. Exposure to oral English and one of the signed systems would not constitute bilingualism, but simply two coding forms of a single language—English.

Several scholars have proffered views on the distinction between bilingualism and second-language learning. Lamendella (1977), for example, argued for the adoption of the following terms: primary language acquisition, secondary language acquisition, and foreign language learning. This researcher referred to primary language acquisition as the normal language learning process occurring up to the age of about 5 years regardless of the number of languages involved and the manner in which they are introduced to the child. Secondary language acquisition, which can also involve the learning of two or more languages, is considered to occur in a naturalistic setting and manner after the period of the primary language acquisition (after about 5 years of age). Lamendella described foreign language learning as that which occurs in the formal classroom setting and is cognitively different from secondary language acquisition.

From another perspective, there seems to be little developmental difference between learning a language in either the classroom or in a naturalistic setting (e.g., McLaughlin, 1985, 1987). In addition, the time frame of Lamendella's primary language acquisition is not widely accepted. This issue, known as the critical period hypothesis, is still being debated (e.g., Crystal, 1987; McLaughlin, 1984). However, there seems to be an optimal period for learning a language or languages (e.g., from birth to about 10 years or so), and this issue has pervasive implications for language and deafness, as discussed later.

A useful, chronological-age distinction between bilingualism and second-language learning has been offered by McLaughlin (1984). This researcher stated that the presence of two languages before the age of 2 years leads to simultaneous acquisition, that is, bilingualism. The acquisition can be described as successive (second-language learning) if the presence of a second language is delayed until the age of 3 years or later. There seems to be some consensus that the learning of a second-language, particularly in later childhood, adolescent, or adulthood, is much more difficult than the learning of two languages in a bilingual situation in early infancy and childhood (e.g., see McLaughlin, 1984, 1985; Wong Fillmore, 1989).

Despite the varying views, it is safe to conclude that bilingualism and second-language learning is not an all-or-nothing phenomenon. Rather, it is a function of degree depending on the age of the individual and the mode of the language (e.g., speaking, reading, writing). This issue is even more complex in considering deaf students. It is true that English is the first language of exposure for the majority of deaf students from English-speaking homes. However, unlike many other majority-language students, most students with severe to profound hearing impairment come to school with minimal or limited competency in their home language and culture. Indeed, these students can be classified as minimal speakers/users of English. This situation has led some researchers to argue for the development of ASL as a *first* language for *all* deaf students, regardless of degree of hearing impairment, parental hearing status, or language spoken in the home (e.g., Johnson et al., 1989; Liddell & Johnson, 1992).

THEORETICAL MODELS OF BILINGUALISM

In addition to variation in definitions of bilingualism and second-language learning, there is a diversity of theoretical models in the literature. There is also diversity in the classification of these theories. This diversity depends on the metatheories, methodologies, and foci of the researchers. For example, there are a number of models dealing with the effects of bilingualism on cognitive and academic achievement (e.g., Cummins, 1977, 1978, 1984; Lambert, 1972; Macnamara, 1966). It is also possible to classify models according to certain disciplines such as linguistics (e.g., Krashen, 1981, 1982, 1985; Selinker, 1972), sociolinguistics (e.g., Hymes, 1974), social psychology (Lambert & Tucker, 1972), neurolinguistic (e.g., Lamendella, 1977), and cognitive (e.g., McLaughlin, 1987, Chapter 6). From another perspective, McLaughlin (1987) described five types of theories in second-language acquisition and process: the monitor model, interlanguage theory, linguistic universals, acculturation/pidginization theory, and cognitive theory.

Despite the preponderant amount of theoretical and research work in the area of bilingualism and second-language learning, there is no coherent theory of bilingualism relative to linguistic, cognitive, and social phenomenon (e.g., see Beardsmore, 1986; Cook, 1991). In addition, the classification schemes mentioned above are not mutually exclusive. Our approach here is to discuss a few of these models in the various categories mentioned above and those which are also discussed in several reviews of the literature (e.g., Beardsmore, 1986; Cook, 1991; McLaughlin, 1984, 1987). With the remarks on classification schemes in mind, two groups of models are discussed below. The first group of models seems to be most related to the effects of bilingualism on cognition and academic achievement whereas the second group focuses mainly on the acquisition process (e.g., as discussed in Beardsmore, 1986, Cook, 1991; McLaughlin, 1984, 1987).

Effects of Bilingualism: Theoretical Considerations

Macnamara (1966) proposed a balance theory, sometimes termed the genetic inferiority or verbal deprivation theory. This researcher asserted that an individual has a fixed amount of language learning ability which must either be divided among two or more languages or devoted entirely to one. It is claimed that most people are unable to learn two languages simultaneously as well as monoglots (monolinguals) learn one by itself. There is a large body of data which demonstrates inferior performance of bilinguals in one language (usually, the majority or dominant language of society) (e.g., see review in McLaughlin, 1984). This suggests that the other language interferes with the learning process. The deficiency in the majority language is purported to be reflected in the lowered performance in all academic areas.

From another perspective, Lambert (1972; Lambert & Tucker, 1972) espoused an interdependence theory. It is argued that, under certain conditions, access to two languages can positively influence the development of some cognitive processes which can consequently lead to higher IQ and academic achievement. For these positive effects to be detected by research studies, certain confounding factors must be controlled, for example, socioeconomic status, gender of subjects, and degree of bilingualism.

The contradictory findings in the literature have been addressed by Lambert (e.g., 1972; Lambert & Tucker, 1972) with an additive/subtractive hypothesis, which is a corollary to his interdependence model. Lambert attributed the contradictory findings to differences between bilinguals in an additive environment and those in a subtractive environment. An additive educational or social environment is one which poses no threat of replacing the first (L1) or home language of the language-user with a second (L2) or majority language of the culture. On the contrary, a subtractive environment aims to supplant the minority, home, or first language with the majority one.

Lambert argued that bilinguals in an additive environment usually possesses a first language which may be the dominant or majority language of the culture (i.e., majority-language users). These students (typically from middle or upper socioeconomic status [SES] classes) become balanced bilinguals when they add another language (either a majority or minority one). Consequently, they perform as least as well as matched monolingual users of either of the two languages involved. Contrariwise, the inferior skills of many of the bilingual subjects reported in other studies were probably due to the fact that these subjects were in a subtractive environment, which posed a threat to the first language. In addition, some of the contradictory findings might be due to studies failing to (1) control for the bilingual subjects' level of competence in either L1 or L2 and

(2) acknowledge that subjects might have had less than nativelike skill in both their languages because they came from low SES environmental backgrounds.

A somewhat similar model to the additive/subtractive one is the societal factor model. Proponents of this model have argued that a home-school language switch results in high levels of functional bilingualism and academic achievement in majority language children; however, it also leads to inadequate command of both languages and poor academic achievement in many minority language children. These scholars have also argued for an emphasis on the determining role of societal factors (e.g., see discussions in Beardsmore, 1986; Cook, 1991; McLaughlin, 1987). In essence, the societal factor model rejects axiomatic statements regarding the medium of instruction and assigns a fundamental causal role to societal or sociocultural factors.

Development of L1 and L2

There are several models that focus on the relationship between the development of the two languages involved. Cummins (1977, 1978, 1984) has proposed a threshold model, which is also offered as an explanation for the contradictory findings in the research literature. It is argued that the cognitive and academic effects of bilingualism are mediated by the levels of competence attained in both languages regardless of whether the subjects possess a majority or minority language as a first language. Cummins further argued that there might be threshold levels of linguistic competence which a bilingual child must attain (i.e., in the two languages) both to avoid cognitive disadvantages and to allow the potentially beneficial aspects of bilingualism to influence cognitive functioning. The threshold model assumes that those aspects of bilingualism which might positively influence cognitive growth are unlikely to come into effect until the child has attained a certain minimum or threshold level of competence in the second language.

Another model, termed the developmental interdependence model, proposes that the development of skills in a second language is a function of skills already established in the first language (Skutnabb-Kangas & Toukoman, cited in Cummins, 1978; McLaughlin, 1984). In situations where the first language is inadequately developed, the introduction and promotion of a second language can impede the continued development of the first. This inadequate development of the first language, consequently, will limit the development of competence in the second language. Contrariwise, a highly developed L1 (prior to the introduction of L2) will contribute to a high level of development in L2 at no cost to L1 competence. The developmental interdependence model emphasizes the importance of the continuing development of the first language.

There are a few models concerned with the development of L1 and the subsequent development of literacy skills, particularly reading, in the second language. The vernacular advantage model asserts that the best medium for teaching a child in a bilingual situation is in the mother language or first language (e.g., Cummins, 1984, 1988; Modiano, 1968; Rosier & Farella, 1976). This model is specifically intended for children whose first language is a minority language. Proponents have argued that instruction through the medium of the first language or mother tongue for minority-language children in the early grades is a prerequisite for equality of educational opportunity. Furthermore, when instruction is through the medium of a second or majority language and the school makes no concessions to either the language or the culture of the minority-language child, the result is frequently low levels of competence in both languages and academic failure.

It is argued that reading should be introduced in the learner's first language (i.e., mother tongue) for which the child has already acquired the sound system, structure, and vocabulary. Subsequently, when the student achieves an independent reading level in L1, the student can then begin to read in the second language. It is reasoned that the acquisition of reading skills in the first language leads to an efficient transfer of skills and, thus, faster acquisition of second-language reading (e.g., Cummins, 1988; Gamez, 1979).

Some scholars have argued that the direct approach to reading is the most efficient approach. That is, reading should be introduced initially in the second language. Most of the evidence for this position seems to be from students whose first language or home language is the majority language or one that is equally prestigious as the second language (e.g., Cummins, 1988; Genesee, 1987; Swain & Lapkin, 1982).

The issue of the most efficient way to transfer skills from one language to another in reading is an area of intense research. It has brought the debate on the theories of first-language reading (see Chapter 5) into the realm of research on reading in the second language. As in first-language reading, it seems that social-cognitive interactive theoretical models have become accepted as plausible explanations of the second-language reading process (e.g., Bernhardt, 1991; Grabe, 1988, 1991).

As is discussed later, several of the models in this section, particularly those that deal directly with the development of L1 and L2, have influenced program models for bilingual education. It seems that these program models have influenced much of the discussion of bilingualism with deaf students (e.g., see discussion in Paul & Quigley, 1987b, in press).

These models have also proffered explanations for the acquisition of a second language, including reading. A summary of the major highlights of these theoretical models is presented in Table 6–1. Other views of the second-language acquisition process are discussed briefly in the next section.

Theories of Second-Language Learning

The models in this section deal specifically with the acquisition of a second language. Not all second-language models are discussed here. Although our selection of the models is primarily subjective, it is based on several reviews of the theoretical and research literature (notably, Beardsmore, 1986; Cook, 1991; McLaughlin, 1987). As in first-language acquisition, the models in this section have been influenced by the prevailing views on language development, for example, linguistic and cognitive (including, cognitive-interactionist and social-interactionist). This is also some influence from the emerging field of neurolinguistics.

Interlanguage

There are a few models that have been motivated by the linguistic thinking of Chomsky (1957, 1965; see Chapter 2). One of these, termed the interlanguage theory (Selinker, 1972), has been labeled a "bottom-up" approach to the problem of second-language acquisition (e.g., McLaughlin, 1987). This is interpreted as an inductive approach to theorizing that attempts to deal with a restricted range of data. Initially, the interlanguage model was used to explain adult second-language acquisition; however, it has also been used to account for the acquisition of a second language by children (e.g., Selinker, Swain, & Dumas, 1975; for a recent discussion of interlanguage, see Davies, Criper, & Howatt, 1984).

The term interlanguage is said "to refer to the interim grammars constructed by second-language learners on their way to the target language" (McLaughlin, 1987, p. 60). Selinker (1972) has proposed this notion to deal with the inadequacies that exist in the weaker language of a bilingual individual who has not achieved fluency in this language. In essence, the learner's knowledge base of the "weaker" language is not commensurate with that of a native speaker of the same language, especially from a transformational generative grammar perspective.

Selinker offered this hypothesis to show also that the spoken productions could not be attributed solely to interference from the first language or to the transfer of first language skills. The researcher stated that the interlanguage is a separate linguistic system which is distinct from both

TABLE 6-1. Highlights of the Theoretical Models of Bilingualism

	Effects of Bilingualism
Macnamara (1966)	The researcher proposes a balance theory, also known as the genetic inferiority or verbal deprivation theory. An individual has a fixed amount of language learning ability which must either be divided among two or more languages or devoted entirely to one.
Lambert (1975 & Tucker (1972)	The researchers propose an interdependence theory. Access to two languages can positively influence the development of some cognitive processes which can consequently lead to higher IQ and academic achievement. An additive educational or social environment is one which poses no threat of replacing the first or home language with the second or majority language of the culture. On the contrary, a subtractive environment aims to supplant the minority or first language with the majority one.
Cummins (1977, 1978, 1984)	The researcher proposes a threshold model. Cognitive and academic effects of bilingualism are mediated by the levels of competence attained in both languages regardless of whether the subjects possess a majority or minority language as a first language. Aspects of bilingualism which might positively influence cognitive growth are unlikely to come into effect until the child has attained a certain minimum or threshold level

(continued)

TABLE 6-1. *(continued)*

Effects of Bilingualism

	of competence in the second language.
Vernacular Advantage Model	The best medium for teaching a child in a bilingual situation is in the mother tongue or first language. The model is intended for children whose first language is a minority language. Reading should be introduced in the learner's first language (L1). Subsequently, when the student achieves an independent reading level in L1, the student can then begin to read in the second language.
Direct Approach to Reading	Reading is introduced and developed in the second language only.

the first language of the speaker and the target (or second) language that the speaker is attempting to learn. This system is the result of the user's attempts (i.e., strategies, hypothesizing) to learn the target language.

Selinker argued further that the interlanguage is a distinct system based on the occurrence of *fossilized* (or frozen) features in the target or second language. That is, the second-language user persists in the use of certain features in the interlanguage despite the seemingly adequate input from or experiences with the second language. Fossilization may occur because the second-language learner has reached communicative competency although not grammatical competency, or it may be the result of other forces (e.g., language transfer). It should be underscored that fossilized features do not appear in the development of the first language.

In attempting to explain second-language acquisition, Selinker proposed that the interlanguage is influenced by five cognitive processes: language transfer, language-teaching effects, learning strategies, communication strategies, and overgeneralization. These components have been described as follows:

1. Language transfer: some items, rules, and subsystems of the interlanguage may result from transfer from the first language.

2. Transfer of training: some elements of the interlanguage may result from specific features of the training process used to teach the second language.
3. Strategies of second-language learning: some elements of the interlanguage may result from a specific approach to the material to be learned.
4. Strategies of second-language communication: some elements of the interlanguage may result from specific ways people learn to communicate with native speakers of the target language.
5. Overgeneralization of the target language linguistic material: some elements of the interlanguage may be the product of overgeneralization of the rules and semantic features of the target language. (McLaughlin, 1987, p. 61)

The notion of interlanguage has evolved, and there are several additional models (e.g., see discussions in Bialystok & Sharwood-Smith, 1985). The notion is considered to be a reaction against behaviorism because of its emphasis on the influence of internal, cognitive factors (e.g., see McLaughlin, 1987). Even more striking is the fact that it is becoming increasing difficult to separate interlanguage theory from others (e.g., Universal Grammar) because of overlapping components (Beardsmore, 1986; McLaughlin, 1987). Although the theoretical merits of interlanguage are open to question, one of its greatest weaknesses is its inability to explain fully why later bilinguals do not achieve a level of competence commensurate with early bilinguals (Beardsmore, 1986). One attempt to deal with this issue has been the Monitor Model, proposed by Krashen (1981, 1982, 1985).

Monitor Model

Krashen's Monitor Model is considered to be mainly a deductive model on which research is based and hypotheses are derived. The model is an attempt at "explanatory adequacy" (see Chapter 2). In this sense, it has been labeled "The most ambitious theory of the second-language learning process" (McLaughlin, 1987, p. 19). Because of Krashen's attempts to elucidate his model, it is widely known by teachers of second-language.

To deal with the differences between late and early bilinguals, Krashen sought to develop a theory that made a distinction between *language acquisition* and *language learning*. Within this perspective, acquisition is considered a natural, unconscious process whereas learning is a contrived, conscious activity. Thus, the truly competent bilinguals are those who "acquire" the two languages in a natural, noninstructional setting.

Krashen also hypothesized that differences can be attributed to the age of the learner, specifically if one is attempting to learn a language after the age of 12. In this view, the potential for using "language acquisition processes" diminishes with the onset of abstract, metacognitive abilities. This is the basis of the *monitor* hypothesis of his overall "Monitor Model." The "language learner" (as opposed to the language acquisitioner) makes use of monitor functions which are similar to the "editing" or "revising" functions of a reader or writer. Because of constraints and difficulties associated with time, and the representation and use of language rules, the "language learner" is not as successful as the "language acquisitioner."

In the further development of his model, Krashen proposed the notion of *affective filter*, which is said to account for discrepancies in the "ultimate" attainment of the two languages between late and early bilinguals (e.g., see Beardsmore, 1986; McLaughlin, 1987). The affective filter contains emotional and other affect aspects such as motivation, anxiety, and confidence. In all, there are five hypotheses associated with Krashen's Monitor Model: monitor, acquisition-learning, affective filter, input, and natural order (for an in-depth discussion of the research merits of these aspects, see Beardsmore, 1986; McLaughlin, 1987).

Despite the few merits of Krashen's model, it has been widely criticized because of its inconsistencies and its broad, sweeping claims (e.g., see McLaughlin, 1987). We do not intend to provide a point-by-point refutation of each aspect of the model. However, it is important to note that there is a growing support for the assertion that little differences exit between the notions of "acquisition" and "learning" (e.g., see research reviews in McLaughlin, 1984, 1985).

Several statements should be made on this issue. First, it is difficult to separate these two entities, that is, an individual who achieves competency in a language probably has engaged in both "processes" (assuming there is a difference). In addition, it is possible to "learn" a language in a classroom setting with a level of proficiency commensurate with that of "acquiring" a language in a natural setting. Finally, this issue tends to "blur" somewhat the distinctions between the debates regarding the "teachability" versus "learnability" of languages and those on the "natural" versus "structural" language-teaching methods (for an in-depth discussion of these issues relative to deafness, see McAnally et al., 1987, in press).

Other Linguistic Approaches

Several other linguistic approaches have been influenced by the work of Chomsky (1965, 1975, 1980, 1988), particularly the notion of Universal

Grammar. Universal Grammar is concerned with first language acquisition. However, this notion has also influenced research on language acquisition and deafness (e.g., Lillo-Martin et al., 1991) and on second-language learning (e.g., see reviews in Beardsmore, 1986; Cook, 1991; McLaughlin, 1987).

Felix (1982) proffered a novel linguistic approach to account for the differences in achievement between early and late bilinguals. This researcher argued that differences between the two groups can be attributed to the use of different cognitive systems. Early bilinguals, particularly children, use cognitive structures that are suited for the acquisition of language. Late bilinguals, particularly adults, are using two systems that compete with each other: language-specific cognitive system and a cognitive system that functions for general problem-solving tasks. Felix labels this process in adults as the "Competition Model."

Because of the notion of separate cognitive systems in the brain, it seems that this researcher and others (notably, Fodor, 1983) ascribed to the principle of modularity (see Chapter 2 of this text). For dealing with linguistic information, the general problem-solving systems are not as efficient as the language-specific cognitive systems. The emergent of the problem-solving system occurs after puberty. Felix's hypothesis asserted the importance of the critical-age hypothesis; however, this importance is not based on physiological criteria. It seems to be related to what is considered age-determined changes in the development of the cognitive system of humans.

Other Approaches

Dissatisfactions with "pure" linguistic approaches have led to the use of approaches that can be termed sociolinguistic, social psychological, neurolinguistic, and cognitive, specifically information processing. For example, the sociolinguistic framework has been influenced by the work of Labov (1972) and the social psychological view by Schumann (1978). The sociolinguistic framework has been used to explain the varieties of language used by deaf individuals (e.g., Bochner & Albertini, 1988). Even more interesting is the influence of this view on determining the nature of ASL. A number of scholars have called into question the "pure linguistic" descriptions of ASL (e.g., see *The Deaf American*, 1990).

In our view, the cognitive models, particularly information processing, have exerted the most pervasive influence on theories of second-language acquisition. The future potential of these models can be found in McLaughlin (1987). Perhaps the most noticeable influence has been on second-language reading, particularly via the use of interactive theories (e.g., Grabe, 1988, 1991). The influence of interactive theories on second-language reading is discussed briefly later in this chapter.

Despite differences between the major theoretical frameworks, there are several critical summary statements that can be made. It has been stated:

> What does seem to be emerging from the different types of argument put forward by various scholars is that bilingual ability, by and large, seems to be affected by the age of initial *prolonged* contact with the second language, that in the process of becoming bilingual the speaker goes through several stages of interlanguage in the L2, that these are partially determined by factors like the nature of the input, interference effects from L1 and other effects independent of L1, that the acquisition of bilingual proficiency partially follows that of native-language acquisition but not completely, that strategic competence seems to play a significant role in the achievement of linguistic goals in the weaker language and that fossilization may set in at different stages of bilingual development, leading to only partial attainment in the L2. (Beardsmore, 1986, p. 135)

A summary of the major highlights of the theories discussed in this section is provided in Table 6–2.

Development in L1 and L2: Similar or Different?

In this section, we discuss briefly whether the acquisition of English as a second language is qualitatively similar to the acquisition of English as a first language for hearing individuals. We also examine this notion relative to the acquisition of English literacy, particularly reading. These issues have wide-reaching implications for instruction and curriculum. Later in the chapter, we explore these issues relative to the acquisition of English by deaf students. In relation to deafness, some insights on this qualitative issue were provided in Chapter 5.

Research on the development of English as a second language has been documented relative to three broad groups: preschool, school-age children, and adults (e.g., see reviews in Cziko, 1992; McLaughlin, 1984, 1985, 1987; Paul, 1985). One of the critical issues seems to be the notion of language transfer. That is, the issue is what effects does the nature of the first or native language of the individual have on the acquisition of the second or target language? This is referring to the notion of interference (McLaughlin, 1984, 1985; Paul, 1985).

In general, it has been documented that the notion of interference, albeit important, does not adequately explain the acquisition process of the second language (e.g., King, 1981; McLaughlin, 1984, 1985). For example, second-language learners of English from different L1 backgrounds make similar errors, and these errors are also similar to individuals learning English as a first language. Although the acquisition process entails the

TABLE 6-2. Highlights of Theories of Second-Language Learning

Interlanguage

- This is a separate linguistic system which is distinct from both the first language of the speaker and the target (or second) language that the speaker is attempting to learn.
- This system is the result of the user's attempts—strategies, hypothesizing—to learn the target language.
- The system is based on the occurrence of fossilized (or frozen) features in the target or second language.

Monitor Model

- The model makes a distinction between language acquisition and language learning.
- Differences can be attributed to the age of the learner, specifically if one is attempting to learn a language after the age of 12.
- There are five hypotheses associated with the model: monitor, acquisition-learning, affective filter, input, and natural order.

Competition Model

- The model attempts to account for the differences between early and late bilinguals.
- The model ascribes to the principle of modularity (Fodor, 1983).
- The model asserts the importance of the critical-age hypothesis, that is, the age-determined changes in the development of the cognitive system of humans.

Source: Adapted from Beardsmore (1986) and McLaughlin (1987).

interaction of both developmental and transfer factors (e.g., transfer of reading skills in L1 to the acquisition of reading in L2), the bulk of the process seems to be explained by developmental factors.

It should be highlighted that "transfer" (or interference) results in the production of some *deviant* structures; that is, structures that are not typically produced by the language learner in either the first or second language development. The production of these structures might be related to the influences of social and psychological factors on language-learning strategies. A greater number of deviant structures have been documented in school-age children, as compared to preschool children. This has been attributed mainly to two major factors: (1) the lack of native language peer models and (2) the use of unsound instructional practices and methods (e.g., McLaughlin, 1985; Paul, 1985). Similar arguments have been made for the "stilted" English written language productions of deaf students (see Chapter 5). A third factor, the learning of a language in a classroom setting, has not withstood the test of time. That is, there is no substantial evidence that learning a language in a classroom setting is developmentally different from learning the same language in a natural setting (e.g., McLaughlin, 1985).

Similar findings have been reported for adult second-language learners. The few interference errors are common in the early stages of the language acquisition process. Most of the "errors" are similar developmentally to individuals learning English as a first language. As is discussed later, the same is true for deaf students learning English as a first or second language (e.g., King, 1981). In essence, it has been remarked that:

> There seems to be little evidence from studies comparing language learning in children and second-language learning in adults that the two groups go through radically different processes. What evidence there is points to the conclusion that the processes involved are basically the same. (McLaughlin, 1984, p. 66)

There is increasing evidence that reading in English as a second language is similar to the process of reading in English as a first language (Bernhardt, 1991; Grabe, 1988; Paul, 1993). This viewpoint can be seen in the shift from the use of both text-based and reader-based models to those based on interactive theories (Grabe, 1988; see also, the discussion in Chapter 5). At this point in time, it appears that research on second-language reading has not been markedly influenced by another group of theories labeled literary critical theories (see Chapter 5).

As discussed previously, it has been documented that the reading acquisition process of deaf students is similar to that of hearing students learning to read English as a first language. A summary of this research on deaf and second-language readers has been provided:

> Second-language readers do not begin reading English with the same knowledge of English language and sociopolitical culture as first-language readers. *Indeed, this describes the condition of many deaf students.* Both second-language readers and many deaf students do not have a large vocabulary or command of basic syntactic structures . . . Like first-language learners, second-language learners experience two major kinds of difficulties: overreliance on text-based processing or overreliance on reader-based processing such as extensive guessing or use of context. Interactive theories also apply to the reading process in a second language. (Paul & Jackson, 1993, p. 137)

RESEARCH ON BILINGUALISM, SECOND-LANGUAGE LEARNING, AND DEAFNESS

As mentioned previously, there is a dearth of theoretical and research literature on the issues of bilingualism, second-language learning, and deafness. Much of the literature contains anecdotal reports, descriptions of a few existing bilingual programs, and proposed models for ASL/English bilingual educational programs for deaf students. The information in this section is organized around five areas: (1) primary bilingual development; (2) effects of ASL on the subsequent development of English; (3) language production and preference of deaf students, including bilingual deaf students; (4) ASL/English instructional programs; and (5) development of L1 and L2 in deaf students, including Spanish deaf students.

Primary Bilingual Development

A review of the literature revealed only two studies on deaf children reared in a bilingual home environment; that is, their parents used both ASL and some form (i.e., speech and/or sign) of English. A more recent study (Philip, 1992) indicated the existence of a "successful" bilingual ASL/ English program at a learning center for more than 5 years; however, little information was provided. It should be emphasized that the type of signing used by deaf parents in the two earlier studies was presumed to be ASL, even though an adequate description of the grammar of ASL did not emerge in the research literature until the late 1970s (e.g., see discussions in Klima & Bellugi, 1979; Lane & Grosjean, 1980; Liddell, 1980; Wilbur, 1987).

Schlesinger and Meadow (1972) described the primary linguistic development of four deaf children, each from a different family with either deaf or hearing parents. Only one child, who had deaf parents and two sets of deaf grandparents, is reported here. The subject, a girl, was diagnosed as deaf (due to heredity) at the age of 3. Her hearing threshold averaged 85 dB (ISO) across the speech frequencies in the better ear. Although no formal assessment of the parents' proficiency either in ASL or English was conducted, Meadow, in reporting this study in a book, remarked that:

> Ann's mother, also the child of deaf parents, used English syntax in her written English and alternated between English and Ameslan syntax in her signed and spoken communications. Ann's father was more likely than her mother to use Ameslan syntax in all his communication. (Meadow, 1980, p. 19)

Schlesinger and Meadow (1972) observed the child from age 8 months to 22 months. At 8 months, the child engaged in vocalization and gestures to convey emphasis and emotions. By the end of 12 months, she executed (approximately) the formal adult signs for *pretty* and *wrong*, and she understood the command "come here." By the 20th month, her sign vocabulary totaled 142, and she knew 14 letters of the finger-spelled alphabet. The researchers concluded that the subject had a sign vocabulary that "compares very favorably with the spoken vocabulary of hearing children" (p. 60).

Schlesinger and Meadow also described the use and meaning of the subject's first individual signs/words which were similar to the one-word utterances of hearing children. A one-word/sign can have one of several functions: (1) It can express a feeling, (2) it can label or name an object, or (3) it can fuse the label with the feeling about the object. This one-word/sign can also be classified according to a single feature. For example, the deaf child appropriately used the sign *dog* for pictures of dogs, real dogs, and the *Doggie Diner Restaurant*. However, the child inappropriately used the sign to refer to all animals, or even to animal objects not resembling the parents. It was reported that the deaf girl did not use all aspects of a sign (i.e., shape, movement, and placement) in the adult form. This finding is similar to that observed for hearing children who must mature in order to reproduce the sounds of language in their more adult forms. The most interesting finding reported was the deaf child's vocabulary of 117 signs at 19 months was greater than the typical range of hearing children's words which has been estimated to be more than 3 and fewer than 50 (e.g., Goodluck, 1991; Ingram, 1989; Lenneberg, 1967).

Collins-Ahlgren (1974) analyzed recorded expressive language samples of a girl, deaf from heredity, from age 16 months to 44 months. The deaf girl's parents were college graduates and were informally judged to be proficient in ASL and English. It was reported that the parents used both a "native language of signs" (p. 486) and English-based signs. The girl was exposed to "ASL-like" signing (i.e., with speech) in the earlier months. After various grammatical and semantic functions became productive through the sign forms, the parents introduced standard English forms (e.g., articles, auxiliaries, and inflections) through the use of "signed" or "manual English" techniques.

The results indicated that the deaf girl's expressive language proceeded through several stages, ranging from invented and imaginative ASL signs to uninflected signs used in English word order to some inflected English-based signs, and finally, to signed standard English. An example is the manner in which the subject demonstrated awareness of the present progressive function. Initially, she used the ASL form *NOW* as in *I GO NOW* (these words are the English glosses for the ASL signs). Then, her parents presented the auxiliaries and *-ing* forms as in *I AM GOING* (in this case, the sign *NOW* would be dropped unless the English sentence is: I am going now). A transitional stage with partial omission occurred prior to the time the full form became productive.

Collins-Ahlgren concluded that the girl was developing a language equivalent to that of her hearing peers. The researcher also argued that the educational signed or manually coded English systems should be taught as a second language to children of both deaf and hearing parents. In essence, these systems can "build on a native language foundation, and it should prove helpful for English reading and for communication with the hearing world" (p. 493).

Effects of ASL on the Subsequent Development of English

There are very few studies dealing with the English linguistic abilities of deaf children who were supposedly exposed to ASL in infancy and early childhood. The focus here is on studies that employ the paradigm of comparing deaf children of deaf parents (DCDP) with deaf children of hearing parents (DCHP). Some of the studies were retrospective (e.g., Brasel & Quigley, 1977; Meadow, 1968) and used various means for determining the form of language used with the deaf children in infancy and early childhood. Even the best techniques, however, leave some doubt when respondents (deaf parents) are reporting on events that occurred as much as 10 to 15 years previously.

The performance of DCDP was compared with that of DCHP on a number of measures, for example, overall academic achievement, intelligence, psychosocial development, reading, vocabulary, written language, speech reading, finger spelling, and signing abilities. A consistent finding emerged across several investigations, namely, that the performance of DCDP was significantly better than that of DCHP (e.g., Balow & Brill, 1975; Meadow, 1968; Quigley & Frisina, 1961; Stuckless & Birch, 1966). Relative to reading, it was observed in some studies that the mean reading level of DCDP was almost two grades higher than that of DCHP. In addition, even having one *deaf* parent was sufficient—that is, this condition correlated with higher achievement scores.

The differences between the two groups of deaf children were attributed to two broad variables: parental acceptance and early use of manual communication (presumably, ASL). There is little doubt that a high level of parental acceptance is an important factor (e.g., see discussions in Levine, 1981; Meadow, 1980; Paul & Jackson, 1993); however, it is not only present in deaf parents or in deaf parents who sign. Some researchers have reported a high level of acceptance in homes where deaf parents used speech with their children and in homes in which the parents were hearing (e.g., Corson, 1973; Messerly & Aram, 1980).

Another common assumption in some of these studies was that the language input was relatively homogeneous—specifically, it was primarily American Sign Language. Obviously, the research cited above on parental acceptance presents contradictory evidence. In addition, interpreting the form of manual communication as ASL must be done with caution since a grammar of ASL has only recently been written. Furthermore, as discussed in Chapter 4, Brasel and Quigley (1977) demonstrated that the *type* of manual communication was important, especially if it corresponds to the structure of English. Brasel and Quigley's findings were supported in a recent study by Luetke-Stahlman (1988a; also discussed in Chapter 4). Luetke-Stahlman asserted that the most important issue was how well or how complete English was represented (as in the SEE systems and cued speech) and whether or not a particular symbol system was a language (as in the use of ASL). Finally, as discussed in the last two chapters, the development of English is such a complex activity that it should not and cannot be attributed to one all-encompassing factor such as ASL or any other manual communication form.

Language Production and Comprehension

There have been a few studies that examined the language production and comprehension of deaf students exposed to ASL and English (i.e., English-based signing). The impetus for these investigations is the hypothesis proffered by Gee and Goodhart (1985, 1988): Deaf individuals have a biological predisposition for manual language, specifically, the language of signs. This "biological disposition" hypothesis is also an argument for the establishment of a cultural paradigm for constructing theories, conducting research, and implementing practices (e.g., Crittenden, 1993).

Much of the evidence for the predisposition to the language of signs, namely, ASL, has come from studies on language preference (e.g., Livingston, 1983; Stewart, 1985; Strong, 1988b; Supalla, 1986). For example, Stewart (1985) examined the signing behaviors of deaf students in high school (Vancouver, British Columbia, Canada). Students were required to retell stories presented on video tapes in both ASL and signed English (SE). Stewart reported that both ASL-dominant students and SE-dominant students preferred to retell the stories in ASL.

Similar findings were documented by Strong (cited in Strong, 1988b) on deaf children between the ages of 4 and 7 years old, inclusive. These children were exposed to both ASL and *the signs* from SEE 2 (signing exact English). Analyses of the spontaneous language samples revealed "an overwhelming majority of ASL over English elements, regardless of situation or skill level and in spite of constant English input from the teachers throughout the year" (p. 120).

The hypothesis of Gee and Goodhart, however, was not confirmed in an investigation by Eagney (1987). Eagney examined the comprehension performances of deaf children between the ages of 5 and 15 years old. Sentences were presented in three modes: standard signed English, simplified signed English, and ASL. No significant differences were reported for the three modes. It should be emphasized that the language proficiency of the students was not determined prior to the comprehension tasks.

ASL/English Instructional Programs

The focus of this section is on instructional activities and programs that incorporated the use of ASL and English in either ESL or bilingual situations. Despite the theoretical and philosophical support for these types of programs, little empirical evidence is available on their use and effectiveness. Nevertheless, some insights can be gleaned from these few studies and descriptions for the future implementation of such programs for students with severe to profound hearing impairment. It should be underscored that many of the more recent studies are only slight variations of the earlier investigations. Because of this situation, we have discussed some of the earlier studies in depth.

Early Investigations

Within the framework of error (i.e., contrastive) analysis, Crutchfield (1972) developed some procedures for teaching English as a second language through the use of ASL. For example, this researcher emphasized count features of both ASL and English. The count features refer to words similar to *much, many, few*, and so on. If the count features in ASL are different from those in English, the first step is to bring the ASL-like features to the students' attention. Consider the following example: *MUCH BOY LEFT SCHOOL.* Even with ASL-like signing, this sentence should be rejected by the ASL-using students. The students should be required to correct these unacceptable utterances using ASL. Thus, students might sign: *MANY BOY LEAVE FINISH SCHOOL.* The English glosses for this is: *Many boy left school.* Next, the teacher can write this sentence on the board and explain that some utterances unacceptable in ASL may also be unacceptable in English. In addition, some acceptable utterances in ASL may also be acceptable in English—providing *boy* is given a plural inflection (which is another lesson). Crutchfield remarked that the main purpose of this lesson (and all initial lessons) is to demonstrate similarities of acceptability and unacceptability in ASL and English. Subsequently, the instructor can proceed to those structures in English which are different from those in ASL and those in ASL which are different from English.

Goldberg and Bordman (1975) described an ESL program offered for deaf students at Gallaudet College (now, Gallaudet University). It was argued that the samples of written language indicated that most students had reached adulthood without a command of English. The deaf students had difficulties in expressing themselves; these difficulties were similar to those of speakers of other languages in ESL classes.

These scholars made two major modifications in their ESL procedures. One, they conducted all language practices in writing (i.e., on the chalk board, overhead projector, paper). Two, they invented steps to compel students to express the concept involved. Goldberg and Bordman argued that English needs to be presented exclusively in the written form to ensure that the students know the *words* that are being addressed. The "sign system" or communication mode preferred by the students was used to *communicate with the student, not to teach the students written English.*

These scholars suggested also that the serious English structure problems of the deaf students are interwoven with the deeper problem of not knowing the concepts which these structures expressed, and not knowing when to use them. Thus, in their attempts to learn English, the deaf students are in a situation similar to that of hearing ESL speakers who do not make certain concepts distinctions fundamental to English. For example, the ESL students may feel no need to distinguish between: *They eat sandwiches* and *They are eating sandwiches.* In sum, Goldberg and Bordman stated that there is a need to design materials which consider the above issues.

Jones (1979) attempted to delineate the interference aspects of a signed language for the purpose of incorporating them in the teaching of written English. The researcher argued that ASL has both nonmanual and manual aspects (see Wilbur, 1987; see also Chapter 1 of this text). In writing nontechnical prose, Jones hypothesized that deaf students tend to translate into English only the manual signs of ASL that they would use if rendering the same passage in their use of English-based signing. The nonmanual aspects, which supply very important linguistic information, are not signed and thus are omitted in the writing of English. Consequently, the written productions of the students do not express enough of the intended message to be comprehensible to a fluent native speaker of English.

Jones further argued that the written language productions of deaf students would become more comprehensible if these productions included information from both manual and nonmanual aspects. To resolve this condition, the students need to become aware that some signed information is absent in their writing. Informal interviews with native and nonnative users of ASL by the investigator indicated that both manual and nonmanual "signs" are important; neither is of primary importance. This is unlike spoken communication (e.g., English) in which nonoral activity (e.g., hand movements) is secondary to oral activity.

Jones hypothesized that the influence of English has caused deaf students to feel that their native language must have only a primary channel. As a result, their writing of English must reflect the fact that English has a primary channel. Thus, the students write only English glosses of the manual signs. This writing style is described as one which is very similar to that of hearing foreign students, who have less-than-adequate proficiency in English.

In conclusion, Jones proposed two techniques for resolving this problem. One, inform the students that they are translating manual signals only and are ignoring the other, nonmanual aspects of a sign which contain important linguistic information. Two, demonstrate to the students that a "signed" version of what they have written contains much more information. It is suggested that the second part of this technique might be more beneficial in helping the students to include the nonmanual information "without making them overly self-conscious about either language" (p. 278).

Recent Investigations

There have been a few bilingual or ASL/English programs that focused on the development of both ASL and English (e.g., Philip, 1992; Strong, 1988b). Relative to English, most of the programs emphasize the development of *written* English. The assumption is that it is possible to proceed from ASL to the written form of English.

One example is the work by Marbury and Mackinson-Smyth (1986), who described the performance of elementary-age ASL-using deaf students. Using an ESL technique known as grammar-translation (e.g., see McLaughlin, 1985), the students attempted to "translate" grammatical features of ASL into English. The content of the translation was taken from an ASL-signed story in which both students and teacher discussed certain aspects such as characters and events. The students were required to focus on the ASL features in the story and to translate these features into English equivalents. Both teachers and students produced a final draft of the story in English.

A number of researchers/educators believe it is important for deaf students to be able to develop an awareness of ASL and English as separate languages. This perception of differences between the two languages is a metalinguistic ability. One of the major goals of Strong's (1988b) project was to develop deaf students's ability to perceive differences between ASL-signed stories and English-based signed stories.

The development of this metalinguistic ability might lead to an improvement in the development of English writing skills. For example, Akamatsu and Armour (1987) examined the performance of deaf students who received grammatical instruction in both ASL and English. The researchers reported that there was some improvement in the English written language productions of the students, particularly at the grammatical level. As discussed in Chapter 5, the grammatical level involves the lower-lever skills of writing. Lower-level skills need to become automatic so that students can use or improve higher-level skills such as organization and intent.

A good model for programs using ASL and written English is the ongoing project of Neuroth-Gimbrone and Logiodice (1992). To participate in this project, deaf students needed to have communicative competency in American Sign Language. One of the goals of the project was to enable students to improve their competency in ASL. This is deemed necessary for the development of metalinguistic skills—specifically, the ability to reflect on ASL. Subsequently, the students should be able to develop skills relative to translating/code-switching and English literacy. The eventual goal of this 3-year project was an adequate development of metalinguistic skills in both ASL and English.

Development of English as L1 and L2

The question posed here is: Is the development of English as a second language similar to the development of English as a first language for deaf students? As discussed previously, the answer to a similar question is *yes*, relative to hearing first- and second-language learners. Much of the work on this similarity issue has been investigated by Quigley and his collaborators on deaf students learning English as a first language, as discussed in Chapter 5 on reading and writing. The common finding has been that the English language development of deaf students is quantitatively reduced, albeit qualitatively similar, to that of hearing students. Chapter 5 also presented similar evidence for vocabulary development (e.g., Paul, 1984; Paul & Gustafson, 1991) and for the acquisition of reading (e.g., Hanson, 1989; Hays & Arnold, 1992).

Few studies have been conducted on the qualitative status of the acquisition of English as a second language by deaf students. One line of research has been to show that English is a *second* language for many deaf students by comparing their performances to second-language hearing learners (e.g., Charrow, 1975; Charrow & Fletcher, 1974). One researcher also examined the qualitative issue in depth with deaf students learning English as a first language and Spanish deaf students learning English as a second language (e.g., King, 1981).

Charrow and Fletcher (1974) explored the possibility that deaf children learn English as a second language. They compared the performance on a test of ESL of two groups of deaf students (DCDP and DCHP) with each other and with a group of hearing students learning English as a second language. Three hypotheses were tested: (1) DCDP should outperformed DCHP; (2) the performance of the hearing students learning English as a second language should resemble the performance of the DCDP group more than it resembled that of the DCHP group; and (3) the performance by the DCDP group on a test of English as a second language and on a standard test of English skills should resemble each other less than should performances by the DCHP group on the same tests. The two tests used were the *Test of English as a Foreign Language* (TOEFL) and the *Stanford Achievement Test* (SAT).

Results supported the first hypothesis: DCDP performed significantly better than DCHP on most of the subtests and on the total score on the TOEFL. In addition, DCDP performed significantly better than DCHP on the Paragraph Meaning and Language subtests of the SAT. Ambiguous results were reported, however, for the second and third hypotheses. Relative to the second hypothesis, it was found, as predicted, that the performances of the DCDP group resembled those of the foreign hearing students more than the DCHP group did on two of the TOEFL subtests, namely, English Structure and Writing Ability. This result was not observed on the other two subtests—Vocabulary and Reading Comprehension. Findings were similar for the third hypothesis. The hypothesis was supported by performances on only some subtests of the SAT.

Charrow and Fletcher (1974) concluded that the issue of whether deaf children typically are learning English like a second language might be too broad to investigate. Based on the mixed results for the second and third hypotheses, they argued that some aspects of English are learned by deaf students like a second language and some are not. In the absence of logical or research support for such differences among various aspects of English, the interpretation should be treated with caution.

In another study, Charrow (1975) attempted to identify and provide normative data for the nonstandard features of English language usage by deaf persons. These features were labeled as "Deaf English" (DE). This term implies that deaf persons might have a dialect of English which is different from standard English. It was argued that deaf individuals have typical patterns of variant structures in their use of English that are consistent (see also, the discussions in Quigley, Wilbur, Power, Montanelli, & Steinkamp, 1976, and Chapter 5 of this text). Charrow argued further that the variances alternated with some standard English features to produce a simplification or pidginization of standard English. In essence, the range of grammatical forms, standard English and nonstandard English, appears to parallel the "pidgin continuum" found in the speech of pidgin English speakers.

Charrow (1975) examined this issue by comparing the responses of three groups—DCDP, DCHP, and hearing subjects—to 50 "Deaf English" sentences written by deaf teenagers and 50 standard English (SE) sentences. The researcher presented the sentences in random order to the subjects, individually. Subjects were required to write the sentences on an answer sheet from memory, one sentence at a time. Results indicated that the deaf subjects found the DE sentences easier to remember and recall than did the hearing subjects. In addition, there was no significant difference in the recall of DE and SE sentences for the deaf subjects. Finally, there were no significant differences between the two deaf groups—DCDP and DCHP.

Charrow (1975) concluded that deaf students acquire most, if not all, the rules of standard English syntax; however, they apply them in an inconsistent manner. The researcher reasoned further that many of the variances from standard English, such as omission of articles and past tense markers, that are found in the written language of deaf students are not the results of interference from ASL. Rather, these "errors" reflect redundant, nonessential features of English that are difficult to learn and easy to overlook. In sum, this study and the one by Charrow and Fletcher (1974) found little evidence that deaf children are learning English as a second language. These are indirect studies of the problem, however, and certainly do not settle the issue.

A more direct study of the issue was conducted by King (1981). Specifically, King was interested in whether the acquisition of English by deaf students is different from or similar to that of hearing children learning English as a first language. The investigation also provided some insights for bilingual education because the researcher used deaf students who were exposed to Spanish as a first language. King examined one component of language (syntax) and one mode of language (reading). The instruments used in the study were the screening test and four individual diagnostic tests of the *Test of Syntactic Abilities* (TSA).

Forty deaf subjects between the ages of 8 and 13 and 40 hearing subjects between the ages of 8 and 11 years old participated in the study. Twenty deaf and 20 hearing subjects were classified as L1 learners—that is, learning English as a first language. The remaining deaf and hearing subjects were classified as L2 learners, that is, learning English as a second language. The L1 subjects were exposed to English in the home and had no formal foreign or second-language instruction. The L2 subjects were Puerto Rican Americans of Spanish descent. The subjects were matched on language, type of school attended, amount of exposure to English, and type of instruction received. That is, all subjects attended schools in which English was the primary language and had received English instruction in content areas.

Results indicated that the order of difficulty on syntactic tasks were similar for both groups of deaf and hearing subjects. The researcher concluded that deaf children acquire syntactic structures in the same order as hearing children. In addition, analyses of errors revealed tentatively that the types of errors were similar for both groups. Table 6–3 illustrates the types of errors in this study and in a selection of others.

The most interesting finding for bilingualism was the effects of knowing more than one language for both hearing and deaf students. King reported that knowing Spanish as a first language appeared to have no effects on the English language abilities of hearing children on a quantitative level. This seems to suggest no positive advantages for bilinguals, at least linguistically in the area of syntax. Contrariwise, the effects of another language on the abilities of deaf children were reported to be equivocal. King proffered two explanations: (1) one of the two deaf L2 groups might have been atypical, and (2) deafness overrides any effect (positive or negative) of being exposed to two languages. It should be pointed out that these students were not in a bilingual program per se, and this might have also influenced the results. Finally, King (1981) remarked that all deaf subjects used little or no English on entering school.

Some support for King's second explanation can be found in a study by Luetke-Stahlman and Weiner (1982). These researchers conducted a study using Spanish deaf students to determine whether or not there is a "first language" that should be used to teach language concepts. They were also interested in determining if the children were homogeneous with respect to their first language (Spanish) and thus could be grouped together in the same classroom using similar teaching methods. Five language/systems (L/S) were delineated: (1) oral English, (2) English and signs, (3) oral Spanish, (4) Spanish and English, and (5) signs only.

Three Spanish deaf females participated in the investigation. Subject 1 was 4 years, 4 months old with a bilateral profound, sensorineural hearing impairment. Subject 2 was 3 years, 5 months old and had a bilateral moderate-to-severe sensorineural hearing impairment. Subject 3 was 4 years, 11 months old and had a moderate-to-severe hearing impairment. The subjects were taught a receptive vocabulary of nouns, verbs, and adjectives in each of the five L/S. Acquisition curves were constructed for each subject's performance on each of the form class of vocabulary words.

Results indicated that Subject 1 performed best in the English and signs, Spanish and English signs, and signs only. The greatest improvement was reported to be in the use of signs. Subject 2 performed best in

TABLE 6–3. Distinctive Structures in the Language of Deaf Students

Distinctive Structure	Environment	Example
Negative outside sentence	Negation	No Daddy see baby.
Negative inside sentence but not correctly marked	Negation	Daddy no see baby.
Nonrecognition of negative marker	Negation	Reads negative sentence as positive.
Object-Object deletion	Conjunction	John chased the girl and he scared. (her)
Object-Subject deletion	Conjunction	The boy hit the girl and (the girl) ran home.
No inversion in questions	Questions	What I did this morning? The kitten is black?
Inversion of object and verb	Questions	Who TV watched?
Overgeneralization of contraction rule	Questions Negation	Amn't I tired? Bill willn't go.
Noun copying	Questions/ Relativization	Who the boy saw the girl? The boy saw the girl who the girl ran home.
Pronoun Copying	Questions/ Relativization	Who he saw the girl? The boy saw the girl who she ran home.
by deletion	Verbs	The boy was kissed the girl.
Unmarked verb in sequence	Verbs	The boy saw the girl and the girl kiss the boy.

TABLE 6–3. (continued)

Distinctive Structure	Environment	Example
Be + unmarked verb	Verbs	The boy is kiss the girl. The sky is cover with clouds.
Confusion of tense markers	Verbs	Tom has pushing the wagon.
Omission of verbs	Verbs	The cat under the table.
be-have confusion	Verbs	The boy have sick. This boy is a sweater.
Omission of be or have	Verbs	John sick. The girl a ball.
Third person marker missing	Verbs	The boy say "hi."
Omission of conjunction	Conjunction	Bob saw liked the bike.
Omission of determiners	Determiners	Boy is sick.
Confusion of determiners (Nonrecognition of definite indefinite distinctions)	Determiners	The some apples. . . . A best friend. . . . He was the bad boy.
Confusion of case pronouns	Pronominalization	Her is going home. This he friend.
Wrong gender	Pronominalization	They packed our lunch. (their) Sue is wearing his new dress today.
Object-Subject deletion	Relativization	The dog chased the girl had on a red dress.

(continued)

TABLE 6–3. *(continued)*

Distinctive Structure	Environment	Example
Relative pronoun + possessive pronoun	Relativization	The boy helped the girl who her mother was sick.
Noun Phrases	Relativization	The boy helped the girl's mother was sick.
Extra *for*	Complementation	For to play baseball is fun.
Extra *to* in POSS-ing	Complementation	Joe went to fishing.
Infinitive in place of gerund	Complementation	Joe goes to fish.
Omission of *to* before second verb	Complementation	Chad wanted go.
Inflection of infinitive	Complementation	Bill like to played baseball.
Adjective following Noun	Relativization	The barn red burned.
For + Ving or For + V for infinitive	Complementation	The boy likes for fishing.
*Surface reading order strategy	Verbs	<u>The boy</u> was <u>kissed</u> by <u>the girl</u>.
	Relativization	The boy who hit the <u>girl ran home</u>.
	Complementation	That the boy hit <u>the girl surprised me</u>.
	Nominalization	The discussion of <u>the party bored Bob</u>.

Source: Adapted from King (1981) and Quigley, Steinkamp, Power, & Jones (1978).
* Only underlined words are read.

oral English and signs only. Subject 3 had mixed results. For the noun category, the greatest improvement occurred in Spanish and English signs and signs only. For the verb category, the greatest improvement occurred in English and signs, Spanish and English signs, and signs only. For the adjective category, the greatest gain was observed using the signs only L/S. Similar to the others, these gains were determined to be due to the effects of training.

The researchers concluded that the choice of a language in educating Spanish deaf children should not be based solely on either heritage or etiological classification. They proposed that the choice of language is dependent on a combination of factors: (1) the language and/or communication system of the principal caregiver, (2) the amount of exposure to sign language and/or systems, (3) the degree of usable aided hearing ability, and (4) the language and/or system demonstrated to be most effective for learning.

BILINGUAL EDUCATION MODELS

In addition to having a variety of theoretical acquisition models, the field of bilingualism has a number of program models. The descriptions and research effectiveness of these models are shrouded in controversies. This is due primarily to the philosophies and goals of specific programs (Cummins, 1988; Reich, 1986). To obtain a better understanding of this issue, it is necessary to discuss type of student and language goals.

Type of Student

Bilingual programs may vary according to the type of student who participates in the program. For example, bilingual programs may be established for majority-language students. Individuals who speak the majority (or main) language of society are labeled majority-language students (Cummins, 1988; Genesee, 1987). In the United States, such students may typically enroll in foreign language or second-language course(s).

On the other hand, a commonly accepted bilingual program model in Canada is the immersion model. This model is employed in an area in which there are two main or heritage languages such as English and French. That is, individuals in these areas who speak either English or French are considered majority-language students. These individuals are expected to acquire communicative competency in both languages and knowledge of both cultures. In an immersion program, students receive instruction in the early grades in a language which is not their native language. Instruction in their native language occurs after a reasonable level of competency is established in the nonnative language (Genesee, 1987; Swain & Lapkin, 1982).

Individuals who do not speak the majority or main language of society are labeled minority-language students. In the United States, most "bilingual" programs are established for or involved students who do not have competency in the majority-language (English) and its accompanying culture. Relative to deafness, individuals may be reared in minority or non-English using homes, for example, homes in which the native language is ASL, Spanish, or German. It is also possible to consider other deaf students as "minority-language" users if they have not acquired an adequate level of communicative competency in the majority-language by the time they begin their formal schooling. This latter group might pertain to most students with severe to profound hearing impairment (King, 1981; Paul, 1990, 1991).

Controversies which have arisen about the appropriate goals and procedures for minority-language students are similar to some of the controversies in the education of deaf students. For example, there is disagreement as to whether the goal should be to make the minority-language student a fully participating member of the majority culture even at the expense of the student's minority culture (assimilation). Some scholars favor the preservation and maintenance of the student's native culture even if this means lessened participation in the majority culture (language and culture separatism).

Language Goals

The various types of programs are related to the language goals. Programs vary from complete submersion in the general educational system with limited or no support in the student's native language and culture to separate education in the student's native language and culture and gradual submersion in the general educational system. There are also programs that maintain a 50/50 model throughout the school years (Navarro, 1985; Cummins, 1988; Reich, 1986).

Relative to bilingual programs, there are three broad language goals: language shift, language maintenance, and language enrichment. The main goal of submersion or transitional programs is to enable minority-language students to learn the language and culture of the majority society. In essence, the students "shift" from their home language to the majority language. Submersion programs are conducted in the majority language only (i.e., English). In transitional programs, the home or native language may be used to ease the "shift" to the majority language. For example, students acquire content and cultural knowledge via the use of their home language while they are attempting to learn L2. It should be underscored that there is no attempt to maintain or promote competency in L1.

In general, language maintenance refers to the maintenance bilingual programs. One type of program is labeled static maintenance, which is similar to the transitional model (e.g., Otheguy & Otto, 1980; Reich, 1986). Static maintenance refers to the process of preventing the loss of minority-language students' L1 skills while promoting proficiency and literacy in L2. In both static maintenance and transitional programs, reading is typically introduced in the second or majority language. Proponents of these models endorse the balance acquisition theory of bilingualism (discussed previously, e.g., Macnamara, 1966). Four basic arguments are presented: (1) instruction in or on L1 subtracts from instruction for developing L2 skills; (2) development of L1 competes with L2; (3) minority-language students already possess competency in their L1; thus, it is not necessary to teach L1; and (4) reading skills are best developed in L2 by employing the language of L2, not L1. In general, these proponents argue that the best way to teach English to limited English users is simply to teach them English (see discussions in Cummins, 1988; Troike, 1981).

Language enrichment can be applied to another type of maintenance program entitled developmental maintenance (Cummins, 1988; Otheguy & Otto, 1980; Reich, 1986). The major aim of developmental maintenance bilingual programs is to develop a high level of competency in both the minority and majority language. These programs can refer to those involving total or partial immersion in a second language or to programs in which the two languages are employed more or less equally (50/50) for instructional purposes. In essence, developmental maintenance programs are considered to be truly "bilingual" programs because of the emphasis on the development and maintenance of *two* languages.

Synthesis of Research

The research effectiveness of the French immersion programs in Canada has been well documented (Cummins, 1988; Genesee, 1987; Reich, 1986; Swain & Lapkin, 1982). Because of its success, there have been attempts to establish "immersion" programs for students in the United States (e.g., see discussion in Cummins, 1984, 1988). One problem with the application is the neglect of considering type of student, that is, majority-language students in Canada and minority-language students in the United States. A major issue is the misinterpretation of the goals and success of bilingual programs in Canada. For example, the success of the French immersion programs has been used as support for English "immersion" (actually, submersion) programs in the United States (Cummins, 1988).

In the United States, four types of "immersion" programs have been identified: L2 submersion, L2 monolingual immersion, L2 bilingual immersion, and L1 bilingual immersion (e.g., Cummins, 1988; see also, Cziko, 1992). Previously, we described briefly some of the tenets of submersion programs. The only difference between submersion and L2 monolingual immersion is that the latter modifies the content and grammar of the majority language in order to facilitate comprehension. Both L2 bilingual immersion and L1 bilingual immersion programs offer instruction in both languages and culture; however, L1 immersion actively promotes the language and culture of the students' home environment.

It has been argued that both L1 and L2 immersion programs are effective for minority-language students. There is some theoretical support (e.g., Cummins, 1988, 1989) and some empirical support (for L2, see Baker & de Kanter, 1981; for L1, see reviews in Cummins, 1984, 1988). The reason for the research effectiveness has been attributed to the fact that there is greater transfer from L1 to L2. This transfer is facilitated by the inclusion of the students' home language and culture.

Bilingual Education Program for Deaf Students: A Model

In advocating bilingual education programs for deaf students, there are a number of questions that need to be resolved. Indeed, differences between proposed models are due to the perspectives on these questions. Some unanswered questions include:

1. Should ASL and English be developed (or taught) concurrently in infancy and early childhood as in a bilingual environment?
2. Should ASL be taught as a first language to all deaf students with English taught as a second language?
3. Should English be taught as a second language only to students who know ASL as a first language or to all deaf students?
4. If ASL is taught as the first language, at what grade or age level should English be introduced?
5. When both ASL and English are used, how much exposure should be allotted to each language? (Paul & Quigley, in press)

Several bilingual models have been proposed for deaf students (e.g., see Luetke-Stahlman, 1983; Neuroth-Gimbrone & Logiodice, 1992; Paul, 1990, 1991; Strong, 1988b). We favor L1 immersion models for two major reasons: (1) deaf students have enormous difficulty in acquiring

English, and (2) ASL does not have the same level of prestige as English in the education of deaf students. Because of pragmatic difficulties (e.g., most deaf children have hearing parents), there is some support for using both ASL and English simultaneously, as in 50/50 programs (e.g., this seems to be similar to the model briefly discussed by Philip, 1992).

For 50/50 models to work effectively, there needs to be an adequate quantity and quality of human interactions with both languages. The use of technology might be a reasonable supplement; however, it cannot supplant these important interactions between the child and significant others. Regardless of the model used, we feel that one of the most important issues—(perhaps, the most important)—is the development of a first language at as early an age as possible. This is clearly not the case for most deaf children of hearing parents (e.g., King, 1981). The late onset of a first language has pervasive negative effects on the subsequent development of academic achievement (see discussion in Chapters 4 and 5). For this reason, it seems that L1 immersion programs might have the greatest potential for most students with severe to profound impairment, despite its pragmatic difficulties.

One L1 immersion model has been described in several publications (e.g., Paul, 1990, 1991; Paul et al., 1992; Paul & Quigley, 1987b, in press). This model is based on the theoretical and research data available for hearing minority-language students in L1 immersion programs (e.g., Baker & de Kanter, 1981; Cummins, 1984, 1988). The model is also based on reading research with both L1 and L2 students (e.g., Bernhardt, 1991, Grabe, 1988).

The L1 immersion model described here has been labeled as a minority-language immersion program for deaf students. The following principles are guidelines:

1. A reasonable level of communicative and grammatical proficiency is established in American Sign Language; a minimum of three academic years is recommended.
2. ASL is used as the medium of instruction for academic content areas.
3. A reasonable level of communicative and grammatical proficiency is established in English via a form of English-based signing; modifications of English input are necessary to match the motivational and cognitive capacities of the students.
4. Development of English literacy skills and use of English to teach academic content areas.
5. Eventually, the amount of instructional time devoted to the use of ASL and English should be more or less equal, depending on the progress and proclivity of students. (Paul & Quigley, in press)

Similar to other L1 immersion models, this model is constructed so that both L1 and L2 are promoted and developed. Although the acquisition of L2 (i.e., English, specifically literacy) is a main goal, it is not an all-encompassing goal. That is, this model recognizes that not all deaf students will be able to achieve a high level of competency in English-based signing or English literacy. Nevertheless, it is hypothesized that most students will, at least, achieve literate thought in ASL (see Chapter 5). In addition, this proficiency in ASL can be used to enable students to acquire knowledge of the educational curriculum, including that of mainstream society.

It should be underscored that the instructional practices used in this model are based on theory and research. For example, we advocate that the teaching of reading should be based on the major principles of interactive theories (see King & Quigley, 1985; Paul, 1993; see also, Chapter 5). Examples of language-teaching procedures can be found in several sources (e.g., Luetke-Stahlman & Luckner, 1991; McAnally et al., 1987, in press).

It cannot be overemphasized that any bilingual program for deaf students needs to be evaluated. This evaluation can take several forms, for example, quantitative, qualitative, and critical (e.g., critical theory). In our view, the evaluation of a program should consider, but not be limited to, the following areas:

1. Identification of deaf students for placement in a bilingual program.
2. Evaluation of teachers' proficiency in both ASL and English *and* in the teaching of both ASL and English.
3. Assessment of students' grammatical and communicative proficiency in ASL.
4. Assessment of students' achievement in academic subjects and sociocultural knowledge via the use of ASL.
5. Evaluation of students' grammatical and communicative proficiency in English.
6. Assessment of students' achievement in academic subjects and sociocultural knowledge via the use of English (i.e., in both the signing and print modes).
7. Evaluation of cognitive and psychosocial developments. (Paul & Quigley, in press)

FINAL REMARKS

The growing advocacy of the establishment of bilingual and/or second-language programs for deaf students has been motivated in part by the growing dissatisfaction with the language, literacy, and educational achievement of most of these students. Not surprisingly, there is much resistance to bilingualism and second-language learning because such programs seem to be based on sociopolitical goals, rather than on educational goals (e.g., see Stuckless, 1991). The sociopolitical goals seem to be influenced by the thinking of critical theorists and some of their fundamental concepts such as enlightenment, emancipation, and empowerment (Gibson, 1986). For example, one rendition of these concepts, particularly emancipation and empowerment, can be seen in the assertion that ASL should be the first language for all deaf children, regardless of degree of hearing loss and family background (Johnson et al., 1989).

We are sympathetic to sociopolitical goals; however, the establishment of bilingual and second-language learning programs needs to consider also the outcomes of theory and research based on the scientific method. In this chapter, we summarized what we considered a representative sample of current thinking on bilingualism and second-language learning. Based on our synthesis, we suggested that a bilingual minority-language immersion model might be most beneficial for some deaf students.

In sum, it should be underscored that any proposed bilingual method should be subjected to a comprehensive evaluation. However, an evaluation is not possible without the establishment and implementation of programs. It seems that the use of ASL in a bilingual or English-as-a-second-language program has not been widely accepted. This chapter provided support for such programs for *some* deaf students. It might be applicable to many, if not most, deaf students if it is accepted that a first language (i.e., any language) should be developed at as early an age as possible.

FURTHER READINGS

Burt, M., & Kiparsky, C. (1972). *The gooicon: A repair manual for English.* Rowley, MA: Newbury House.

Delgado, G. (Ed.). (1984). *The Hispanic deaf: Issues and challenges for bilingual special education.* Washington, DC: Gallaudet University Press.

Erickson, J., & Omark, D. (Eds.). (1981). *Communication assessment of the bilingual bicultural child.* Baltimore, MD: University Park Press.

Gaarder, A. (1977). *Bilingual schooling and the survival of Spanish in the United States.* Rowley, MA: Newbury House.

Omark, D., & Erickson, J. (1983). *The bilingual exceptional child.* San Diego, CA: College-Hill Press.

Wode, H. (1981). *Learning a second language: An integrated view of language acquisition.* Tubingen, Germany: Narr.

C H A P T E R 7

LANGUAGE INSTRUCTION

Learning a language takes practice, and practice takes time, at least as much time as learning any other skill, such as the ability to play a musical instrument. If little time can be devoted to language learning, the most suitable method may be the one with the minimum learning load and the maximum range of meaning and expression, in other words, the one with the greatest relative productivity. (Mackey, 1965, p. 328)

The child's exposure to language should not be called "teaching." He learns the language, but no one, least of all an average mother, knows how to teach it to him. He learns the language because he is shaped by nature to pay attention to it, to notice and remember and use significant aspects of it. (Miller, 1965, p. 178)

Despite the fact that these quotes appeared about 30 years ago, the issue of whether language can be "taught" or whether it is "learned" is again the focus of intense debate (e.g., Rice & Schiefelbusch, 1989). However, this debate did not begin 30 years ago; it can be found in analyses of the philosophies of Plato and Aristotle (e.g., Snyder, 1984). It should be clear that this issue is not merely an academic one. It has enormous implications for the establishment and implementation of research and practice. If language can be taught—is there a "best" method or are there "effective" methods? If language must be "learned" or "acquired"—what conditions are necessary to foster this learning? Is there a middle ground in this debate?

The main purpose of this chapter is to provide an overview of language-teaching methods and practices that have been used or can be used with deaf children and adolescents. The notion, language instruction, is interpreted broadly. That is, it refers to the teaching of a first or second language and to the teaching of literacy (reading and writing) in a first or second language. The emphasis here is on the teaching of English. The acquisition and teaching of American Sign Language (ASL) as a first or second language is in its infancy and some details can be found in other sources (e.g., Lucas, 1990; Strong, 1988a; Wilbur, 1987).

In addition to providing definitional and historical perspectives, we present some examples of language-teaching procedures. Many of these procedures have been influenced by the broad language theories discussed in Chapters 2 and 3 and in Chapter 6 on bilingualism. The examples related to literacy (reading and writing) are based on the information in Chapter 5. The reader is reminded that this chapter provides a brief introduction to language instruction. More detailed information on the teaching of language and literacy to deaf individuals can be found elsewhere (e.g., King & Quigley, 1985; Kretschmer & Kretschmer, 1988a; McAnally et al., 1987, in press).

THE TEACHABILITY/LEARNABILITY OF LANGUAGE

To provide some insights into the methods and materials used to teach language, reading, and writing, it is important to present a few highlights of the current debate between the learnability of language versus the teachability of language (e.g., Ingram, 1989; Rice & Schiefelbusch, 1989; Stevenson, 1988). In essence, the debate revolves around the question of whether language can be "taught." It is also not uncommon to encounter such debates in the fields of reading and writing, including second-language literacy (e.g., see discussions in Bernhardt, 1991; Dechant, 1991; King & Quigley, 1985; Paul, 1993). For example, King and Quigley (1985) have described this issue relative to reading—that is, can reading be "taught" or must it be "caught?"

Relative to deafness, the "teaching" of language and literacy is a critical area because it is often stated that most deaf students come to school not knowing *any* social-conventional language and some deaf students know ASL as a first language (e.g., Johnson et al., 1989; Paul & Jackson, 1993). Thus, the discussion centers on whether English can be "taught" either as a first or second language, either in the primary (speech and/or sign) or secondary form (print).

The notion of learnability—most notably, the learnability hypothesis in linguistics—refers to the specification of conditions and constraints that contribute to or enable the "learning'"of a first or second language (e.g., see discussion in Pinker, 1989). Despite their influence on the development of language methods and materials, the linguistic theories, specifically those motivated by Chomsky's thinking (e.g., 1975, 1988), ascribe to the condition of learnability (see Chapter 2). Based on the innate hypothesis (e.g., the Language Acquisition Device), Chomsky viewed language as an innate process within a maturational framework. That is, the linguist attempts to arrive at explanatory adequacy in describing how and what is acquired, not how and what should be taught. As discussed in Chapter 2, this is primarily a mentalistic, rationalistic view of language development.

On the other end of the continuum are the behavioristic theories, which view language as a verbal, observable, empirical behavior (see Chapter 2). The teaching of language depends on the specification of conditioning, specifically operant conditioning within a stimulus-response (S-R) paradigm. The behaviorist's approach epitomizes the teachability of language, indeed the teachability of all observed behaviors. As discussed in Chapter 2, this approach, along with logical positivism in philosophy, has influenced "descriptive" language views, for example, structural linguistics.

The third broad group of theories—interactionist, particularly social-interactionist—represents a "balanced" view of language development with a focus on interactions among language, cognition, and the social-environmental conditions. Some interactionists place more emphasis on innate, or nature, factors whereas others favor nurture, or social-environmental, factors. A similar analogy can be made relative to the continuum of interactionists' views on the teachability/learnability dichotomy. For example, some proponents stress the teachability notion whereas others emphasize learnability. If teachability is emphasized, then this can be interpreted to mean that a great deal of language can be taught. On the contrary, if learnability is emphasized, then only some aspects of language can be taught.

Teachability/Learnability and Literacy

The teachability/learnability debate can also apply to the implications of theories of literacy (see Chapter 5). It should be clear that literary-critical theories are not concerned with the improvement or "teaching" of reading and writing. Rather, these theories focus on the value and uses of literacy within a particular society or context.

The teachability/learnability issue is most applicable to theories of reading comprehension. For example, there are three broad categories of models within reading-comprehension theory: bottom-up, top-down, and interactive. It should be recalled that bottom-up models place much emphasis on the text of the reading process. The text refers to structures such as letters, words, and sentences. The assumption is that readers need to know—specifically taught—the "alphabet system," namely, the system on which written English is based. Aspects of this knowledge include an understanding of letters, letter-sound correspondences, and, essentially, a deep knowledge of the morphophonological and syntactic system of English.

In some top-down models, particularly a very popular model known as the "whole language" approach, reading is viewed as a language-learning process—namely, a psycholinguistic guessing game (e.g., Goodman, 1985). Within this framework, individuals are said to acquire reading in the same manner as they acquire language—mainly by engaging in the "act" of reading. The knowledge of language and culture in the readers' heads should be sufficient for the ongoing development of reading proficiency.

As we discussed in Chapter 5, the "balanced" approach to the teachability/learnability issue appears to be social-cognitive interactive theories of reading, which can also be applied to the development of written language. Within this framework, some aspects of reading and writing can and should be taught (e.g., word identification and meaning vocabulary); however, a substantial amount of the higher-level features of literacy must be acquired or developed by individuals. Nevertheless, it is possible to "teach" (i.e., model, show examples of) some aspects of higher-level skills such as making inferences or using metacognitive skills.

Teachability/Learnability: An Interactive Perspective

In general, it is possible to characterize our view of the teachability/learnability situation concerning language and literacy as interactive (see discussions in King & Quigley, 1985; Paul, 1993; Paul et al., 1992; Paul & Quigley, 1990). We believe that it is important to teach some aspects of language and literacy or, at least, to construct exemplary situations in which individuals can acquire or develop proficiency in certain areas (see also, Quigley & Paul, in press). Although we place more emphasis on learnability, it is critical to attempt to improve the language and literacy proficiency of individuals with severe to profound hearing impairment. This is true especially when hearing-impaired students have had difficulty "acquiring" skills in these areas.

As is discussed later, any type of language and literacy intervention—natural, structural, combined, or eclectic—can be viewed as favoring "teachability." Instructional examples based on this interactive framework can be seen in the discussion of combined approaches (natural and structural) of language instruction and in discussion of literacy activities, especially those in the section on the use of ASL to teach English as a second language.

APPROACHES TO LANGUAGE INSTRUCTION

Historically, there have been two major approaches to language instruction, structural and natural, as well as "combinations" of these approaches (see also, McAnally et al., 1987, in press). In many cases, it is possible to state that structural approaches adhere to the concept of teachability whereas natural approaches adhere to that of learnability. However, relative to deafness, the teachability/learnability distinction becomes blurred due to the fact that many deaf children come to school not knowing a social-conventional language or have not acquired the social-conventional language of the home environment. Within a learnability framework, it can be argued that many deaf children have not "acquired" a first language under natural, typical circumstances. Thus, the natural approaches in school might involve constraints and conditions (e.g., intensive and extensive exposure to linguistic stimuli within a planned format) that are different from those that exist in the home for typical, first-language or bilingual-language learners.

The ensuing sections present information relative to the two broad "language-teaching" approaches: structural and natural. The reader is reminded that these approaches are "broad" and that there have been attempts to clarify and refine the meaning of terms such as approach and strategy within the language learning/teaching framework (e.g., see McAnally et al., 1987, in press; Marton, 1988). In general, instructional strategies are associated with an approach such as structural or natural. For example, McAnally et al. (1987, in press) stated that teaching strategies associated with the structured or combined (structural and natural) approach include *correct-incorrect, completion, replacement, combination, scrambled sentences,* and *revision.* Nevertheless, our goal is to adopt and describe the general terms, structural and natural, because they are most familiar to researchers and teachers of deaf individuals (see discussions in King, 1984; McAnally et al., 1987, in press; Moores, 1987).

Descriptions and Some Historical Perspectives: Structural Approaches

Advocates of structural (or structured) approaches assert that language can and needs to be taught to students with hearing impairment. Students are required to analyze and categorize the grammatical aspects of the language, for example, parts of speech such as nouns, verbs, and objects. The grammatical aspects are typically represented by patterns via a metalinguistic symbol system. Metalinguistic symbols refer to symbols such as noun phrase (NP), verb phrase (VP), subject, or other symbols and words used to describe the language. Students demonstrate their understanding by writing sentences that correspond to previously taught patterns. As noted by McAnally et al. (1987; see also in press):

> Structured methods treat language analytically and prescriptively, emphasizing knowledge of structure as embodied in rules of grammar. Through processes of direct imitation, memorization, and drill, usually within the framework of a strictly sequenced curriculum, the deaf child is expected to acquire a grammatically accurate version of the general language of the society. Examples of users of structured approaches to language development have been de l'Epee and Sicard in France in the second half of the 18th century, Clerc and Gallaudet in the United States in the early to late 19th century, and Barry and Fitzgerald in the United States in the first half of the 20th century. (p. 78)

Historically, in the United States, the use of structured approaches and the language of signs occurred simultaneously, as evident in the first residential school for the deaf in Hartford, Connecticut. Influenced by the work of de l'Epee and Sicard, teachers constructed diagrams, or line drawings, to represent the various grammatical features of English. Subsequently, a number of metalinguistic symbol systems were developed during the late 19th and early 20th centuries. Examples include Barnard (straight-line and curved-line symbols), Storrs (symbols above words), Wing (numbers, letters, and other metalinguistic symbols above words), and Barry (five slates or tablets of materials used for writing only, similar to the approach used by Sicard).

Two examples of structured approaches (and materials) are highlighted here: the Fitzgerald Key, developed during the early 20th century, and APPLE TREE, developed during the late 20th century. The Fitzgerald Key is probably the most widely known structural approach and one that is still used in a number of programs (McAnally et al., 1987, in press). The Key was developed by Edith Fitzgerald (1929), who was a deaf teacher at the Wisconsin School for the Deaf. With some modifications and refinement, the Key is based on the Barry Five Slate System. There are six columns, and each column is headed by words or symbols as follows: subject (*who, what*), verb and predicate words, indirect and direct objects (*what, whom*), phrases and words denoting place (*where*), other phrases and word modifiers (e.g., *how often, how much*), and words concerning the concept of time (e.g., *when*). The structure of the Key is illustrated in Table 7–1.

In general, Fitzgerald (1929) asserted that the purpose of this approach is to help deaf children learn some of the English structures and to construct and evaluate their own *written* compositions. A good discussion of the implementation of the Key can be found in Pugh (1955; see also the discussion in McAnally et al., 1987, in press).

The APPLE TREE is an acronym for A Patterned Program of Linguistic Expansion through Reinforced Experiences and Evaluations

TABLE 7-1. A Sample of The Fitzgerald Key

Column 1	Column 2	Column 3	Column 4
Who: Whose: What:		What: Whom: ( ) Whose: Whom: What:	Where

Column 5	Column 6
How much: For: How often: From: How long: How:	When:

Source: Adapted from Pugh (1955).
NOTE:
Column 1 contains subjects as noun phrases and is labeled with the interrogative terms: *who* and *what.*
Column 2 contains verb phrases, subject complements, predicate nouns, predicate adjectives, and predicate pronouns. There is no heading for this column; it uses symbols which are placed below the words.
Column 3 contains the direct and indirect objects and is marked by the interrogatives, *whom, what,* and *whose* for direct object. The *what* and *whom* with the parentheses ( ) indicates indirect object.
Column 4, 5, and 6 contains adverbials or phrases modifying the main verb. Column 4 represents adverbial of place and is marked by the term, *where.* Column 5 contains frequency and causal modifiers of the main verb and is marked by terms such as *how much, how often, how long, for, from,* and *how.* Column 6 represents adverbials of time and is represented by the heading, *when.*

(Anderson, Boren, Caniglia, Howard, & Krohn, 1980). This program consists of pre- and posttests, workbooks, and a teacher manual designed to teach 10 sentence patterns as shown in Table 7–2.

The exercises in the workbooks consist of comprehension, manipulation, substitution, production, and transformation activities. Transformations include only negation and question forms. These exercises are considered fundamental steps and as part of instructional procedures (Caniglia, Cole, Howard, Krohn, & Rice, 1975). For example, the first step, comprehension, refers to the development of vocabulary, concepts, and form of the structure. The APPLE TREE program was designed to introduce the sentence patterns in a sequenced, spiraling manner, that is, proceeding from the easiest to the hardest structure.

As a supplement to the basic APPLE TREE materials, a series of short story books have been developed, using only the sentence patterns depicted

TABLE 7–2. Sentence Patterns and Examples for APPLE TREE

Sentence Pattern	Example
N1 + V (be) + Adjective	The boy is short.
N1 + V (be) + Where	The girls are in school.
N1 + V (be) + N1	I am a student.
N1 + V	The boy is running.
N1 + V + Where	The children are running to school.
N1 + V + Where + When	Mother went to work this morning.
N1 + V + N2	The woman bought a car.
N1 + V + N2 + Where	The boys took their bats to the game.
N1 + V + N2 + Where + When	I will take my wife to the doctor tonight.
N1 + V + N3 + N2	Jill gave me a toy.

NOTE:
N1 = noun phrase one (i.e., subject or predicate nominative)
N2 = noun phrase two (i.e., direct object)
N3 = noun phrase three (i.e., indirect object)
Adjective = word or words that modifies noun phrase
V = verb phrase
V (be) = be verb (i.e., linking verb or copula)
Where = adverbial phrase of place
When = adverbial phrase of time

in Table 7–2. Supplementary activities in the form of additional workbooks are also available. It should be obvious that this language approach is structural. To complete the exercises in the workbooks successfully, the deaf students need to know and understand the metalinguistic terminology used throughout the materials.

In essence, the structured approaches epitomize the teachability of language, especially via the use of written language. There are numerous principles associated with the use of structured approaches in both first- and second-language teaching (e.g., see discussions in McLaughlin, 1985; Rice & Schiefelbusch, 1989; Wiig & Semel, 1980). Some of these principles include the following (Wiig & Semel, 1980):

- Unfamiliar words and sentence formation rules should be presented according to normal language developmental sequences or established orders of difficulty.
- The words featured in the phrases, clauses, and sentences used for intervention should be highly familiar. They may be selected from vocabulary lists for age or grade levels at least 3 years or grades below the child's current vocabulary age or grade level.
- Sentence length in number of words should be kept to an absolute minimum. This may be achieved by limiting sentence length to five to 10 words and by keeping phrase or clause length to two to five words.
- Unfamiliar words or sentence formation rules should be introduced in at least 10 illustrated examples. The examples should feature different word selections.
- The knowledge and use of words and sentence formation rules should be tested in at least 10 examples that feature vocabulary not previously used. (pp. 122–123)

The structured approach is also associated with the concept of direct instruction (e.g., McAnally et al., 1987, in press; Schirmer, 1994). Some of the basic tenets of direct instruction include: explicit teaching of rules and strategies, selection of examples, sequencing of examples, and the principle of covertization (i.e., internalizing the rules and principles). The beginning stages of direct instruction require explicit instruction of the application of rules. The thinking process is made overt and observable (e.g., Carnine et al., 1990). Next, a series of examples are used for guided practice and the teaching of the rule. The examples are similar enough to foster generalization to future similar examples. The use of leading questions and overt steps enable the teacher to know whether students are following a specific thinking process. Other instructional strategies associated with direct instruction are similar to those discussed previously for structured approaches (e.g., correct-incorrect, completion, replacement, and so on).

Examples of Lessons Using APPLE TREE

As mentioned previously, the instructional procedures of this program includes five steps: comprehension, manipulation, substitution, production, and transformation (see McAnally et al., 1987, in press). Because we discussed the comprehension step already, the intent here is to provide examples of the other steps as indicated in McAnally et al. (1987). It is assumed that the deaf child has acquired or learned a number of vocabulary-words-concepts.

During the second step, manipulation, the deaf child attempts to apply the knowledge of words-concepts. The child is exposed to a variety of "visual" patterns relative to the structures of the program. In essence, the goal is to enable the child to understand when the specific words can be used in the specific structures and when they cannot be used. For example, students might be required to arrange word cards into patterns such as the following (McAnally et al., 1987, p. 123):

Mary/   is/   happy.
John/   is/   sad.
Harry/   is/   lazy.

Subsequently, the students manipulate the following word-phrase cards:

John and Mary/   went/   to their grandmother's house.
Did John and Mary/   go/   to their grandmother's house?
Where/   did/   John and Mary go?

The third phase is substitution. Adhering to the examples above, the lesson looks like the following (McAnally et al., 1987, p. 123):

Mary is happy.
She is happy.
John is sad.
He is sad.

John wants to work.
Mary wants to stay home.
I want to watch TV.

With these exercises, the students gain an understanding of the relationships of words within the sentences and across sentences, particularly the notion of pronominalization, or pronoun reference.

During the fourth phase of the process, students are required to produce, or write, spontaneously, using their knowledge of sentence patterns and vocabulary. The impetus for these activities might be pictures, objects, field trips, and so on. Reinforcement and enrichment exercises are also present in the workbooks, which accompany the program.

The last phase deals with the transformation of the basic kernel sentences. As mentioned previously, there are two transformations: negation (i.e., the word *not*) and the question form. An example of each activity is as follows (McAnally et al., 1987, p. 124):

Negation

> The apple is red.
> The apple is not red.
> John is sad.
> John is not sad.
>
> We will go to the store this afternoon.
> We will not go to the store this afternoon.
> Ms. Pat sang a song at the party.
> Did Ms. Pat sing a song at the party?
> Ms. Pat did not sing a song at the party.

Question Form

> Mr. Brown ran in the Boston Marathon.
> Mr. Brown did run in the Boston Marathon.
> Did Mr. Brown run in the Boston Marathon?

Other examples of instructional strategies and activities associated with APPLE TREE and other structured approaches can be found elsewhere (McAnally et al., 1987, in press; Schirmer, 1994).

Descriptions and Some Historical Perspectives: Natural Approaches

Advocates of natural approaches assert that language should be "acquired" in a holistic manner. With intensive and extensive exposure to a language-rich environment, students with hearing impairment should be able to discover and internalize rules and principles associated with the grammar of English. It is not necessary—indeed, it is counterproductive and unnatural—to teach specific grammatical features. As remarked by McAnally et al. (1987; see also, in press):

> Development is planned to parallel the sequence of language acquisition in hearing children. The deaf child is expected to acquire language principles inductively and unconsciously through constant exposure to appropriate language patterns in situations that are designed on the basis of the child's needs and interests. . . . Some of the foremost proponents of natural approaches have been Hill in Germany in the early and mid-1800s, Greenberger and Groht in the United States from the late 19th to the mid-20th century, and many individuals in many countries in the present era. (p. 78)

The natural approach commanded a substantial amount of attention with the publication of *Natural Language for Deaf Children* by Groht (1958). Groht stated several principles, which seem to be common across all natural approaches. These include:

1. The content of language lessons should be dictated by the needs of the child rather than by vocabulary lists or language rules.
2. The child learns natural language via meaningful situations rather than by drills and exercises.
3. The functions of language can be taught best through conversations, discussions, writing, and the academic subjects.
4. Language principles should be introduced incidentally in natural situations, possibly explained by the teacher in real meaningful situations, and practiced by the children in numerous activities such as games, stories, and conversations.

If the structured approach is synonymous or nearly synonymous with direct instruction, then the natural approach is often associated with the inquiry method (e.g, McAnally et al., 1987, in press; Schirmer, 1994). Synonymous labels for the inquiry method include holistic teaching, holistic constructionism, and even the scientific approach (e.g., Bateman, 1990; Schirmer, 1994). The teacher is often viewed as a "facilitator" or "consultant," rather than an expert who imparts knowledge. Much of the theoretical support for this approach comes from Piaget's work on the cognitive development of children and adolescents (see Chapter 3).

Models of the inquiry method utilize some of the basic steps of the scientific method. Although there are several variations, some possible steps are as follows:

1. Identification and definition of the problem.
2. Formulation of hypotheses.
3. Gathering of data via the use of experimentation or observation.
4. Analysis and interpretation of the data.
5. Formulation of conclusions and generalizations.

It is also possible to have a step which deals with a reflection on this process, that is, metacognition. This is considered to be an analysis of the inquiry process itself (e.g., Joyce, Weil, & Showers, 1992) similar to other activities that involve thinking about language (metalinguistic) or thinking about comprehension in reading (metacomprehension, metamemory). In essence, the focus is on the use of a method that is similar to that used by scientists and researchers in attempting to understand and solve a problem or condition. This approach emphasizes strongly that science is not merely the accumulation of knowledge; rather, it is a process that involves critical and reflective inquiry in which there is little separation between the knower and the knowledge attained (for an interesting perspective, see Piaget, 1971).

Examples of Lessons Using Natural Approaches

It should be recalled that natural approaches focus on developing language in meaningful, natural, communicative situations. The development of language is not divided into parts such as form (e.g., vocabulary, syntax), content (e.g., meaning), and use (e.g., pragmatics). Rather, these components of language are an integral part of every lesson (McAnally et al., 1987, in press; Schirmer, 1994). The following two examples are taken from McAnally et al. (1987, pp. 98-99). These activities serve as exemplars for instructional activities within any natural approach.

PRESCHOOL LEVEL

Sample Goal: To develop the concept of apple.

Lesson 1: Pre-visit preparation

Objective:	• Prepare children for field trip.
Strategy:	• Planned situation as opposed to "teaching to the movement."
	• Communicative interaction between teacher and learners in speech/sign.
	• Questioning.
	• Discourse.

Procedure:
- Teacher shows a picture (preferably a photograph) of an apple tree and asks: "What is this? Do you know? Can you tell me? What is this?"
- Children: "Tree."
- Teacher: "You're right—this is a picture of a tree! (points to apple) What's this?"
- Children: (Some may respond *apple*, some may respond *eat*, some may not respond at all.)
- Teacher: "Yes, this is an apple. Look in my bag here—what is in the bag?"
- Children take turns peeking in the bag. Responses may be: *apple, eat,* or no response.
- Teacher takes an apple out of the bag and compares it to apples on the tree in the picture. Teacher: "Tomorrow, we will go somewhere. You will come to school in the morning. Then we will ride a bus. We will see many apple trees. We will buy some apples and bring them back to school. Maybe we will eat apples tomorrow. Do you like to eat apples?"
- All children have an opportunity to respond.
- Teacher and children find "tomorrow" on calendar and mark by drawing an apple on calendar.

Lesson 2: Trip to orchard

Objective:
- See apple trees.
- Pick apples off the trees.
- Buy apples in the orchard store.

Strategy:
- Field experience.
- Communication.
- Discourse.
- Questioning.

Procedure:
- The teacher or teacher aide should take instant-developing photographs during the trip, so children see the pictures together with the real thing.
- When the children are approaching the orchard, the teacher should comment about what they see (e.g., many trees, apples on the trees, size and colors of apples). Each child could pick an apple and the teacher could discuss "good apples" and "bad apples."
- Teacher and children go into the orchard store and see and discuss the apples.

- Most orchard stores offer samples of different kinds of apples so the children can taste the different ones.
- Teacher and children buy apples and juice to take back to school.

Lesson 3: Teacher and children develop written experience story by discussing each photograph. They eat apples and drink juice.

Additional examples of instructional activities related to natural approaches can be found elsewhere (e.g., Luetke-Stahlman & Luckner, 1991; McAnally et al., 1987, in press; Schirmer, 1994).

THE USE OF COMBINED APPROACHES

In the second half of the 20th century, several special language materials have been developed and a number of combined approaches have been advocated. The combined approaches entail the teaching of language in a natural manner via the use of a structured approach (King, 1984; McAnally et al., 1987, in press). This approach seems to be a balanced approach, 'combining' the best features of both natural and structured approaches (e.g., see materials and procedures in Blackwell, Engen, Fischgrund, & Zarcadoolas, 1978; Quigley & Power, 1979; van Uden, 1977).

Three approaches are highlighted here. van Uden (1977) developed a method called the maternal reflective method. It contains a "natural" component because of its emphasis on the development of the mother tongue— "the language first learnt by the speaker as a child" (van Uden, 1977, p. 93)—via oral conversational methods based on the experiences of the children. van Uden argued that contrived experiences and language patterning are not successful. Children do not learn questioning techniques by being presented isolated sentences such as "The box is on the table" and by being requested to produce a Wh- question based on these sentences. van Uden also asserted that children learn language by participating in dialogue that is meaningful and by listening to the conversation of others. Thus, it is reasoned that teachers of deaf children should not only engage in meaningful dialogue with their students, but should also direct the attention of their students to the conversations of others in the classroom. The influence of social-interactionist theories can be seen in this method, particularly within the framework of pragmatics (see Chapters 1 and 2).

Blackwell et al. (1978) developed the Rhode Island Curriculum designed for students at the Rhode Island School for the Deaf. This approach is primarily structural and is based on the assumptions of early transformational-generative grammar theory (Chomsky, 1957). Relative to linguistic principles, students are initially introduced to five sentence patterns—kernel sentences—as illustrated in Table 7–3.

The curriculum contains three levels. The first level is designed for children in preschool and kindergarten. This level consists of activities for exposure, recognition, comprehension, production, and writing of the linguistic principles. The second level is labeled the simple sentence stage, whereas the third level is the complex sentence stage. These latter two levels include activities for each of the areas identified for Level 1 with the addition of activities for sentence analysis. Although syntax serves as the unifying factor of the linguistic portion of the curriculum, it should be stressed that Blackwell et al. have included provisions in their approach for the development of cognition, semantics, and pragmatics.

The Blackwell et al. (1978) curriculum also contains the coordination of the language goals with the content area goals. Thus, language is not to be "taught" in isolation. Because language should be used to convey information in content areas such as social studies and mathematics, it is important for teachers to consider not only their students' abilities to understand the content, but also, their abilities to understand the language through which the information is conveyed.

The *Test of Syntactic Abilities Syntax Program* (TSA) was designed to assist deaf students in the comprehension and production of the nine major syntactic structures discussed in Chapter 5 (see also Chapter 8). For

TABLE 7–3. Sentence Patterns and Examples for the Rhode Island Curriculum

Sentence Pattern	Example
NP + V	The bird flies.
NP1 + V + NP2	The bird eats worms.
NP + LV + Adjective	The bird is small.
NP + LV + NP	The bird is a sparrow.
NP + LV + Adverbial	The bird is in the nest.

NOTE:
NP = noun phrase
NP1 = noun phrase one (i.e., subject or predicate nominative)
NP2 = noun phrase two (i.e., direct object)
V = verb
LV = linking verb or copula
Adjective = word or words that modifies noun phrase
Adverbial = phrase of time or place

each major structure, there is a teacher's manual, which provides descriptions of the structures, information on the acquisition of the structures by both deaf and hearing students, objectives for teaching the nine structures, diagnostic guides for assessing students' performances on the TSA, and suggestions for additional activities to reinforce the students' learning of the structures. There is also a set of 20 workbooks, which correspond to the linguistic components assessed by the TSA, and which consist of programmed activities related to each major structure. It is not necessary for students to know metalinguistic terminology in order to complete the activities.

The TSA Syntax Program is based on a large body of information gained by research conducted by Quigley and his associates between 1968 and 1978. The research was motivated by the linguistic thinking of Chomsky (1957, 1965) and its variations. As with any structured program, one of the weaknesses might be that students cannot generalize their "understanding" to spontaneous productions. As a result, the authors have suggested the use of more natural activities in the teachers' guides to assist students in the generalization process. It should be remembered that the materials covered only the syntactic component of English. Thus, Quigley and Power (1979) have remarked that this program should be used as part of a language program which includes all major components of English. It is implied that any language program should be well supported by theory and research.

LANGUAGE INSTRUCTION AND BEST METHOD

One of the most controversial and long-standing issues in the teaching of language to deaf children and adolescents is the notion of "best method" (Luetke-Stahlman & Luckner, 1991; Moores, 1987; Paul & Quigley, 1990). An extensive review of research on this notion, relative to language, has been provided by the work of McAnally et al. (1987, in press). To illuminate the results of this research review, we discuss the survey research of King (1984), which serves as an exemplar study. Finally, we provide a brief overview of the recent work on the notion of "best method" (e.g., Prabhu, 1990).

King (1984) sent questionnaires to 576 programs of students with hearing impairment throughout the United States. The questionnaire requested information on the materials and techniques teachers used in their language programs. This survey is considered the first generally available rendition of this issue since 1949.

The respondents were requested to describe the language program as structural, natural, combined, or eclectic. King defined these terms as follows:

Structural approaches
>   Language teaching requires students to study syntax and grammar.
>   A symbol system is used to represent the structure of language.
>   Other labels for structural approaches include scientific, formal,
>   logical, analytical, and systematic.

Natural approaches
>   The emphasis is on the development of colloquial and idiomatic
>   expressions. No symbol systems are used. Other labels for these
>   approaches include mother tongue, informal, synthetic, and devel-
>   opmental.

Combined approaches
>   These approaches combine aspects of the structural and natural ap-
>   proaches. The relative use of structural or natural approaches varies
>   from program to program.

Eclectic approaches
>   The approach to language development is the decision of the in-
>   dividual teacher. The type of approach or combination of ap-
>   proaches may vary from classroom to classroom within the same
>   program. This approach can be described as: "Anything and ev-
>   erything that works." The effectiveness of the approach is decided
>   by the individual teacher.

Results reveal that, at all levels (preschool, primary, intermediate, junior high, and high school), the combined approaches were the most frequently used approaches. Percentages of use range from 36% at the preschool level to about 56% at the intermediate level. In addition, at the preschool level, 34% of the respondents indicated the use of natural approaches. The use of the natural approaches at other levels ranged from 1.5% at the junior-high level to 6.2% at the primary level. With the exclusion of the preschool level, the second most frequently reported approach was the eclectic approach with percentages ranging from a little more than 27% at the primary level to more than 39% at the high-school level.

King (1984) reported that a majority of the programs used some type of metalinguistic symbol system in the teaching of English. The various systems ranged from traditional/structural approaches to those based on transformational generative grammar (see Chapter 2). Many programs employed more than one symbol system. Additional research on the effectiveness of these systems is needed.

In essence, it was reported that preschool programs classified their language curricula as natural or combined whereas those for older students (i.e., primary through high school levels) described their programs as combined and eclectic. In addition, it was stated that most respondents felt that it is better to combine several methods rather than rely exclusively on a single, all-encompassing approach.

The works of King (1984), McAnally et al. (1987, in press), and others (e.g., Luetke-Stahlman & Luckner, 1991) seem to indicate that there is no overall best method. For many teachers, including those who work with deaf children, this might not be an earth-shaking conclusion. The notion of "best method" has been studied and, at least, three broad interpretations have been proffered (Prabhu, 1990):

1. Different methods are best for different teaching contexts;
2. All methods are partially true or valid; and,
3. The notion of good and bad methods is itself misguided. (p. 161)

Some theorists and researchers have argued that it is nearly impossible to use objective, experimental (i.e., quantitative) research to evaluate items 1 and 2 above. The assumption is that there is a complex web of interactions within the teaching/learning situation that causes the results of experimental research to be limited or impractical. In addition, the traditional definition of a method has also been limited because it fails to consider the complex array of interactions between teachers and students. Thus, the notion of best method is misguided; the best we can hope for is an understanding of the teacher-learner situations via the use of qualitative research approaches (Brumfit, 1984; Prabhu, 1990).

With these considerations in mind, Quigley and Paul (in press) have reasoned:

> It seems that a combination of natural and more structured language development practices relative to the involvement and skill of the teacher and the reactions and responses of the students is the most productive approach. As in communication approaches, the field in theory, although perhaps not in practice, keeps swinging from one approach to the other, from natural to structured and back again. This alone is usually a strong indication that each approach, by itself, holds only part of the answer.

THE INSTRUCTION OF LITERACY

In this section, we present our views regarding the teaching of literacy skills in English as a first or second language. In Chapter 5, we argued that both reading and writing are interactive processes which entail the interactions between the individual and a text whose meaning needs to be constructed. Both reading and writing involve the application of lower-level and higher-level skills. The lower-level skills of reading are word identification skills whereas those of writing are spelling, grammar, and capitalization. The higher-level skills of reading are labeled comprehension skills and those of writing are organization, intent, and audience. The lower-level skills of the reader/writer need to become automatic so that higher-level skills can be used to compose a model of what the text means.

Regardless of whether one uses the direct instruction or inquiry approach—or basal readers or children's literature—it is generally assumed that a reader/writer should acquire or learn the lower-level skills as early as possible, preferably by grade three (e.g., Adams, 1990; Anderson et al., 1985; Lipson & Wixson, 1991). The acquisition of the lower-level skills is facilitated by the higher-level ones and vice versa.

It has been argued that, for example, for many poor readers, including those in special education programs, it is necessary to utilize direct instruction procedures in the teaching of word-identification skills (e.g., Carnine et al., 1990; Lipson & Wixson, 1991). There is a substantial amount of research showing also that knowledge of the alphabet system is critical and that such knowledge is facilitated by activities that focus on the sound system (e.g., phonics and structural analysis; Brady & Shankweiler, 1991; Chall et al., 1990; see also, Chapter 5).

Much of what we know about first-language reading and writing seems to be applicable to second-language reading and writing (e.g., Bernhardt, 1991; Paul, 1993; Paul & Jackson, 1993). Thus, as discussed in Chapter 6, the social-cognitive interactive theory has important implications for the teaching of literacy skills in English as a second language. In addition, this information pertains to deaf students, including those who know ASL, who are or might be learning English as a second language. For deaf students and even some hearing second-language learners, controlled readers such as *Reading Milestones* (Quigley & King, 1981-1984) and *Reading Bridge* (Quigley et al., 1990, 1991) are also beneficial.

Instructional Activities: General Comments

There is a great need for research on the effectiveness of instructional practices and materials related to reading and writing (King & Quigley, 1985; Paul & Quigley, 1990; Schirmer, 1994). Much of the information regarding instructional activities has come from research on hearing children. This information is still applicable because research has shown that the reading process for deaf children is essentially similar to that for hearing children (e.g., see reviews in Hanson, 1989; Paul, 1993; Paul & Jackson, 1993; see also, Chapter 5). The activities depicted in this section are based on the social-cognitive interactive framework. Additional information can be found elsewhere (Paul & Quigley, 1987b, 1990).

Instructional Activities and Materials: Reading

Our focus here is on the areas of vocabulary and comprehension (i.e., prior knowledge and metacognitive activities). It has been argued that vocabulary instruction needs to enable students to bridge what they know with what they do not know (e.g., Paul & O'Rourke, 1988; Pearson, 1984). Traditionally, teachers have used what can be called a definition approach (e.g., arrogant means proud) or a definition-and-sentence approach (Jane is an arrogant person). There needs to be a move away from these approaches because they have not been very effective (see Paul & Gustafson, 1991; Paul & O'Rourke, 1988). To bridge the known with the unknown, the focus should be on semantic-elaboration techniques such as semantic maps, semantic feature analysis, and word maps (for a good description of these techniques, see Heimlich & Pittelman, 1986; Mason & Au, 1986; Pearson, 1984). A word map is illustrated later.

Comprehension is or should be the most important focus of reading. The reader needs to be able to infer a great deal of information during reading. This inferential ability depends on the store of prior knowledge and the reader's ability to apply this knowledge (metacognition). As a result, teachers might need to develop prereading questions to activate and enrich prior knowledge. In addition, the construction of good postreading questions enable the reader to develop and apply inferential skills. As we indicated previously, it is difficult to teach inferential skills directly—in fact, relative to this issue, we tend to believe in the "learnability" of such skills.

Example—Story (taken from Paul & Quigley, in press)

It is a beautiful Saturday morning. Joan decided that it is a good day to go fishing. However, she can't make up her mind where to fish. Should she go to the lake? The stream? The river? Well, because it is going to be a hot day, Joan ruled out the lake. She wanted to go barefoot, and the beach would get too hot for her feet. Finally, Joan decided to go to the river. She knew of a perfect spot. In her mind, she could picture this huge tree with branches hanging over a part of the bank of the river. A great place to fish!

Important word—bank

Discussion of *bank* centers around three questions: (1) What is it?, (2) What is it like?, and (3) What are some examples? Additional meanings of *bank* can be obtained by asking additional questions: (1) What else is it?, (2) What else is it like?, and (3) What are some more examples?

. . . the teacher can ask additional questions about the word *bank*: What is it not? What is it not like?

Comprehension Activities—Postreading Questions

1. What day is it?
2. What did Joan decide to do?
3. Where did Joan go fishing? Why?
4. The story says *It is a beautiful Saturday morning*. What does this sentence mean?
5. Where can you find a beach?
6. Where else (i.e., besides bodies of water) can you find a bank?
7. Did Joan like to fish?
8. Do you like to fish?
9. What kind of fish can you catch in a river?

Special Materials

Because of the great difficulty deaf students have with the language, particularly vocabulary, syntax, and figurative language (see Chapter 5), of reading materials, it has been recommended that special materials be developed (see discussion in King & Quigley, 1985; Quigley & Paul, 1989). It should be emphasized that special materials should be used only when it is ascertained that students are having difficulty with the use of regular, grade or age appropriate materials. At least three methods have been discussed relative to constructing special materials: (1) simplify the language of existing materials; (2) modify the instructional strategies used with existing materials; and (3) construct original, special materials. Despite the controversies surrounding the use of special materials, it needs to be stressed that the ultimate goal is to enable deaf students to read eventually the regular materials of mainstream society.

Special materials control the introduction and use of certain language structures such as vocabulary and syntax. These structures are often introduced in a spiraling fashion, that is, proceeding from easiest to most difficult. Special materials are often recommended for students who are learning English as a second language. Relative to deaf individuals, both special language (see the section on structured approaches) and reading materials have been created. Special reading materials include *Reading Milestones* (Quigley & King, 1981–1984) and *Reading Bridge* (Quigley et al., 1990, 1991).

In a study of basal readers used with deaf students, LaSasso (1985) reported that *Reading Milestones* was used in nearly half of the programs. In a later study (1987), LaSasso remarked that the basal reader is the most commonly used material at the elementary and intermediate levels. Nearly 20 basal readers have been reported in educational programs for students with hearing impairment. The four most common readers are *Reading Milestones, Reading Systems and Systems Unlimited* (Scott, Foresman),

Ginn 360, and *Ginn 720* (Ginn & Co.), and additionally, the *Houghton Mifflin Readers* (Houghton Mifflin). In this study, respondents were also asked to rate the basal series relative to certain variables such as vocabulary, syntax, figurative language, and content. It was found that *Reading Milestones* was rated higher than all other series in all areas except interest level and diagnostic materials. These concerns have been addressed in the second edition of *Reading Milestones*.

Discussion of Writing Activities

As discussed in Chapter 5, the current research and instruction of written language emphasizes writing as a process approach. Within this perspective, it is still important to teach both lower-level and higher level skills of writing. However, the major instructional framework entails thinking of the writing process relative to three broad stages: planning, composing, and revising. The following description is taken from Paul and Quigley (1990, p. 199). Additional discussion of writing strategies can be found elsewhere (e.g., Bereiter & Scardamalia, 1987; Chall et al., 1990).

Example—Description of the Three Stages of Writing Instruction

Planning. Planning activities are similar to prereading activities. The teacher should enrich and activate the prior knowledge of students. . . . Through the use of questions and semantic elaboration techniques . . . , the teacher can help students choose a topic, generate and organize ideas, identify an audience, and establish a purpose for writing.

Composing. . . . students write the first draft of their composition, using their outlines or semantic maps to guide the organization and content of their papers. Teachers can also prompt students with questions and comments. . . . Students also may receive additional support and insights from their peers.

Revising. . . . writers attempt to polish, alter, expand, and clarify their manuscripts . . . teachers may decide that some students need more specific instructions in lower-level skills . . . Instruction may be necessary and meaningful because students are having difficulty rewriting or combining sentences or selecting more appropriate words.

TEACHABILITY AND TWO MAJOR GUIDELINES

If the goal is to teach language and literacy, there are several major guidelines relative to the teachability aspect. We emphasize two salient guidelines here. One, there needs to be a stronger interrelationship among theory, curriculum, instruction, and assessment. We discuss the role of assessment in this interrelationship and the special relationship of assessment to instruction in Chapter 8. Our point here is that any language program, utilizing strategies and materials, should be based on a well-defined theory. This theory should drive the development of the language curriculum and language assessment. As discussed previously, we recommend a social-cognitive interactionist framework with a strong emphasis on the learnability of language.

Relative to literacy, this theoretical framework has been labeled a social-cognitive interactive approach. It has been argued that the development of literacy assessments—as well as curricula and instructional practices—have not keep pace with emerging theoretical views of literacy for both hearing (e.g., Nystrand & Knapp, 1987; Pearson & Valencia, 1986) and deaf (see discussions in King & Quigley, 1985; Paul, 1993; Quigley & Paul, 1989) children. Examples of this problem in reading have been described by Pearson and Valencia (1986):

> Prior knowledge is a major determinant of reading comprehension, yet we mask any relation between knowledge and comprehension on tests by using many short passages about unfamiliar, sometimes obscure, topics.
>
> To accomplish the goals of reading, readers must orchestrate many so-called skills, yet many of our reading assessment schemes fragment the process into discrete skills, as if each was important in its own right. (p. 4)

The second major guideline concerns the educational preparation of teachers of deaf students in the areas of language and literacy. Several surveys have revealed that many teachers are not well educated in these areas, particularly if number of university-level courses are used as an indication. It is not uncommon to find that many teachers have only taken one or two courses (see reviews in King & Quigley, 1985; Moores, 1987; Paul & Quigley, 1990).

In essence, it seems that teachers of deaf individuals need more training in language and literacy. To paraphrase Russell et al. (1976), a good teacher of literacy needs to know as much about literacy as say a teacher of chemistry or physics is expected to know about these content areas. This education should involve, at least, a very strong background in theoretical frameworks and a general familiarity with a number of instructional strategies.

A general familiarity of strategies is recommended due to our present understanding of instructional approaches—including the concept of "best method"—and our current thinking on the learnability/teachability situation. In addition, there is very limited research on deaf children in the area of instruction for both language and literacy. The crux of the matter here is similar to what we have stated emphatically elsewhere (Quigley & Paul, 1989):

Instructional methods which have been proven successful with normally-hearing students should be explored with deaf students. It is also beneficial for trainee teachers to become aware of those methods, based on current thinking in linguistics and reading, that have been developed for other language-impaired student populations. In addition, *owing to the lack of conclusive findings, trainee teachers should not perceive the use of the various approaches as either-or situations; that is, natural or structural, bottom-up or top-down.* Finally, prospective teachers should receive adequate training in assessment and research methodology so that they can participate in evaluating the merits of their practices. (emphasis added; p. 17).

FINAL REMARKS

One of the most controversial, long-standing issues in the education of deaf children and adolescents is the manner in which English can be taught most effectively. This issue presumes that language can be taught and that there are methods of teaching that are better than others. Indeed, within this framework, there might be a "best" method.

To provide a better understanding of this situation, we discussed the recent debate in linguistics and elsewhere on the teachability/learnability dichotomy. This dichotomy also exists in theories and research on reading and writing. Major highlights of teachability/learnability were related to the information on theories of language in Chapter 2, theories of literacy in Chapter 5, and theories of bilingualism in Chapter 6.

Our views on teachability/learnability can be best characterized as "interactive." For example, relative to theories of language acquisition, we tend to favor interactionist perspectives with a heavy emphasis on learnability. That is, it is possible to teach some aspects of language; however, most of language is acquired and, indeed, may depend on innate qualities.

Relative to literacy, we support the interactive framework also. In other words, we view literacy as an interaction between the individual and the text she or he is trying to compose. This interaction depends on both bottom-up and top-down processes. In this chapter, we argued that our position on teachability/learnability represents a "balanced" view.

With the background on teachability/learnability, the reader should have obtained a deeper understanding of the various approaches to language instruction. In addition to providing historical perspectives, examples were provided on the two overall approaches: structured and natural. In our view, the "balanced" approach is the combined approach, which utilizes the best elements of both structured and natural approaches.

A synthesis of the research on the use of the various language-teaching approaches revealed that there is no superior approach. In many instances, practitioners either used a combined approach or thought it was best to use more than one approach. In addition, we discussed the notion of best method. Due to the complex interactions between teacher and students and the complicated description often associated with a method and its assessment, we agree with others that it is difficult to state one best method or several best methods.

Although it is difficult to describe a best method, we argued that it is possible to provide guidelines for the teaching of language and literacy. In our view, these guidelines should focus on the interrelations among theory, research, curriculum, instruction, and assessment. We presented some techniques that should be used in the teaching of reading and writing. It was also suggested that teachers of deaf students need to improve their knowledge of the processes of language and literacy. Finally, on the basis of research syntheses on both hearing and deaf students, we recommended that teachers become familiar with a wide variety of theory-based instructional strategies. More important, teachers and educators should avoid what can be construed as either-or instructional decisions.

FURTHER READINGS

Cazden, C. (1988). *Classroom discourse: The language of teaching and learning*. Portsmouth, NH: Heinemann.

Herriot, P. (1971). *Language and teaching: A psychological view*. London: Methuen.

Huckin, T., Haynes, M., & Coady, J. (Eds.). (1993). *Second language reading and vocabulary learning*. Norwood, NJ: Ablex.

Maria, K. (1990). *Reading comprehension instruction: Issues and strategies*. Parkton, MD: York Press.

Mason, J. (Ed.). (1989). *Reading and writing connections*. Boston, MA: Allyn & Bacon.

Oller, J., & Richard-Amato, P. (Eds.). (1983). *Methods that work: A smorgasbord of ideas for language teachers*. Rowley, MA: Newbury House.

C H A P T E R   8

LANGUAGE
ASSESSMENT

Language testing is central to language teaching. It provides goals for language teaching, and it monitors, for both teachers and learners, success in reaching those goals. Its influence on teaching (the notorious "backwash" or "washback" effect) is strong—and is usually felt to be wholly negative. It provides a methodology for experiment and investigation in both language teaching and learning/acquisition. So potent an influence, so salient a presence, deserves much closer attention and study than it typically receives. Compared with writings about language teaching, whether methodology, syllabus, materials or theory, those about language testing are very small beer indeed. (Davies, 1990, p. 1)

The passage above underscores the close relationship between language assessment and language instruction. Indeed, one of the goals of language assessment is to delineate areas that need attention for the purpose of improving the language development of individuals via language-teaching methods (e.g., Baker, 1989; Davies, 1990; Harrison, 1983). Assessment is not only related to instruction, but also, it is or should be related to language theory and curriculum. That is, a particular language theory should determine the *what* and *how* of curriculum, instruction, and assessment. As discussed in Chapter 2, all of these variables are driven by a specific metatheory (Ritzer, 1991).

The passage above also states that not enough attention is often given to language assessment, which focuses on the *why* and which can be compared to the cornerstone of a building. Relative to the total structure of a building, the cornerstone occupies a limited amount of space. However, in light of its function, the cornerstone can be viewed as an extremely critical component of the building. This analogy applies to the notion of language assessment, which is a critical aspect for the broad areas of language instruction or language therapy.

A carefully constructed language assessment program should occupy only a small portion of the designated time for classroom instruction or clinical therapy. The program should also provide teachers and clinicians with sufficient information on students' language skills and progress toward the achievement of instructional or clinical goals. Without assessment, there is no barometer on whether students' language needs are being met. In addition, there is no way to determine the efficiency of instructional or clinical methods.

The chapter provides a brief overview of several important issues in the area of language assessment. After presenting some general principles on the relation of language and assessment, we discuss the purposes and types of assessment, including some influences from the areas of language development and measurement. The next section of the chapter deals with some qualities of a good test, namely, reliability, validity, and the characteristics of the norming sample. Some consideration is also given to other critical issues such as selection, administration, interpretation, and the use of informal measures. Subsequently, we synthesize information on methods of assessment, including a discussion of several selected assessments used with individuals with hearing impairment. The importance of these issues have been espoused:

> To obtain useful assessment results, an examiner must thoroughly understand the type of information that various tests and assessment procedures can provide, as well as the limitations of the information that is obtained. Furthermore, with students who have a physical impairment, such as a hearing loss, one must be familiar with procedures that can circumvent a handicapping condition and understand how the handicap may affect a student's behavior. This knowledge is necessary to ensure that results accurately reflect a student's aptitude and achievement. (Bradley-Johnson & Evans, 1991, p. xi)

Because of the growing support for American Sign Language (ASL)/ English programs, we also provide some background on the language evaluation of students in bilingual or second-language learning programs. Finally, the chapter ends with our reflections on further research in language assessment. Information on language-teaching procedures and language materials are not discussed in this chapter; however, a good treatment of these issues can be found elsewhere (e.g., McAnally et al., 1987, in press).

LANGUAGE AND ASSESSMENT

In assessing and explaining language acquisition, one common area of agreement across recent theoretical models (e.g., linguistic and interactionist; see Chapter 2) is the distinction between knowledge possession and its use, that is, from the learning and the performance points of view (e.g., see discussions in de Jong & Verhoeven, 1992; Ingram, 1989; Medin & Ross, 1992). This is analogous to other terms, for example, the competence and performance notions of Chomsky (1957; 1965), the linguistic knowledge and channel control notions of Carroll (1961), or the notions of language as action versus language as system (Baker, 1989). These views should be kept in mind relative to the four skills or domains often used to discuss language development: listening (or observing, in the case of signs), speaking (or signing), reading, and writing. Listening (observing) and reading are considered to be receptive skills whereas speaking (signing) and writing are labeled expressive skills. These two groups of skills present different types of assessment problems. For example, it is not possible to observe receptive skills directly. In addition, although expressive skills are observable, they may not be indicative of underlying competence or "all that is observed in performance data is not necessarily skill related" (de Jong & Verhoeven, 1992; p. 8).

Relative to language assessment, several dichotomous models or assessment perspectives have been discussed in the literature (e.g., Baker, 1989; Davies, 1990; de Jong & Verhoeven, 1992; Duchan, 1984; Harrison, 1983). We are interested in those viewpoints which not only have exemplified the distinction between language knowledge and language performance but also have influenced the development and use of controlled and free methods with deaf individuals. In addition, this information is also relevant to the discussion of language assessment and bilingualism (e.g., Beardsmore, 1986; Cummins, 1984; McLaughlin, 1985). Pertinent to our purposes, two dichotomies are discussed: direct versus indirect procedures and discrete-point versus integrative measures.

Direct Versus Indirect Procedures

Direct procedures refer to the emphasis on the use of language to communicate or convey information in a natural manner. The language user is presumed to use language rules intuitively to express a message, for example, in spontaneous speech. One of the main goals of this method is to obtain a language sample, either spoken or written, which can be subsequently analyzed. Direct procedures are related to the use of free methods, as discussed later.

Indirect procedures refer to the conscious reflections of the language user on the language rules that are required to perform or complete a particular linguistic task. These procedures often are indicative of actual "testing situations" such as paper-and-pencil tasks. The focus is on gathering information about the individual's language proficiency without specific reference to use or purpose. Most language tests fall into this category via the use of test formats such as fill-in-the-blanks or multiple choice items. Indirect procedures are related to the controlled methods, discussed later.

A more detailed discussion of this dichotomy and related issues, such as reliability and validity, can be found elsewhere (e.g., Baker, 1989; Davies, 1990; de Jong & Verhoeven, 1992). It should be added that both direct and indirect procedures can be used to assess language knowledge and language use.

Discrete-Point Versus Integrative Measures

Discrete-point measures focus on the evaluation of certain important language elements or skills (e.g., vocabulary, syntax, distinctive features). In conjunction with a test format such as multiple choice, these measures are termed "objective" and "analytic" (e.g., Baker, 1989; de Jong & Verhoeven, 1992). Relative to the test formats of these measures, it has been remarked that:

The kind of questions (usually termed "items") which were used included:

Multiple choice items
Sentences with gaps to be filled
Sentences to be transformed in various ways

All of these item types have the following characteristics:

1. There is usually only one possible correct answer for each item.
2. Each item samples a particular element through the use of one skill.
3. Items are not dependent on one another—changing one item does not change the testee's performance on the other items of the test—cf. cloze testing. (Baker, 1989, p. 34)

Integrative measures were developed because of debates on the validity of the discrete-point measures—for example, the superficial, unnatural, decontextualized, and mechanical foci on language use (e.g., de Jong & Verhoeven, 1992). The goal of integrative measures is to obtain a global understanding of the language performance of the individual. This involves the use of holistic scoring methods and the focus on the use of language in natural, meaningful situations. One strong influence of these measures can be seen in the emerging paradigm of writing as a process approach (e.g., Bereiter & Scardamalia, 1987; see also, the discussion in Chapter 5). Besides being time consuming, integrative measures are subject to problems of reliability and validity (these concepts are discussed in a later section).

GENERAL ISSUES OF ASSESSMENT AND DEAFNESS

There are several general issues that should be considered prior to, during, and after the testing situation (Anastasi, 1982; Salvia & Ysseldyke, 1991). These issues impact the selection, administration, and interpretation of a test. The examiner should be well informed on the characteristics of both the test and the subject who is planning to take the test.

Relative to deafness, there are certain background demographics that are important to obtain, such as degree of hearing impairment, age at onset of impairment, etiology (cause), mode of communication, family background information, use of audition and vision, ethnic and cultural status, and the presence of additional disabilities (Bradley-Johnson & Evans, 1991; Paul & Jackson, 1993; Vernon & Andrews, 1990). These characteristics are important in determining whether a particular test is appropriate for the deaf individual. That is, it needs to be determined whether the characteristics of the sample (e.g., on normed tests) reflect the characteristics of the individual taking the test.

Paul and Jackson (1993) have listed several variables that should be considered to ensure that formal (and in many cases, informal) evaluations are fair, objective, and useful: "background information on the client or test taker; ethical considerations; definition and purpose of the test; standardization of procedures; technical quality—reliability and validity; and representativeness of the sample" (p. 240). It is also important to utilize information from other sources to supplement the results of the test (Moores, 1987; Vernon & Andrews, 1990). Such sources can include files, results of interviews, and data from observations.

CHARACTERISTICS OF ASSESSMENT

Three of the most important characteristics of assessment are reliability, validity, and practicality (Anastasi, 1982; Borg & Gall, 1983; Harrison, 1983; Salvia & Ysseldyke, 1991). These concepts apply to all measures: formal, informal, and unobtrusive observational assessment. It is important for teachers and clinicians to seek objective information about the reliability and validity of a particular test. The criteria used for evaluating practicality depends on the needs of teachers, clinicians, and administrators.

Reliability

Reliability is concerned with the consistency of test results regarding the performances of students (Anastasi, 1982; Borg & Gall, 1983; Salvia & Ysseldyke, 1991). That is, reliability refers to the degree to which an assessment measures what it was designed to measure. For formal, norm-referenced tests, the most common procedures for determining reliability are alternate (or parallel) form, test-retest, and internal consistency. For informal assessments, the commonly used procedures are interexaminer and intraexaminer procedures.

If there are two equivalent forms of the same test, the alternate or parallel form procedures can be used to determine reliability. The reliability coefficient is based on the computation of a correlation coefficient between the two forms of the test (see discussion of calculations in Borg & Gall, 1983; Salvia & Ysseldyke, 1991). This is the most commonly used estimate of reliability for standardized tests.

The concept of equivalent or parallel forms is not without its difficulties. The two tests might differ significantly in content to such an extent that the concept of equivalence would not be valid. In this case, the reliability coefficient might be underestimated. On the other hand, the two forms might be so closely matched in content that the estimated correlation coefficient might represent an overestimation of reliability. Thus, teachers and clinicians should seek the test-developer's justification of "equivalency." In addition, it should be ensured that a sufficient amount of time has elapsed between the administration of the first and second parallel forms.

Test-retest procedure refers to the administration of the same test (i.e., the same form) twice. The correlation coefficient for this procedure is typically higher than that obtained for alternate form procedure (Anastasi, 1982; Borg & Gall, 1983; Salvia & Ysseldyke, 1991). One reason for the higher correlation might be the students' recall of their answers to specific items. On the other hand, a lower correlation might result if test-takers become annoyed by the familiarity of the test. Thus, it is important to ensure that a sufficient time has elapsed between the two administrations. However, this does not guarantee an accurate correlation score.

To save time and to minimize the problems associated with repeated testing, several methods can be used to determine the reliability of an test based on a single administration. These measures are considered internal consistency measures. Typically, the procedures entail the dividing of a test into two equal parts and comparing the students' performance on both parts. In this case, it must be ensured that both parts of the tests are equivalent in some fashion.

Additional measures of internal consistency include the use of analysis of variance computations, for example, the method of rational equivalence involving the Kuder-Richardson (K-R) 20 and 21 formulas and the use of Cronbach's (1960) coefficient alpha (Borg & Gall, 1983; Salvia & Ysseldyke, 1991). The use of the K-R 20 and 21 formulas require that items be assessed dichotomously, that is, as right or wrong. Cronbach's coefficient alpha is considered a general form of the K-R 20 formula which can be used on tests with items that are not dichotomous.

Relative to informal assessments, including direct, integrative or spontaneous language samples, it might be necessary to assess reliability based on the extent to which independent analyses concur relative to the students' responses or levels of achievement. Interexaminer procedure refers to the degree of agreement between different evaluators' judgments of the same data (Anastasi, 1982; Borg & Gall, 1983; Salvia & Ysseldyke, 1991). Because these evaluators are exposed to the same training procedures, it is expected that there will be a high correlation between their conclusions. This agreement aids in the interpretation of the results. Interexaminer procedures are analogous to the notion of internal consistency procedures for standardized tests.

Another procedure for informal tests, intraexaminer, is analogous to the test-retest procedure for standardized test discussed previously (Borg & Gall, 1983; Salvia & Ysseldyke, 1991). The evaluator judges two sets of either highly similar or identical data after a period of time has elapsed (e.g., 1 week). The purpose is to compare the correlation between the two interpretations of the data. If there is a high correlation or substantial agreement, it can be concluded that the examiner applied the same criteria for his or her interpretations. If there is no substantial agreement, it might be concluded that the examiner has analyzed the data in an arbitrary fashion.

Validity

The concept of validity refers to the question of whether a test measures what it is designed to measure (Anastasi, 1982; Borg & Gall, 1983; Salvia & Ysseldyke, 1991). It is also possible to assess validity by comparing the findings of a test with those from observational and clinical situations. There are several types of validity; the ones discussed here are face, content, construct, concurrent, and predictive.

Face validity is concerned with the appropriateness of a specific test for the individual. For example, the test-takers should understand the purpose of the test and the manner in which they should respond (i.e., directions). One of the most important aspect of face validity is students' attitude toward the test. As discussed previously in test-retest procedures, this aspect can affect the reliability of the test.

Content validity is also known as rational or logical validity (Borg & Gall, 1983; Salvia & Ysseldyke, 1991). It is important to be aware of the assumptions of the test developers and the literature that is relevant to the variables of interest. Thus, content validity involves a comparison of the representativeness and appropriateness of the content of the test in question with the content of other, similar tests that have been used.

Construct validity refers to the degree to which the test in question is representative of a specific theoretical construct. For example, suppose that a theory maintains that the syntactic development of deaf students is qualitatively similar (i.e., manner of acquisition is similar) to that of hearing students. If a particular measurement verifies this similarity for structures such as negation and relative clauses, then construct validity has been established for hearing status relative to these two syntactic variables.

Concurrent validity can be ascertained via the evaluation of one measure by another one which represents the same criterion (Borg & Gall, 1983; Salvia & Ysseldyke, 1991). This type of validity is important for the adoption of new assessments. In essence, the scores on the 'new' test are compared to the scores on another, older test, which contains different items but is said to measure the same behavior.

Predictive validity refers to the degree to which a test can predict an individual's performance in a future situation (Borg & Gall, 1983; Salvia & Ysseldyke, 1991). This type of validity is critical for assessments that are employed to classify or select persons for specific areas, for example, entrance into college or a special-education program.

Some highlights of the concepts of reliability and validity are presented in Table 8–1.

Practicality

There are several issues relative to practicality, such as the amount of time for test administration, special equipment needs, costs of test materials and scoring procedures, and special arrangement needs (e.g., for individual testing, for individuals with special needs). The issues of practicality should not be underestimated. For example, test developers might have a highly reliable and valid test, but it might be impractical for some classrooms because of the amount of time required to administer it. In essence, practicality is important for the "marketability" of a specific test. It has been stated:

TABLE 8-1. Highlights of the Concepts of Reliability and Validity

Reliability

- The concept is concerned with the consistency of test results. Reliability refers to the degree to which an assessment measures what it was designed to measure.
- For formal, norm-referenced tests, the most common procedures are alternate (or parallel) form, test-retest, and internal consistency. Alternate form involves the computation of a correlation coefficient between the two forms of the test. Test-retest refers to the administration of the same test. Internal consistency includes the use of analysis of variance computations, for example, the method of rational equivalence involving the Kuder-Richardson 20 and 21 formulas and the use of Cronbach's coefficient alpha.
- For informal assessments, the commonly used procedures are inter-examiner and intraexaminer procedures. Interexaminer procedure refers to the degree of agreement between different evaluator's judgments of the same data. In the intraexaminer procedure, the evaluator judges either two sets of highly similar or identical data after a period of time has elapsed.

Validity

- This concept refers to the question of whether a test measures what it is designed to measure.
- Validity can be assessed by comparing the findings of a test with those from observational and clinical situations.
- There are several types of validity—face, content, construct, concurrent, and predictive. Face validity is concerned with the appropriateness of a specific test. Content validity involves a comparison of the content of a test in question with that of other, similar tests. Construct validity refers to the degree to which a test is representative of a specific theoretical construct. Concurrent validity can be ascertained by evaluating one measure against another measure which represents the same criterion. Predictive validity refers to the degree to which a test can predict an individual's performance in a future situation.

Source: Adapted from Borg & Gall (1983) and Salvia & Ysseldyke (1991).

In brief, tests should be as economical as possible in time (preparation, sitting and marketing) and in cost (materials and hidden costs of time spent). This sounds a very obvious statement to make, but it is easy to lose sight of overall efficiency in the detailed work required to prepare appropriate and useful tests. (Harrison, 1983, p. 13)

PURPOSES AND TYPES OF ASSESSMENT

The selection of a test or a battery of tests is influenced markedly by several factors. For example, we have discussed the important factors of reliability, validity, and practicality. Test examiners also have to decide whether they are interested in assessing only one component of language, for example, syntax, or all of language, that is, the four or five major components. In addition, they need to decide how language should be assessed; this was the focus of the information discussed previously in models of language assessment. Another area of concern is whether the test or battery of tests is appropriate for the population being assessed, in this case, individuals with severe to profound hearing impairment. It is obvious that there is no "cookbook" for the selection of a test or a battery of tests; however, the information presented thus far should be considered guidelines.

Perhaps, one of the most important factors to consider in the selection of a test or a battery of tests is the purpose of the evaluation. This issue, in turn, affects the type of assessment. Type of assessment also determines the method that will be employed to collect the data. For example, norm-referenced and criterion-referenced tests typically employed the use of controlled methods (discussed in the next section). The use of observations might entail the use of free methods (also discussed later); it is also a type of informal assessment.

Several conceptualizations exist relative to types (i.e., functions) of assessment (e.g, Baker, 1989; Davies, 1990; Harrison, 1983). For example, Davies (1990) categorizes test types as achievement, proficiency, aptitude, and diagnostic. Harrison (1983) uses the terms placement, achievement, proficiency, and diagnostic. In this chapter, we focus on three labels: achievement, diagnostic, and proficiency. The differences among these types can be discussed relative to the variables of time and content (Davies, 1990; Harrison, 1983).

Achievement

An achievement test can also be labeled as an attainment or summative test (Harrison, 1983). The achievement test is typically used at the end of a particular period of time or of learning. The information on the test is supposed to be a representative sample of the content covered during that time frame. The time frame might be associated with a school year, an academic course, or high-school or college career.

The achievement test is typically manifested as a standardized (i.e., norm-referenced) test (Anastasi, 1982; Borg & Gall, 1983; Salvia & Ysseldyke, 1991). Borg and Gall (1983) described the standardized test as "one . . . that produces very similar results when different persons administer and score the measure following the instructions given and . . . for which normative data are present to describe how subjects from specified populations perform" (p. 272). In essence, the student's overall performance is compared with other students at the same age or grade level.

The use and development of "standardized" tests for deaf students have been long-standing controversial issues in the education of these students (e.g., Moores, 1987; Paul & Quigley, 1990; Vernon & Andrews, 1990). One major problem has been the accuracy (i.e., validity) of the norms—particularly as they relate to the content of the test and the type of student taking the test. As described by Harrison:

> The conditions for setting an achievement test . . . brings up problems of sampling, since what has been learnt in a year (for example) cannot all be assessed in one day, yet the test must reflect the content of the whole course. Decisions therefore have to be made about what should be included in the test, and whether assessing one thing can be assumed to include another. For example, if a student can cope with the form and meaning of the past perfect tense, does that imply a similar mastery of the present perfect, since the normal sequence of learning deals with the second of these before the first? (Harrison, 1983, p. 7)

Diagnostic

An achievement test attempts to indicate the "overall" achievement of the student (compared to other students); however, to obtain information about specific strengths and weaknesses, a diagnostic test should be used (Anastasi, 1982; Borg & Gall, 1983; Salvia & Ysseldyke, 1991). Davies (1990) remarked that a diagnostic test can be considered the flip or reverse side of an achievement test. That is, an achievement test is concerned with the success of a student whereas a diagnostic test is concerned with the failure, so that it can be remedied.

A diagnostic test can be labeled as a progress or formative test (Harrison, 1983; Salvia & Ysseldyke, 1991). The test typically focuses on an individual's performance in a particular domain or area, such as language, reading, or mathematics. The diagnostic test is manifested as a criterion-referenced test. Students' scores are not compared with those of other students; rather, they are compared to an absolute standard, which is arbitrary determined. In other words, the test score purports to reflect the extent to which a student has mastered the content of a particular domain.

It should be kept in mind that many tests are both norm-referenced (i.e., achievement oriented) and criterion-referenced (i.e., diagnostic oriented). It has been argued that the distinction between the types is often misleading, causing problems with the interpretation of the results (e.g.,

Carver, 1974). Carver (1974) maintained that "all tests, to a certain extent, reflect both between-individual differences and within-individual growth. Because of their design and development, however, most tests will do a better job in one area than the other" (p. 512).

Proficiency

A number of theorists and researchers have argued for the assessment of language proficiency, as opposed to language competence as defined by Chomsky, especially for bilingual or second-language students (e.g., see discussions in Cummins, 1984; McLaughlin, 1985; Verhoeven, 1992). In one sense, proficiency is related to the performance or use of language (and other skills). The goal of a proficiency test is to ascertain the ability of an individual to apply what he or she has learned in real, meaningful situations. Unlike the achievement test, a proficiency test does not constrain the time frame or exhibit control over the previous learning experiences of the individual (e.g., Davies, 1990). Although the test is not specifically concerned with the individual's present level of competence, it is interested in the future performance of the individual in similar real-life situations. These conditions of a proficiency test might contribute to what is often called the "vagueness" of the test with respect to prior learning or knowledge. Proficiency tests can be related to the use of free methods in language assessment.

Controlled Methods

There are a number of advantages to using controlled methods in the assessment of language. For example, with controlled methods, language researchers can examine certain linguistic structures that might appear infrequently or never appear in a spontaneous language sample. Without a sufficient number of examples, it is not possible to determine whether an individual has acquired or has competency in specific language structures such as relative clauses or the use of pronouns. Of course, the converse is true, it cannot be ascertained that an individual does not have knowledge of a particular grammatical structure. These problems have been discussed in the work of Taylor (1969) and Quigley and his collaborators (e.g., Quigley et al., 1976). Using controlled methods, investigators can construct test items that permit the study of an individual's use or understanding of specific linguistic units.

Another advantage of controlled procedures is that they permit investigators to develop tests that address specific language domains such as phonology, syntax, and semantics. It is obvious that the information from such tests would be of great assistance to teachers and clinicians. Because of the nature of language, test-makers need to concentrate on developing an adequate assessment of one domain. That is, it is not possible to construct a test that would provide sufficient information on all language components. Thus, to provide detailed evaluation of a student's skill, it is best to concentrate on one language domain per assessment. This necessitates that students take several language tests.

One of the biggest advantages of controlled methods is the degree of objectivity in the analyses of test results compared to the analyses of data using free methods. Relative to the characteristics of standardized tests discussed previously, this objectivity is due to uniform procedures for administering, scoring, and interpreting the tests (Anastasi, 1982; Borg & Gall, 1983; Salvia & Ysseldyke, 1991). In addition, the interpretation of the tests also depends heavily on whether the characteristics of students taking the test are similar to those who were part of the norming procedures.

Because of standardized procedures, it is easy to compare the obtained results from controlled measures to other results of students or clients with similar characteristics. It cannot be overemphasized that test developers should specify and teachers/clinicians should be aware of the characteristics of the population on whom the tests were normed. Perhaps, it is not possible to develop a test for all students with hearing impairment, due to the discrepancies in achievement across the various subgroups (e.g., see discussions in Paul & Jackson, 1993; Vernon & Andrews, 1990).

Another advantage associated with controlled methods is that the conditions of reliability and validity can be satisfied without much difficulty. By controlling the test stimuli the available responses, and the characteristics of the normative sample, the amount of variance related to external factors can be reduced. The reduction of the variance should result in the enhancement of reliability and validity for the particular test (e.g., Anastasi, 1982; Salvia & Ysseldyke, 1991).

Controlled methods are not above criticism; they do have several limitations or disadvantages. Although it is possible to obtain detailed information on a specific domain of language, it might be difficult to obtain an evaluation of an individual's overall language ability. For example, a test on syntax does not yield information on an individual's understanding of pragmatics. To obtain a comprehensive evaluation of language, it is important not only to use several controlled assessments, but also, to use spontaneous language samples.

Another major limitation of controlled procedures can be seen in the nature of the test. For example, in a test-taking situation or a "laboratory" situation, the examiner attempts to control several areas such as test stimuli, test environment, and the test responses. Due to this nature of control, the investigator cannot assume that the results are reflective of an individual's language behaviors in more naturalistic settings (e.g., see discussions in Baker, 1989; Davies, 1990; Shohamy & Walton, 1992). Thus, it is important to compare the results obtained from the controlled measures with those obtained in a more naturalistic manner.

Test Instruments

In this section, we discuss a few tests and set of procedures that have been used with individuals with hearing impairment. It is still true that most tests and procedures used with hearing-impaired students have been normed on or adapted from those used with hearing students (Bradley-Johnson & Evans, 1991; Moores, 1987; Paul & Jackson, 1993; Vernon & Andrews, 1990). It should be kept in mind that our selection is representative, not exhaustive, of the type of method employed, that is, controlled. Relative to the characteristics of good assessment discussed previously, we attempt to discuss the kind of information that the selected test is purported to convey. A more-detailed, recent discussion of the strengths and weaknesses of a number of tests and good discussions of the selection and use of tests and procedures with students with hearing impairment can be found elsewhere (Bradley-Johnson & Evans, 1991; Luetke-Stahlman & Luckner, 1991; Thompson, Biro, Vethivelu, Pious, & Hatfield, 1987).

Berko Morphology Test. *The Berko Morphology Test* (Berko, 1958) was designed to evaluate children's knowledge of the morphological structure of English. The sample included 56 children who were unevenly divided across seven age levels ranging from 4 to 7 years in 6-month increments. For example, there were 14 subjects between the ages of 4 years and 5 years, 6 months (preschool), but 42 subjects between the ages of 6 and 7 years (first-grade age). No norms are available; however, it is possible to compare a student's score with the respective correct percentage scores for preschool and first-grade children in Berko's study.

The test contains 27 picture cards with accompanying sentences. The morphological structures assessed include plurals, singular and plural possessives, past tense, present progressive and derivational morphemes. For example, there is one item that shows a picture of an animal with bird-like characteristics. Underneath this picture is another picture with two of these creatures. The examiner remarks "This is a wug. Now there is another one. There are two of them. There are two _____ ." Although the test stimuli were closely controlled, the subjects' responses were not constrained.

Subjects were also required to explain (i.e., describe, define, etc.) 14 compound words. For example, given the following item: "A birthday is called a birthday because _____ ," the subjects were expected to provide an explanation.

Modifications of the *Berko Test of Morphology* resulted in the development of the *Exploratory Test of Grammar* (Berry & Talbot, 1966). Modifications include an increase in the number of pictorial stimuli from 27 to 30 and a change in the age range from 4–7 years to 5–8 years. Nevertheless, the limitations associated with the original test remained. For example, approximately 60% of the items on the newer test assess plural nouns and past-tense verb forms whereas only 40% of the items assess structures such as third-person singulars, possessives, derived adjectives, comparatives and superlatives, and the progressive aspect.

With adaptations of the procedures, the "morphology" test has been used to assess hearing-impaired children's knowledge of the morphological rules of English. Adaptations consist of presenting language stimuli in visual modes such as writing and forms of manual communication instead of the oral form. Results have been reported by Cooper (1967; see also, the discussion in Chapter 5) and Raffin (1976; see also, the discussion in Chapter 4).

Northwestern Syntax Screening Test. Lee (1969) developed the *Northwestern Syntax Screening Test* (NSST) to assess the receptive and expressive skills of children between the ages of 3 years and 7 years, 11 months. The NSST contains items that focus on prepositions, personal pronouns, noun-verb agreement, tense, possessives, present progressives, active and passive voice, and wh- questions. There are two parts, receptive and expressive.

The receptive portion of the NSST contains 20 items. Each item has four pictures with stimulus sentences designed to assess the structure under consideration. For example, if the focus is on prepositions, the examiner would hold the appropriate pictures and remark: "On one of these pictures the cat is behind the chair, on another, the cat is under the chair. Now show me the cat is behind the chair." The subject is expected to point to the picture that represented the second stimulus sentence, that is, "behind the chair."

The expressive portion of the NSST is based on an imitation task. The subject is shown 20 pairs of contrasting pictures with accompanying sentences. Consider an item that contains two pictures of babies, one is awake and the other is sleeping. The examiner would remark: "The baby is sleeping. The baby is not sleeping. Now what's this picture?" Subsequently, the examiner points to one of the two pictures and the subject is expected to say (imitate) the previous sentence associated with that picture. Failures to imitate the stimulus sentences are counted as errors for the expressive portion of the NSST.

Norms are available for children between the ages of 3 years and 7 years, 11 months. However, nearly half of the subjects are in the 5-year-old range whereas the other 1-year spans (e.g., 3 to 4 years; 4 to 5 years; etc.) only contains from 10% to 18% of the total sample. These subjects were from middle to upper income families from the midwest. Despite these norms, the test-developer did not report reliability and validity scores. In all fairness, Lee (1969) has remarked that the test should be used primarily as a screening assessment. To obtain a more detailed assessment of the syntactic development of young children, Lee recommended the use of additional assessments.

The use of the NSST with children with hearing impairment has been reported in a study by Pressnell (1973). Pressnell studied children with moderate hearing impairment and greater. Analyzing spontaneous language samples and the results of the NSST, it was concluded that the performance of the students were qualitatively similar but quantitatively reduced when compared to hearing norms. The predictability or explanatory adequacy of the NSST has been questioned by Wilbur et al. (1989) (see also, Chapter 5).

Carrow Elicited Language Inventory (CELI). Carrow (1974) stated that the purpose of the elicited imitation task of the CELI is to measure "a child's productive control of grammar" (p. 4). It is assumed that children's imitations of adult utterances reflect their grammatical competence, especially if there is sufficient emphasis on the use of immediate memory capabilities (e.g., see the discussions in Ingram, 1989; Menyuk, 1977).

The CELI consists of 51 sentences and one phrase, ranging from 2 to 10 words. Forty-seven of the 51 sentences are presented in the active voice whereas the other 4 sentences are presented in the passive voice. Sentences can be classified as affirmative, negative, declarative, interrogative, and imperative. Among the grammatical features assessed are articles, adjectives, nouns, pronouns, verbs, negatives, contractions, adverbs, prepositions, demonstratives, and conjunctions. The test task requires the examiner to present the stimulus sentences and the test-taker to imitate the items. The examiner records the deviations from the test items. Errors can be categorized into five types: substitutions, omissions, additions, transpositions, and reversals.

The CELI was standardized on 475 children between the ages of 3 years and 7 years, 11 months. The children came from middle class homes and attended daycare centers and church schools in Houston, Texas. The reliability of the CELI has been demonstrated using test-retest and inter-examiner techniques. The test-retest procedure was conducted on 25 children, five each at the ages of 3, 4, 5, 6, 7, who were administered the test after a two-week interval. Carrow (1974) reported a correlation coefficient of .98. The two interexaminer tests resulted in coefficients of .98 and .99.

The CELI was shown to have both concurrent and congruent validity. Relative to concurrent validity, it was found that the scores of the standardization (norming) sample increased significantly with age. In addition, the results of the CELI differentiated between children with typical language development from those with atypical or delayed language development. Relative to congruent validity, Carrow found that there was a significant correlation between the CELI and the Developmental Sentence Scoring techniques (Lee & Canter, 1971).

Test of Syntactic Abilities. *The Test of Syntactic Abilities* (TSA; Quigley et al., 1978) is a comprehensive battery of 20 diagnostic tests and two forms of a screening test which assesses deaf students' ability to either select or comprehend grammatically correct English sentences, involving nine syntactic structures (see Chapter 5). The 20 diagnostic tests of the TSA were normed on a sample of 411 students who met the following criteria:

1. Between the ages of 10 years and 18 years, 11 months.
2. Had at least an average IQ score on the performance scale of tests typically used with hearing-impaired students.
3. Possessed a hearing impairment of 90 dB (ISO) in the better ear averaged across the speech frequencies (see Chapter 1).
4. Acquired the hearing impairment prior to or at the age of two years.
5. Had no other educational disabilities.

Data have also been collected on students with normal hearing, Australian deaf children, college level deaf students, and hearing-impaired students from Canada.

Table 8–2 depicts the nine structures assessed by the TSA, the type of task associated with each of the 20 diagnostic tests, and the internal consistency reliability coefficients for 19 of the 20 tests. Table 8–2 shows that the internal consistency relability scores range from .94 to .98. Because these coefficients are higher than the sufficient criterion of .80, it is possible to provide specific diagnostic information regarding the student's performance on the tests. In addition, content validity has also been demonstrated (Owens, Haney, Giesow, Dooley, & Kelly, 1983; Quigley et al., 1978).

Each of the 20 diagnostic tests of the TSA contains 70 multiple-choice items written, in terms of vocabulary, at approximately the first-grade level. The time required for administering a single test ranges from about 35 minutes to 1 hour. Because administering the total battery would take about 10 to 20 hours, the TSA developers constructed two forms of a screening test which requires about 1 hour to administer.

TABLE 8–2. Structures, Types of Tasks, and Internal Reliabilities for the Test of Syntactic Abilities.

Structure	Type of Task	K-R 20
Negation	Recognition & Comprehension	.98
Conjunction		
Conjunction	Recognition & Comprehension	.97
Disjunction & Alternation	Recognition & Comprehension	.96
Determiners	Recognition	.96
Question Formation		
Wh-questions	Recognition	.96
Answer environments	Comprehension	.96
Yes/No questions	Recognition	.97
Verb Processes		
Verb sequence in conjoined structures	Recognition	.97
Main verbs, linking verbs, & auxiliaries	Recognition	.95
Passive voice	Recognition & Comprehension	.97
Pronominalization		
Possessive adjectives	Recognition	.96
Reflexives	Recognition	.96
Possessive Pronouns	Recognition	.96
Forward & backward pronominalization	Recognition	.97
Relativization		
Comprehension	Comprehension	.94
Relative pronouns & adverbs	Recognition	.93
Embedding	Recognition	.96
Complementation		
That-complements	Recognition & Comprehension	.94
Infinitives & gerunds	Recognition	.94
Nominalization	Recognition & Comprehension	—

Source: Adapted from Quigley, Steinkamp, Power, & Jones (1978).

Each screening test contains 120 items, which is representative of the nine syntactic structures contained in the diagnostic tests. The internal consistency reliability coefficients (KR-20) for the two tests are .98, and the coefficients for each of the nine structures ranged from .80 to .87. The reliability indices for each of the nine structures on the screening tests are sufficient for that purpose only—screening. It is suggested that the screening test be administered initially to determine those structures with which test takers have difficulty. On the basis of these results, the examiner can select the relevant diagnostic tests to administer in order to obtain detailed data on a particular structure.

After administering the diagnostic battery, it is possible to engage in both formal and informal interpretation procedures. Relative to formal procedures, the examiner can determine the student's percentile rank, percentile range, and age equivalent scores. Informally, the investigator can calculate the percentage of correct responses for the types of tasks associated with each structure, that is, recognition and comprehension. The same can be done for the types of substructures associated with each of the nine major syntactic structures. For example, the examiner can determine the percentage of correct responses on the Question Formation test for yes/no questions (e.g., *You ate the cookie, didn't you?*) and wh- questions (e.g., *What is your name?*).

There is another interpretation feature of the TSA which provides additional information on deaf students' understanding of syntax. The distractors (incorrect responses in terms of standard English usage) are representative of structures found to appear consistently in the language production of deaf individuals. Thus, by analyzing the incorrect responses, the investigator can ascertain if a particular student consistently selects a deviation from standard English usage that is commonly found among deaf students of comparable age. Along with other diagnostic information on the specific syntactic structure, information on the use of common deviant usages is important for development remediation instructional programs.

Grammatical Analysis of Elicited Language. *The Grammatical Analysis of Elicited Language* (GAEL) was developed at the Central Institute for the Deaf in St. Louis, Missouri. The GAEL has three different levels: the presentence level (GAEL-P; Moog, Kozak, & Geers, 1983), the simple sentence level (GAEL-S; Moog & Geers, 1979), and the complex sentence level (GAEL-C; Moog & Geers, 1980).

With the GAEL-P, the investigator can assess the language-readiness skill of the student. In addition, it is also possible to assess up to three-word combinations in comprehension, production, and imitation tasks with the use of adequate prompts. The GAEL-P was administered to hearing children between the ages of 2 years, 6 months and 3 years, 11 months. It was administered and normed on 150 children with hearing impairment between the ages of 3 years and 5 years, 11 months. Based on the results of 20 hearing-impaired students, the test developers reported test-retest reliability coefficients as follows: .97 for the comprehension task, .95 for the prompted production task, and .93 for the imitation task. The hearing-impaired subjects were identified as "educationally hearing-impaired"; that is, the subjects were too young to provide reliable audiological data reflective of a particular degree of hearing impairment.

With 94 pairs of identical sentences, the purpose of the GAEL-S is to assess the student's ability to produce and imitate specific syntactic structures given adequate prompts. The structures for the GAEL-S were selected from the *Lee Developmental Sentence Scoring* (Lee, 1974) and from *Language Sampling and Analysis* (Tyack & Gottesleben, 1974). Among the structures included were articles, adjectives, quantifiers, possessives, demonstratives, conjunctions, pronouns, nouns in subject and object positions, wh- questions, verbs and verb inflections, copulas and their inflections, prepositions, and negatives.

The GAEL-S was normed on both hearing and hearing-impaired children. The hearing sample included 200 children between the ages of 2 years, 6 months and 5 years old who resided in the St. Louis, Missouri area. The hearing-impaired sample included 200 children between the ages of 5 and 9 years from 13 oral programs for hearing-impaired children in the United States. The children with hearing impairment met the following criteria:

1. Had a hearing impairment greater than 70 dB in the better ear across the speech frequencies (see Chapter 1).
2. Incurred the hearing impairment prior to the age of 2 years.
3. Possessed no additional, educational handicapping conditions.

The test developers reported high reliability and validity scores. To establish validity, the test-developers use statistical analyses to substantiate the effects of age on the specific language variables that were assessed. They also reported a test-retest reliability coefficient of .96 for both the prompted and imitated tasks. The test-retest procedures involved 20 subjects with hearing impairment who were retested after a 30-month interval.

With 88 pairs of identical sentences, the purpose of the GAEL-C is to assess students' production and imitation of complex sentences with the use of adequate prompts. The GAEL-C contains structures such as articles, noun modifiers, nouns in subject and object position, noun plurals, personal pronouns, indefinite and reflexive pronouns, conjunctions, auxiliary verbs, other verbs and verb inflections, infinitives and participles, prepositions, negatives, and wh- questions.

The norming sample of the GAEL-C involved three groups of children. One group was 240 hearing subjects between the ages of 3 years and 5 years, 11 months. There were two groups of children with hearing impairment. One group had 120 children who had hearing losses between 70 and 95 dB and who were between the ages of 8 years and 11 years, 11 months. The second group included 150 children who had hearing losses greater than 95 dB and who were also between the ages of 8 years and 11 years, 11 months.

Using test-retest procedures, 20 children with hearing impairment were retested after a 2-month interval. The test-developers reported reliability coefficients of .96 for the prompted (or production) task and .95 for the imitation task. A sample of 26 hearing children were also retested. The coefficients were .82 for the prompted task and .81 for the imitation task. The test-developers also established statistical validity by correlating the scores with those of other tests which assess both receptive and expressive skills. The test-developers used the subtests of the *Illinois Test of Psycholinguistic Abilities*, the *Northwestern Syntax Screening Test*, the *Peabody Picture Vocabulary Test*, and the *Test for Auditory Comprehension of Language*. Correlations with the subtests of tests assessing receptive skills ranged from .45 to .68. The correlations of the GAEL-C with the tests assessing expressive ability ranged from .83 to .87.

Table 8–3 illustrates a list some tests used to assess the communication skills (e.g., oral, manual, and simultaneous) and achievement areas (e.g., reading and written language) of students with hearing impairment. A good discussion of the strengths and weaknesses of these tests can be found in Bradley-Johnson and Evans (1991).

Free Methods

It is important to obtain information on children's spontaneous use of language through the use of elicitation or prompting procedures such as pictures or video tapes. The goal is to record a large corpus of utterances, typically about 50 to 100. The utterances should be collected in as naturalistic a setting as possible. Several researchers have provided guidelines for collecting informal language samples (e.g., Luetke-Stahlman & Luckner, 1991; Thompson et al., 1987). For example, some suggestions offered are as follows:

- Obtain a sample of each student's language at least two times per year, at the beginning and end of the year.
- Obtain eight to ten utterances of each student's language for 5 days, for a total of 40 to 50 utterances. Make every effort to obtain samples of running discourse.

TABLE 8-3. List of Tests used to Assess Achievement Areas of Students with Hearing Impairment

Achievement Tests

Test	Brief Description
Carolina Picture Vocabulary Test	Can be used with students, age 5 to 12 years old; focuses on vocabulary skill; norm-referenced (Layton & Holmes, 1985)
CID Phonetic Inventory	Can be used with children at any age; focuses on the ability to produce phonemes; results can be used as part of program planning (Moog, 1988).
Rhode Island Test of Language Structure	Can be used with students, age 5 to 17 years old; focuses on syntax; norm-referenced (Engen & Engen, 1983).
Test of Early Reading Ability —Deaf and Hard of Hearing	Can be used with children age 3 to 12 years old; focuses on a selection of reading skills; norm-referenced (Reid, Hresko, Hammill, & Wiltshire, 1991).
Total Communication Receptive Vocabulary	Can be used with students, age 3 to 12 years old; focuses on reception of vocabulary; norm-referenced (Scherer, 1981).
Written Language Syntax Test	Can be used with students age 10 to 17 years old; focuses on syntax; scores can be used for program planning (Berry, 1981).

Source: Adapted from Bradley-Johnson & Evans (1991).

- Each day obtain the eight to ten utterances at different times when the student is communicating with different people in different circumstances so that you sample *use* of language in different contexts.
- Always record some continuous dialogue because this will help you to evaluate discourse strategies the student is using.

- Don't talk too much yourself. The goal is to get the student to do the talking.
- Use questions like "What happened next?" "What do you think will happen?" or "That's interesting. What else can you tell me?"
- Be sure to use the Pragmatic Checklist, the Kendall Communicative Scale, or any other scale, checklist, etc. that will supplement your grammatical analyses of the language sample and assist you in reviewing how your student *uses* language. (Thompson et al., 1987, pp. 103–105)

Strengths and Weaknesses

Perhaps the greatest advantage of free method procedures is the assumption that if a child consistently produces a specific structure, then she or he must have knowledge or competency of that structure. Another advantage is that the interpretation of the data is based on the student's own linguistic features in comparison with other student's language productions rather than with norms (e.g., percentile, age, or grade equivalent scores).

There are a number of limitations associated with the use of free methods. These limitations should be interpreted from the framework of the scientific method, which strives for the condition of objectivity. For example, one limitation is the amount of subjectivity or idiosyncracy. There is a danger of "reading into the data" those factors that are of interest to the examiner; this is much more evident than with the use of more controlled methods. To limit the effects of subjectivity, it is recommended that the examiner who performs the analyses undergo extensive training.

Another difficulty involves the notion of reliability. With the small number of subjects, it is impossible statistically to assess reliability using test-retest, equivalent forms, or internal consistency coefficients. Examiners must rely on the concepts of inter- and intrarater reliability coefficients, which are often used in single-subject designs.

The use of free methods with children with hearing impairment present additional difficulties. For example, it is difficult to record the utterances of children with severe to profound impairment. There is the likelihood that their speech would be unintelligible, rendering the data difficult to analyze. It is possible to record the signing utterances of the individuals. However, because of the nature and use of signing in the home and schools, the analysis of this phenomenon is no less problematic (see discussion of signing behavior in Chapter 4).

The substitution of written language samples for spoken or signed utterances does not resolve this difficulty. Although useful information can be gleaned from analyses of written language productions (see Chapter 5), this information is not the same as that which is obtained from spoken or signed utterances. In addition, the written language samples of both hearing and deaf individuals are typically more limited in scope than the primary mode utterances (spoken and/or signed).

Analysis Procedures

There are several analysis procedures that can be used. It is possible to use terms that have been employed in describing the written language of deaf students, specifically within the paradigm of the "products" of writing (e.g., Cooper & Rosenstein, 1966; see also, the discussion in Chapter 5). These terms include productivity, complexity, flexibility, distribution of parts of speech, and grammatical correctness. Other analysis procedures, designed for analyzing spoken utterances, include mean length of utterance (MLU), developmental sentence types (Lee, 1966, 1974), developmental sentence scoring (Lee, 1974), and others (e.g., Bloom and Lahey approach; Kretschmer spontaneous language analysis procedure).

We have discussed what can be called traditional grammar analysis procedures relative to written language productions in Chapter 5. For example, productivity (Heider & Heider, 1940; Myklebust, 1960) refers to two measures: the average number of words written in a sample and the mean length of the sentences in the sample. The notion of complexity has three measures: (1) ratio of simple sentences to compound, complex, and compound-complex sentences (division procedures); (2) the number of subordinate clauses per main clause; and (3) the T-unit—defined as "one main clause plus all subordinate clauses attached or embedded in it" (Hunt, 1965, p. 141; see discussion of the works of Marshall and Quigley, 1970, and Taylor, 1969, in Chapter 5). Another example is flexibility which involves the use of a type-token ratio for assessing vocabulary diversity. This ratio is calculated by dividing the total number of different words by the total number of words in a 50-utterance sample. The distribution of parts of speech refers to the use of different parts of speech, obtained by dividing the number of occurrences of a part of speech (e.g., verbs) by the total number of words in the sample.

The last category to be discussed is correctness. This category refers to the errors or deviations from standard English usage. Two approaches have been developed. The first approach entails the use of frequency counts for the types of errors found in the written language samples of children with hearing impairment (e.g., Myklebust, 1960). This approach does not have much theoretical or educational significance.

The second approach is an extension of the first one and is more informative and useful because of the attempt to describe the types of errors. For example, Taylor (1969; see also the discussion in Chapter 5) described "the rules violated in the production of any deviant or nongrammatical structures" (p. 45). The researcher noted that deaf students frequently omitted direct objects. However, Taylor also analyzed this phenomenon relative to the linguistic environments in which the omissions occurred at different grade levels. She reported the omissions at the third-grade level appeared, primarily, in simple sentences containing transitive verbs. At the fifth- and seventh-grade levels, however, the omissions of direct objects occurred most frequently in conjoined sentences. At the ninth-grade level, the deaf students produced omissions in complementized sentences, which are more complex structures. Thus, it was found that the frequency of occurrence of direct-object omissions did not decrease as the students advanced in school grades. Nevertheless, the analysis of the linguistic environments in which the omissions occurred did indicate that the student's levels of syntactic complexity were increasing and this contributed to the errors.

Mean Length of Utterance (MLU). The MLU refers to the average number of morphemes per utterance in a sample of 100 utterances (see Brown, 1973). A morpheme is the minimal unit of meaning in language. For example, the word *cat* contains one morpheme, whereas the word *cats* contains two morphemes—*cat* and the plural *-s*. Guidelines for calculating the MLU include (see discussion in Brown, 1973):

1. Compound words (e.g., bluebird, hot dog) and proper names (e.g., Joe, Jane, Jeremiah) count as single morphemes.
2. Irregular past tense verbs (e.g., ran, saw) count as one morpheme.
3. Auxiliaries (e.g., can, must, should) and inflectional morphemes (e.g., possessives, plurals, third-person singulars, regular past-tense verb endings, and progressive aspect endings) count as separate morphemes.

For children with MLUs of five or less, this procedure is a good index of syntactic development. For example, Miller (1981) has reported on predicted chronological ages from the MLU for hearing children. Thus, it is possible to compare the MLUs of children with disabilities, including deafness, with those provided by Miller.

There are several problems, however, with using the MLU procedure in other situations. For example, it is not a reliable index of syntax for children with MLUs over five. With the emergence and frequency of conjoined structures, it is possible to overestimate children's MLUs relative to their language development. Blackwell et al. (1978) have reported additional difficulties. One, the length of the utterance measures obscure differences in syntactic and semantic complexity. Two, the MLU does not provide information regarding children's functional use of the language.

Three, relative to children with hearing impairment, it is debatable to assume that a deaf child with a MLU of 2.3 (Brown's Stage II) displays the same linguistic features as a hearing child at the same stage of development (see discussions in Chapters 4 and 5).

Developmental Sentence Types (DST).   The DST is used to assess the "pre-sentence" stage of language development (Lee, 1966, 1974). It should be used when less than 50% of the child's utterances contain both a subject and a predicate. After collecting a language sample consisting of at least 50 utterances, the utterances can be described relative to a chart which contains three "horizontal" dimensions and five "vertical" dimensions. The three horizontal dimensions are single words, two-word combinations, and multiword constructions. The five vertical dimensions are noun phrases, designative phrases, predicative sentences, subject-verb sentences, and fragments. The DST is based on the debatable assumption that children first learn simple active, affirmative, declarative sentences and then learn to apply transformations to these sentences (see discussion in Kretschmer & Kretschmer, 1978).

Developmental Sentence Scoring (DSS).   The DSS is used when more than 50% of the child's utterances contain both a subject and a predicate (Lee, 1974; Lee & Canter, 1971). In general, the utterances are rated relative to eight grammatical categories: indefinite pronouns or noun modifiers, personal pronouns, main verbs, secondary verbs, negatives, conjunctions, interrogative reversals, and wh- questions. The test-developers constructed a scale of 1 to 8 for the categories. For example, the examiner assigns one point for first- and second-person pronouns. For pronouns such as *oneself*, the examiner assigns seven points. The total number of points for the utterances are divided by 50 (number of utterances). This score can be compared with the norms available for children between the ages of 2 to 6 years. Similar to the DST, the DSS does not consider semantic and pragmatic aspects.

Bloom and Lahey Approach.   Bloom and Lahey (1978) developed procedures which focus on both syntactic (form) and semantic (content) features. The researchers identified 21 semantic features which interact in a hierarchical manner with eight syntactic features within a "phase" framework. For example, Phases 1 and 2, which correspond approximately to one- and two-word utterances, contain the semantic features of existence, nonexistence, recurrence, rejection, denial, attribution, possession, action, and locative action. Phase 3 utterances include the semantic features in Phases 1 and 2 as well as locative state, state, and quantity. Phase 4 utterances include the semantic features of notice and time, and Phase 5 includes the features of coordinate, causality, dative, and specifier. Phases 6 through 8 contained complex sentences, syntactic connectives, modal verbs, and relative clauses in this order. The semantic features of these phases include epistemic, mood, and antithesis. For complete descriptions of all categories, the reader should consult Bloom and Lahey (1978). With this procedure, it is possible to obtain a fairly complete picture of the child's language development (pragmatics included). Nevertheless, this procedure demands a great deal of time because of the number of utterances required (200).

Kretschmer Spontaneous Language Analysis. Kretschmer and Kretschmer (1978) have developed a very extensive and comprehensive procedure for studying the free spontaneous language samples of children with hearing impairment. The procedures can be used for both spoken and signed utterances as well as for written language samples. Although similar in many respects to Bloom's and Lahey's procedure, there are three notable differences: (1) this technique is not dependent on the quantitative measures of MLU; (2) there is a more extensive treatment of semantic categories in Kretschmers' procedure; and (3) there are strategies for describing the atypical language performance of children with hearing impairment.

There are six sections of the Kretschmer and Kretschmer analysis protocol. Each section is described as follows:

1. Descriptive information on the preverbal level of the student.
2. Tallying syntactic and semantic features for the one- and two-word stage.
3. Syntactic and semantic descriptions for single prepositions.
4. Syntactic descriptions for complex sentences.
5. Communication competence of the child.
6. Isolation of structures that differ from standard English.

Similar to the Bloom and Lahey procedure, the procedure by Kretschmer and Kretschmer can be used to obtain a fairly complete description of the language development of children with hearing impairment. The two main limitations are (1) the amount of time required to complete the assessment, and (2) the amount of linguistic knowledge required of the examiner.

Teacher Assessment of Grammatical Structures (TAGS). To accompany the GAEL tests, discussed in the section on Controlled Methods, Moog and Kozak (1983) have developed procedures for analyzing the spontaneous language productions of children with hearing impairment. Thus, there is a protocol for each of the three GAEL tests. The analysis protocol indicates whether the student has acquired or is in the process of acquiring a particular structure under consideration, relative to specified levels of competence. With the exception of the presentence level, each rating form (i.e., analysis protocol) contains levels of imitated, prompted, and spontaneous productions.

The TAGS procedures for each level (i.e., TAGS-P; TAGS-S; TAG-C) consist of analyses of six grammatical categories described as follows: TAGS-P: single words, two-word combinations, three-word combinations, wh- questions, pronouns, and tense markers; TAGS-S: noun modifiers, pronouns, prepositions, adverbs, verbs, and questions; and TAGS-C: nouns, pronouns, verb inflections, secondary verbs, conjunctions, and questions. The six categories of each TAG procedure are also divided into six levels, indicating increasing syntactic complexity.

Other Procedures

Relative to elicited and spontaneous language samples, a number of investigators have described procedures that focus on the widely quoted Bloom and Lahey terms, namely, form, content, and use (e.g., Luetke-Stahlman & Luckner, 1991; Thompson et al., 1987). Despite attempts to use both formal and informal assessments in describing the language performance of students with hearing impairment (e.g., Moeller, 1988), there seems to be a strong movement toward the use of informal, context-bound pragmatics assessments. As eloquently described by Duchan:

> Like Buffalo chicken wings, pragmatics can be bought in its mild, medium, or hot versions. The mild version takes pragmatics as a new aspect of language which needs to be assessed along with our traditional assessment approaches . . .
>
> Those with medium tastes . . . will willingly abandoned their standardized procedures and look at the child's language in light of its intentions, and listener and situational appropriateness. However, they still hold to the idea that language is what they are studying, and context is what is influencing it.
>
> The hot version . . . opt for overthrowing our previous conceptions that language is what we are assessing, and propose that we move toward a new conceptualization which examines communication and context, and if called for, the language within it. The hot view is the one that must be embraced if we are to take seriously what the literature in pragmatics has to tell us. (Duchan, 1984, pp. 177–178)

ASSESSMENT ISSUES FOR BILINGUALISM AND SECOND-LANGUAGE LEARNING

In this section, we provide a brief overview of assessment issues for students in bilingual or second-language learning programs. This information is based on theory and research with hearing individuals (e.g., Beardsmore, 1986; Cummins, 1984; McLaughlin, 1985, 1987; Verhoeven, 1992). As indicated in Chapter 6, there is a compelling need to develop language assessments for deaf children, particularly those students who might be candidates for a bilingual and/or English-as-a-second-language learning program. It is also important to develop an assessment for individuals who desire to become teachers in bilingual programs. Relative to deaf students and interested teachers, the major focus has been on the development and implementation of programs that entail the use of ASL and English. There is a need to consider the establishment of programs for other types of minority-language deaf students, for examples, students who reside in homes in which Spanish or German is the native language.

Approaches to the Assessment of Language

Similar to the approaches to language assessment in the first language, second-language or bilingual assessment has also been influenced by theories of language acquisition (see Chapter 6). These influences have engendered a number of controversies regarding the types, purposes, and methods of assessment, for example, the use of discrete-point versus integrative measures (e.g., McLaughlin, 1985).

A number of tests have been developed to determine degree of bilingualism in hearing individuals (see discussions in Cummins, 1984; McLaughlin, 1985, 1987). These tests can be described according to the categories used previously for first-language assessment, for example, direct versus indirect measures. Nevertheless, research reviews reveal that many of these tests suffer from difficulties in reliability and validity (Beardsmore, 1986; Cummins, 1984; McLaughlin, 1985).

A good example of these difficulties has been provided by McLaughlin (1985). This description refers to some tests designed to measure language dominance.

> For example, the Crane Oral Dominance Test consists of a memory task in which children are given 8 words, 4 in English and 4 in Spanish. The children are to recall the words, and if they recall more Spanish words, they are regarded as Spanish-dominant; if they recall more English words, they are thought to be English dominant. However, it is questionable to assert that recall for vocabulary items measures language dominance. (McLaughlin, 1985, p. 204)

Language Dominance

Although the trend is toward the use of language proficiency tests within the framework of interactionist theories (see Chapter 2), much of the debate has focused on the distinction between language dominance and language proficiency (Cummins, 1984; McLaughlin, 1985; Verhoeven, 1992). In any case, there is no wide agreement on what constitutes language dominance and language proficiency.

The concept of language dominance seems to be concerned with the degree of bilingualism. That is, researchers attempted to compare the individual's levels of skills in two or more languages. As illustrated in the example by McLaughlin (1985) discussed previously, one goal is to determine which language is dominant. The overall goal is to ascertain degree of bilingualism based on an assessment of the individual's ability on certain language elements in the languages involved.

Historically, the preoccupation with the notion of language dominance was considered to be important for the development and implementation of bilingual programs (e.g., see discussion in McLaughlin, 1985). That is, ascertaining language dominance was critical for identification of students and faculty for bilingual programs, the initial language for further testing and possibly instruction, and the requirements for funding, such as program evaluation and needs assessment.

In addition to the general characteristics of tests used, a number of theorists and researchers have proffered several criticisms on the concept of language dominance (e.g., see discussions in Cummins, 1984; McLaughlin, 1985; Verhoeven, 1992). In essence, the notion of dominance is not a one-language-or-the-other-only phenomenon. For example, consider the case in which an individual is exposed to both English and French. It is possible for the individual to be English dominant in some situations and French dominant in other situations. In addition, the individual might be English dominant in the use of syntax, but French dominant in the area of pronunciation. This major criticism has led to the growing use of the term, language proficiency, and the development of more pragmatic-oriented assessment (e.g., see Cummins, 1984).

Language Proficiency

As with language dominance, there is little consensus regarding the nature of language proficiency (e.g., McLaughlin, 1985, 1987; Verhoeven, 1992). It seems that language proficiency refers to the individual's degree of competence in one language, that is, the relative proficiency in both languages (e.g., Cummins, 1984). The current debate on language proficiency seems to center on the question of whether language proficiency is a unitary concept.

Oller and his collaborators (Oller, 1979; Oller & Perkins, 1978, 1980) have argued for a global language proficiency factor, analogous to Spearman's *g* factor in intelligence testing. This global factor is said to account for variance in a wide variety of language measures. It can be measured via the use of tasks that involve listening, speaking, reading, and writing and is correlated with measures of academic achievement and IQ tests, both verbal and nonverbal measures. Most of Oller's data comes from literacy-related tasks, for example, written cloze tests.

A number of theorists and researchers have argued against the global language proficiency model (e.g., Cummins, 1984; see also, the discussion in Verhoeven, 1992). A widely cited "dichotomous" model has been the one developed by Cummins (1984). This model has been used also in discussions of bilingual programs for deaf students (e.g., Luetke-Stahlman & Luckner, 1991).

Cummins categorized the performances of language learners into two groups, which were originally labeled as cognitive/academic language proficiency (CALP) and basic interpersonal communicative skills (BICS). CALP referred to general cognitive or academic skills, for example, knowledge of vocabulary and syntax. BICS referred to the use of language and interpersonal communication. This dichotomous model is the basis for the theoretical foundation of Cummins' interdependence hypothesis, discussed in Chapter 6. In essence, Cummins argued that surface features developed separately in the two languages; however, there is an underlying cognitive/academic proficiency that is common across the languages.

Cummins' CALP/BICS distinction has been misinterpreted as a distinction between cognitive and communicative aspects of language proficiency. This misinterpretation has led to Cummins' disuse of the terminology (e.g., see McLaughlin, 1985). The intent of Cummins' model was to make a distinction between proficiency in communicative-related tasks (as in face to face contextualized conversations) and proficiency in literacy-related tasks as in reading, writing, and academic subjects.

Cummins' thinking on language proficiency, particularly the dichotomous model, is applicable not only to the establishment of bilingual programs for deaf students, but also to account, in part, for their low academic achievement levels. For example, most students with severe to profound hearing impairment do not possess an adequate level of language proficiency in English on entering school and, in many cases, on graduation from high school (King & Quigley, 1985; Moores, 1987; Paul & Quigley, 1990). In essence, deaf students are expected to acquire academic knowledge via the use of a language of instruction (i.e., English) in which they might have little or no communicative competence. That is, they are expected to engage in the extremely difficult task of learning the academic language and acquiring academic content simultaneously.

In sum, despite the lack of a general consensus on the nature of language proficiency, this concept has engendered changes in the field of second-language instruction and assessment. It has become clear that assessing the language of bilingual children is much more difficult than assessing that of monolingual children. Whether the new conceptual framework for assessing language proficiency is on the right track is currently being debated. The remarks by McLaughlin (1985) are still relevant today (e.g., see discussion in Verhoeven & de Jong, 1992):

> The point was made earlier that the increased interest in integrative tests, the development of communicative competence models, and the influence of sociolinguists and ethnographers on language assessment all reflect a common *Zeitgeist*. In the last decade or so, many researchers and teachers have become convinced that traditional approaches to measuring language proficiency are not fair to many children, especially those from minority-language backgrounds. Whether these developments in assessment will provide practitioners with the tools they need to assess minority-language children fairly remains to be seen. (McLaughlin, 1985, p. 223)

FINAL REMARKS

This chapter attempted to establish the importance of language assessment to language instruction and curriculum. The teacher and clinician should not only employ the use of language assessment, but also they should ensure that there is a strong interrelationship among theory, assessment, instruction, and curriculum. It is also important for teachers and clinicians to receive training in assessment so that they can effectively evaluate the merits of their instructional practices and materials.

The chapter provided an overview of the types, purposes, methods, and characteristics of assessment. The controversies on types and methods are related strongly to the controversies on the nature of language acquisition. Relative to the characteristics of a good assessment, we discussed issues such as reliability, validity, and practicality.

A considerable portion of the chapter was devoted to the use of controlled and free methods, including the strengths and weaknesses and a discussion of a representative sample of tests in each area. This presentation should have emphasized the danger of using only *one* test for language acquisition (or for any other domain). Thus, the teacher and/or clinician should use combinations of controlled and free methods and a wide variety of tests and techniques.

There is an urgent need to develop language assessments for deaf students and teachers who might be candidates for a bilingual education program. Such tests are useful not only for evaluating the languages used, but also for evaluating the effectiveness of a program, as discussed in Chapter 6. It needs to be underscored that the development of any assessment should be based on the prevailing thinking on language development.

Relative to developing tests, there is a great need for tests that are normed on individuals with severe to profound hearing impairment. The construction of such tests is not an easy matter, given the fact that this population contains a number of subgroups with varying characteristics. Nevertheless, further research is needed in this area. One of the overall goals of this research effort has been eloquently stated:

It is hoped that significant improvements will be made in the psychoeducational assessment of hearing-impaired students so that it will be possible to make a more helpful contribution to the education of these students. (Bradley-Johnson & Evans, 1991, p. 218)

FURTHER READINGS

Carroll, B., & Hall, P. (1985). *Make your own language tests: A practical guide to writing language performance tests.* Oxford: Pergamon.

Lincoln, Y., & Guba, E. (1985). *Naturalistic inquiry.* Beverly Hills, CA: Sage.

Oller, J. (Ed.). (1983). *Issues in language testing research.* Rowley, MA: Newbury House.

Owen, D. (1985). *None of the above: Behind the myth of scholastic aptitude.* Boston, MA: Houghton Mifflin.

Phillips, J. (1988). *How to think about statistics.* New York: Freeman.

Worthen, B., & Sanders, J. (1987). *Educational evaluation: Alternative approaches and practical guidelines.* White Plains, NY: Longman.

CHAPTER 9

CONCLUSION

But what are these fundamentals? One and one only! Language, and then language-spoken, spelled, or written-and the power to read, and the power to understand what is read. Other requirements will then follow more easily and with greater results than now attained. (Johnson, 1916, p. 95)

A number of inferences can be made regarding the passage above. Only three are stated here, and these provide the conceptual framework for our discussion in this concluding chapter. First, there is an intricate reciprocal relationship between language (conversational and written) and cognition. Second, the development of English reading and writing skills is dependent, in part, on a deep knowledge of the alphabet system—the system on which written language is based. This knowledge entails, at least, an understanding of the morphophonological system of English. Finally, it is important, perhaps critical, to achieve a high level of proficiency in the conversational form of a language at as early an age as possible. This is due to the pervasive effects of language on all subsequent aspects of cognitive, social, and academic developments.

In this text, we attempted to address these three inferences relative to students with severe to profound hearing impairment. These students represent the subgroups of the population of hearing-impaired students who have had the most difficulty in acquiring a spoken language such as English—the language of mainstream society in the United States. As stated in Chapter 1, it is important to define the sample under consideration to avoid overgeneralizations of research results and to develop relevant and effective instructional practices and curricular materials (see also, Quigley & Kretschmer, 1982).

Relative to our three inferences, we can provide tentative answers to two broad questions, which are motivated by the ones asked by King (1981):

1. How do deaf students learn the conversational form of a language?
2. How well do deaf students learn both (a) the conversational forms of English and American Sign Language (ASL) and (b) the written form of English?

In addition to addressing these questions, we provide our reflections on the development of literate thought in deaf individuals, an issue we raised in Chapter 5 on literacy. Literate thought refers to the development of critical and reflective thought.

The *How Do* question refers to both the acquisition of the conversational form of English (speech and/or sign) and of ASL (manual and nonmanual aspects). In the *How Well* question, we attempt to discuss and compare the development of English literacy skills in deaf students with that of hearing students. Related to these questions is the notion of a critical period for learning a language. Relative to this notion, we address whether it is possible to state that either English or ASL should be the "first" language for most, perhaps all, deaf students. Finally, in dealing with the notion of literate thought, we discuss briefly the interrelations among language, literacy, and literate thought. This discussion is influenced by our support of a social-cognitive interactive perspective of language comprehension. This perspective was discussed briefly in Chapter 7 and was the impetus for the examples of language and literacy activities presented in that chapter.

HOW DO

The *HOW DO* question refers to the development and use of language intervention systems with deaf students in infancy, early childhood, and during the school years. As indicated in Chapter 1, this pertains to the representation of English in some form or to the use of ASL. This does not refer to the use of language-teaching methods, for example, natural, structural, and eclectic (McAnally et al., 1987, in press; Quigley & Paul, in press). The main goal is to enable fluent and intelligible communication to occur between deaf students and significant others. This in turns leads to the internalization of a language for communication, thought, and expression.

Language and Communication Intervention Systems

As indicated in Chapter 4, there appears to be three ways to enable deaf students to develop a self-controlling, communication system. Descriptions of the three ways have been provided:

> The first way would be to repair the defective auditory component to the extent that the auditory-articulatory mechanisms would be a functional communication system. The second way would be to use the auditory-articulatory mechanisms as much as possible and to supplement them with the visual-manual mechanisms. The third way would be to substitute other physiological mechanisms for the auditory-articulatory mechanisms, such as vision for audition and manual for articulation. This would result in a communication system based on visual-motor mechanisms. Each of these three ways is the basis for a majority of approaches to educating deaf children—oral-aural, total communication, and American Sign Language. (Quigley & Paul, in press, p. xxx)

Both the oral and total communication (TC) methods are concerned with the representation and development of the conversational form of English. Oral methods employ the use of speech, speech reading, and residual hearing and can be grouped into two broad categories: unisensory and multisensory. In general, unisensory refers to the use and reliance on one sense, typically, audition, whereas multisensory approaches employ the use of two or more senses, which include, at least, audition and vision. Cued speech can be labeled as a multisensory oral approach. The "manual" system of cued speech was designed to represent the phonological system of a language (i.e., vowels and consonants), whereas the various signed systems were designed to represent the morphosyntactic aspects of *written* standard English in the United States (Paul & Quigley, 1990; Wilbur, 1987).

Although many public-school programs employ the use of oral methods, the exemplary programs seem to be those that exist at comprehensive, intensive oral-education schools such as the Central Institute for the Deaf and the St. Joseph School for the Deaf, both in St. Louis, Missouri (Connor, 1986; Ogden, 1979; Paul & Quigley, 1990). It has been hypothesized that the oral components of these programs—that is, speech training, speech reading training, and the exploitation of residual hearing—are much more focused, extensive, and comprehensive than those which have been reported in "typical" oral education programs in regular public schools. It might also be that students who attend these "exemplary" oral programs represent a select group, with higher-than-average IQs, high socioeconomic backgrounds, and highly motivated and involved parents. Nevertheless, both of these points are controversial and debatable (e.g. see discussions in Geers & Moog, 1989; Luetke-Stahlman, 1988a; Quigley & Kretschmer, 1982).

Most educational programs for deaf students adhere to the philosophy of total communication, which has been the dominant philosophy since the early 1970s (Moores, 1987; Paul & Quigley, 1990). TC approaches entail the use of two forms, oral and manual, and aspects of two languages, English and ASL. These forms and languages can be combined in various ways to produce manually coded English systems such as the Rochester method, the SEE systems, and Signed English. The various signed systems are supposed to be used in conjunction with speech. Despite the elements common across the systems, each system operates according to its own set of rules for forming and using signs. Although the signed systems use signs from ASL, the ASL syntactic and semantic constraints of these signs are violated in order to represent the written language structure of English. As discussed later, the critical issues are: how well English can be represented manually and the quality of this representation as compared with the use of speech.

There is a sign communication system which does not specifically adhere to a set of rules: English-like signing, also known as Pidgin sign English, sign English, manual English, signed English, and simultaneous communication. Essentially, this is the use of ASL-like signs in an English word order. English-like signing seems to be the most prevalent form of sign communication used in the schools. Similar to other "pidgins," this sign communication form does not, nor was it intended to, represent the complete grammatical structure of the two languages on which it is based: English and American Sign Language.

The third way refers to the use of ASL as a language-intervention system, particularly in a bilingual or English-as-second-language program. Some deaf students are reared in homes in which ASL is either the "mother tongue" or is used as one of the primary conversational language as in bilingual homes. However, it is suspected that most students with severe to profound hearing impairment acquire ASL via interactions with other native- or near-native student users. This is most likely to occur at residential schools which are the bastion of Deaf Culture and ASL. In any case, there is some evidence that deaf residential students are more proficient in ASL than their public-school peers (e.g., Luetke-Stahlman, 1984).

There is no question that some deaf students know ASL as their primary conversational language, and that many others, perhaps most, acquire ASL by the time they reach adulthood. The debate centers on whether ASL-using deaf students can learn English as a second language or achieve a higher proficiency in English than non-ASL using deaf students. Even more debatable is the "radical" position espoused by some researchers (e.g., Johnson et al., 1989) that ASL should be the "first" language developed in *all* deaf students—that is, *deaf* is defined as all students with hearing impairment. The focus of the Johnson et al. group is on the notion of "accessibility." In other words, the school curriculum is inaccessible to deaf students because of their difficulty with the conversational and written forms of English. Via the use and development of ASL, it is argued that deaf students can access the school curriculum and develop English as a second language. These issues are discussed further in the HOW WELL section of the chapter.

Other Issues

Another perspective on this "how do" issue, especially in relation to the use of manually coded English, can be obtained from a discussion of the notion of "world of vision versus world of audition." Educational and clinical experience have shown that beyond some level of hearing impairment (modified by the interaction of other factors such as IQ and SES) even the best amplification and utilization of residual hearing provide only extremely limited feedback in speech production. Hearing impairment is certainly a continuum as measured on a decibel scale. However, at some point on that continuum an individual ceases to be linked to the world of communication, to any useful extent, primarily by hearing and becomes linked to it primarily by vision. At this point, the term deaf can be usefully applied to individuals who must process the language by eye. This term should distinguish this group from the vast majority of hearing-impaired individuals who can, with appropriate amplification and training, process it by ear.

This is a critical distinction, and it is not always made. Furthermore, this distinction begs the question of whether a spoken language such as English can be processed by the eye—that is, by visual-manual mechanisms. In addition, it can be asked whether it is possible to represent English via the use of visual-manual mechanisms such as the use of manually coded English systems. It has been remarked that:

> Whether an individual is linked predominantly to the world of audition or to that of vision may be instrumental in explaining many of the research findings on language, cognition, and academic achievement. For example, one of the most important educational questions . . . is: Can students connected predominantly to the world of vision learn a spoken language in any form—that is, in the primary (speech and/or sign) and/or secondary (literacy) modes? . . . . Does the type of linkage, audition or vision, have important implications for the acquisition of a particular form of language at as early an age as possible? (Paul & Jackson, 1993, p. 29)

Finally, to shed more light on this distinction, it is necessary for future researchers to focus on providing an "explanation" (i.e., explanatory adequacy) of the language development of deaf students and of the representativeness of the language-intervention system. This was the focus of Chapter 2. Much of the research on language and deafness has been focused on a description of the language development relative to the various communication systems. Although this type of information is important, it is not sufficient for developing sound instructional practices and curricular materials.

HOW WELL

A synthesis of the information presented in Chapters 3 to 6 provides some insights for the "how well" issue. These insights can be presented relative to the development of the conversational form of English via the use of oral and TC approaches and via the use of ASL. We also discuss the acquisition of English literacy skills, either in English as a first language or English as a second language.

Language and Communication Approaches

One of the themes of this book is that the primary language development of deaf children can only be considered in terms of the communication form by which it is developed and through which it finds expression. This means that primary language development has to be considered in terms of oral English (OE), manually coded English (MCE), including English-like signing, or PSE, and American Sign Language (ASL). Much of the material in Chapter 4, relative to language development and deafness, is organized in this manner. It is obvious from the presentation that there is only a very limited amount of data on the effectiveness of these forms. In addition, there is limited information on the use of these communication forms by members of different ethnic groups which constitutes either bilingualism or multilingualism (see discussion in Chapter 6).

Oral English

The studies cited in OE (including cued speech) involved those deaf students in indisputably oral programs or those integrated into the regular classroom. In general, it was found that the conversational (and written language) development of these students is qualitatively similar to but quantitatively slower than that of hearing students. However, a good number of these deaf students performed on grade level with their hearing peers.

It might be difficult to generalize these results to other deaf students on two counts, at least: (1) an active, comprehensive oral approach to language development might be present only in a few educational programs; and (2) deaf students in these problems might be members of a more select group, especially in relation to IQ, socioeconomic status, and highly educated and motivated parents than deaf students in other programs. Despite these two points, these studies do indicate that deaf students in incontestably oral programs or those select few integrated into regular classrooms develop superior language and academic skills compared to those in the general school population. It should be underscored that very few deaf students can acquire a high level of English proficiency in oral programs. It seems that this language-intervention approach does not enable most deaf students to develop and use an automatic, self-controlling auditory-articulatory system similar to that of normal-hearing students (Quigley & Paul, in press). It might be that case that improvements in instructional techniques need to occur in tandem with improvements in technology for the perception of speech stimuli (e.g., cochlea implants, regeneration of the auditory nerve).

Manually Coded English

Most of the MCE approaches cited in this text have been in use for 20 years or longer. Nevertheless, very little educational success has been reported. Almost all the studies indicate that certain aspects of English grammar, for example, morphology, can be taught through a particular approach. The studies demonstrating the most success (e.g., Babb, 1979; Brasel & Quigley, 1977; Luetke-Stahlman, 1988a; Washburn, 1983) indicate that certain conditions are necessary for this level of achievement, for example: (1) active involvement in the home and school; (2) instruction which adheres to the developmental patterns of hearing children; and (3) the use of a manual form that is considered a more complete representation of English, such as the SEE systems—seeing essential English and signing exact English.

Relative to condition 3, it seems that educational programs should consider the adoption of systems such as seeing essential English (SEE I) or signing exact English (SEE II) because these are considered most representative of English in the manual mode. In addition, there have been some impressive results from students exposed to these systems. Nevertheless, it is surprising that most programs for students with hearing impairment use a form of signing that could be labeled English-like signing (or pidgin sign English), even though this form of signing has not been supported by recent research (e.g. see reviews in Luetke-Stahlman & Luckner, 1991; Paul & Quigley, 1990). The use of this system, commonly referred to as simultaneous communication, might be based on reasons other than research effectiveness.

From another perspective, it is difficult to evaluate the usefulness of approaches most representative of English (e.g., SEE I, SEE II) because it has been reported that many practitioners do not adhere strictly to the rules of the systems for forming and using signs (e.g., Kluwin, 1981; Marmor & Petitto, 1979; Strong & Charlson, 1987). This situation is said to be due to the incompatibility of signing and speaking simultaneously, resulting in the omission of signs and/or sign markers. This results in an impoverished language model for deaf students and calls into question the usefulness of the MCE systems (e.g., Luetke-Stahlman, 1991; Maxwell, 1990).

A number of other criticisms have been made concerning the English-based signed systems, for example, the lack of a community of users outside the school system and the presence of processing constraints for many deaf students. Relative to the last criticism, Gee and Goodhart (1988) have reported that deaf students alter the grammatical (morphological and syntactic elements) of the various MCE systems. These alterations occur because the rate of sign execution within the MCE systems is much slower than both the expressive and receptive capacities of deaf students.

In essence, these criticisms seem to suggest that the acquisition of ASL (or any sign language) is easier than the acquisition of any signed system based on a spoken language such as English. In addition, they seem to call into question whether English can be acquired at a proficient level by most students with severe to profound hearing impairment. We agree with Johnson et al. (1989) that one critical issue is that of accessibility. There needs to be a better understanding of how much and what deaf children and adolescents are accessing (or "acquiring") when they are exposed to either the oral or manual forms of English.

Developing models of accessibility might be the next progressive step in obtaining a more comprehensive picture of the language acquisition process. Insights gained from the accessibility models should complement what is known about language development based on the language acquisition models. Relative to individuals with hearing impairment, the accessibility issue is concerned with specific types of "linguistic" information that is or can be captured by the ear or the eye and what is meant by the perception of linguistic information presented simultaneously (i.e., speaking and signing simultaneously).

The work of Maxwell (see the brief discussion in Chapter 4) seems to imply that the presentation of English via a simultaneous mode (i.e., speaking and signing) is complete when it is analyzed at the semantic or meaning level, even though there are gaps at the morphologic and syntactic level. That is, some practitioners tend to omit certain signs with morphological and syntactic properties. Assuming the correctness of Maxwell's conclusion, it is still not clear what deaf students perceive when they are exposed to simultaneous presentations. Much of the research has been on the comparisons of sign systems on a global level (e.g., reading and educational achievement). For example, it is still not known how much and what information deaf students are acquiring relative to the major components of English: phonology, morphology, syntax, and semantics via the use of the various signed systems. Are deaf students acquiring or internalizing the necessary suprasegmental information such as intonation and stress? It is often forgotten that an intuitive knowledge of the phonology of English means an intuitive knowledge of both segmentals (phonemes) and suprasegmentals. According to social-cognitive interactive theories of literacy, this knowledge is important for acquiring high-level literacy skills (see discussion in Chapter 5). Similar analogies can be made about deaf students' intuitive knowledge of the other major English components.

One of the most important inferences that can be drawn from these criticisms of the signed systems is the need for an ongoing assessment of the language development of deaf students. In essence, we are referring to the acquisition of *a* language at as early an age as possible. There is substantial evidence indicating that most hearing children develop a first language by the age of 5 or 6 years (see Chapter 4). If English is the first language of choice, the goal should be to develop proficiency as soon as possible. If English is not developed by age 7 or so in deaf children, perhaps an alternative route such as bilingualism (e.g., ASL and English) should be considered. It is unacceptable to require 10 to 15 years for a high-level development of a first social-conventional language. Or, as is the case for many deaf children, no completely adequate social-conventional language is developed by the time they graduate from high school. As is discussed later, a high-level development of the primary form of English at as early an age as possible is important for the subsequent acquisition of high-level text-based literacy skills.

American Sign Language

If English is a very difficult, or perhaps, impossible, language for most deaf students to acquire, perhaps the focus should be on the acquisition of a bona fide sign language such as ASL. The development of any language is critical, albeit not sufficient, for the development of literate thought.

Only a representative sample of the research studies on the acquisition of ASL was presented in this text. It is clear that ASL is a bona fide language with a grammar different from that of English (e.g., Klima & Bellugi, 1979; Lucas, 1990; Wilbur, 1987). Psycholinguistic research indicates that the acquisition of ASL is essentially similar to and parallel to that of spoken-language acquisition. For examples, strategies and features such as overgeneralization and markedness have been observed in both ASL and English (see Chapter 4). Another example is that certain semantic relations and pragmatic functions observed in hearing children have also been reported in the early acquisition stages of deaf children. Certain areas of syntactic development need further investigation, for example, sign order and nonmanual cues. Perhaps, one of the most interesting and far-reaching finding on ASL development has been the documentation of "manual" babbling in deaf infants (e.g., Petitto & Marentette, 1991).

As discussed in Chapter 6, there seems to be a growing consensus for the development and implementation of ASL/English bilingual programs. The impetus for this approach is that it should be easier for deaf students to learn English if teachers use ASL as the medium of instruction for content courses as well as for teaching English as a second language. Nevertheless, knowledge of ASL is not sufficient for the acquisition of English literacy skills any more than knowledge of French is. Most of the bilingual models discussed in Chapter 6 seem to overlook the major tenets of reading-comprehension theories as summarized again in the next section.

English Literacy

As indicated in Chapter 5, the English literacy achievement of many students with severe to profound hearing impairment who graduate from high school has been reported to be at the fourth-grade level. Our understanding of this problem is best described relative to the research findings on short-term memory (Chapter 3) and those on the relationship between the conversational and written forms of English within the purview of social-cognitive interactive theories (Chapter 5). Not surprisingly, these research efforts have also provided insights into the development of literacy skills in deaf students learning English as a second language (Chapter 6).

As noted in Chapter 7 on language instruction, interactive reading models seem to represent a balanced approach that incorporates both bottom-up and top-down processing skills (Adams, 1990; Anderson et al. 1985). Bottom-up, or decoding, skills pertain to the perception of linguistic aspects of a text such as letters, syllables, and words. Top-down, or comprehension, skills involve the knowledge-based aspects of a reader such as prior (topic or world) knowledge, use of metacognitive skills, and knowledge of the language of print. Adequate bottom-up skills lead to the development of rapid, automatic word identification (decoding) skills, and well-developed top-down processing facilitates the understanding of the text.

Word identification facilitates comprehension and comprehension facilitates word identification. This reciprocal relationship for reading and writing activities is dependent on the overall reciprocal relationship between the conversational and written form, which is activated by the association between phonology and orthography (e.g., Brady & Shankweiler, 1991; Templeton & Bear, 1992).

Understanding the link between the phonemes of speech of a phonetic language and the graphemes of print is critical for reading an alphabetic system such as English. That is, there needs to be an awareness that speech can be segmented into phonemes, which are represented by an alphabetic orthography. As discussed in Chapter 4, this is not a natural, unconscious process; it is a learned behavior.

Fluent word reading is also dependent on the use of a phonological-based code in short-term working memory (STM or WM). The efficient use of STM is dependent on the use of this code, and this efficiency allows the reader to expend more energy on the important top-down processes. The use of a phonological-based code in STM is best for processing verbosequential (or temporal-sequential) information which characterized primarily the structure of a phonetic language such as English.

> It should not be inferred that the: nature of short-term memory is the *only* factor accounting for the English language and literacy difficulty of these students. However, it may be a major one, especially if the tasks or materials require verbal (i.e., phonological) encoding. Within this perspective, the problem seems to be a task- or material-specific one. The problem does not indicate a memory impairment. (Paul & Jackson, 1993, p. 270)

The link between the conversational and written forms of English is also important for students learning English as a second language. Second-language students, including ASL-using deaf students, typically do not begin the reading of English with the same level of English language and cultural knowledge as native first-language learners (e.g., Bernhardt, 1991; King & Quigley, 1985; Paul, 1993). These students also do not possess adequate knowledge about the written language of English, for example, vocabulary, syntax, and the alphabetic principle.

It is possible for second-language learners to learn about English culture for the purpose of reading via instruction in their native language. This is the impetus for some minority-language immersion programs, as discussed in Chapter 6. Nevertheless, both hearing and deaf second-language learners still need a deep understanding of the alphabetic principle of English, which facilitates and permits the effective use of higher-level comprehension processors during literacy tasks.

Relative to English literacy, the major problem of hearing second-language students can be characterized as one of knowledge. In other words, they need to learn the alphabetic principle, as well as other written

English variables. For most typical deaf students—including ASL-using students—and, possibly, some hearing second-language students, this can be characterized as both a knowledge and processing problem (e.g., see the research of Lillo-Martin et al., 1991, 1992; Quigley, Wilbur, Power, Montanelli, & Steinkamp, 1976). The processing aspect might entail one or two conditions: (1) difficulty in accessing segmentals and suprasegmentals of the phonology of English, as well as its other grammatical components; and/or (2) difficulty in processing phonological information in STM working memory as evident in poor readers who are fairly adequate speakers-listeners of English (Brady & Shankweiler, 1991; Templeton & Bear, 1992). The two conditions described above might be related in some, perhaps many, deaf students (e.g., King & Quigley, 1985; Paul & Jackson, 1993).

The discussion above is based on the major tenets of social-cognitive interactive theories of literacy. However, it is possible to present a few assumptions common across all three broad groups of reading-comprehension theories. These brief statements should show why text-based literacy is difficult for many hearing second-language learners and for deaf students, including those who know ASL as a first language.

The three broad groups of reading-comprehension theories, bottom-up (text-based), top-down (reader-based), and interactive, assert that a working knowledge of the language of print is important prior to beginning reading activities. This knowledge also includes knowledge of the culture (e.g., world knowledge; school knowledge) associated with the language. It is, of course, possible to learn about the language of print while reading; however, this reciprocity is limited if individuals do not have a "working" knowledge of the language. Consider the 3-year-old hearing child who attempts to scribble or to read some items. This "emerging literacy" phase is supported by a fairly extensive intuitive understanding of the language at this age.

With respect to the assumption of Johnson et al. (1989), it is possible to use ASL to teach the necessary school curricula and other content knowledge that are critical for understanding the language of print. However, ASL-using deaf students—as well as other second-language users—still need a high level of English, particularly the alphabetic code. Without this knowledge and relying only on their first language (i.e., not English), ASL-using deaf students will depend too heavily on the use of top-down skills (e.g., prior knowledge via ASL) which can lead to misinterpretations of the texts.

It should be emphasized that there is no compelling evidence that second-language students can learn to read in the second language via exposure to the print of that target language and explanations in their native or first language (e.g., see Bernhardt, 1991). As stated previously, this is the impetus for several of the ASL/English bilingual models discussed in Chapter 6. Most of these models seem to be influenced by a top-down perspective of literacy, particularly reading. However, even top-down theorists assert that it is important to possess a "working" knowledge of the language in which one is trying to read (e.g., Goodman, 1985). For typical hearing students, this means a working knowledge of the primary, or spoken form, of the language.

Finally, it is important to provide a few remarks on the acquisition of bottom-up, or word identification, skills, which was discussed at the beginning of this section. The debate seems to center on whether these skills need to be taught, *not whether they are important for the reader*. As stated by Paul and Jackson (1993):

> Two of the three groups of reading theories (text-based and interactive) assert that bottom-up skills must be taught. The third group (reader-based or top-down) *assumes* that readers have an intuitive knowledge of sound-letter correspondences and other bottom-up skills because of their command of the language *prior to the reading task*. Because of the importance of phonological coding, knowledge and use of the alphabet code (i.e., sound-letter correspondences) is important for beginning reading. This, along with the continual development of higher-level comprehension skills, leads to the development of competent readers. (p. 139)

Literate Thought

In Chapter 5, we remarked that if reading and writing are difficult for deaf students, perhaps other viable means of developing literate thought should be pursued. This statement is motivated by the growing support for acceptance of a second group of "literacy" models labeled literary critical theories. As discussed in Chapter 5, literary critical theories are not concerned with the improvement of literacy; rather, the focus is on how literacy is used and valued within a particular context. Relative to this group of theories, we are concerned with two questions:

1. Is it possible to develop literate thought without possessing high-level skills in text-based literacy, that is, the ability to read and write printed materials?
2. Is literate thought sufficient for participation in a scientific, technological society such as the United States?

In relation to the first question, Olson (1989) has synthesized much of the debate in the literature regarding the relationship between text-based literacy (i.e., reading and writing skills) and literate thought. He argued that text-based literacy does not seem to be critical for the development of highly complex thought processes such as logic or reasoning. Rather, the ability to read and write well is a manifestation of an individual who can think and reason well. Thus, it is still possible for individuals to develop the ability to think critically and reflectively about complex topics such as law and philosophy despite their inability to access the same information in printed and written materials.

Support for this contention comes from at least two sources. First, Olson (1989) cited historical research which indicates nontext-based literate individuals engaged in reflective and logical discussions of texts or printed materials that were read or orally presented to them. This was during the time when text-based literacy was not common or when texts were not abundant. The "reader" or "speaker" was merely an individual responsible for transmitting the information to the audience. Members of the audience were responsible for interpreting or debating the issues.

A second line of recent research has shown that presenting information in the primary mode (speaking or signing) can be as complex, logical, or deliberate as the information that is presented in printed texts (e.g., see discussions in Olson, 1989; Wagner, 1986). One example of this complexity can be seen in "talking books" or other complex recorded materials for individuals with varying levels of visual impairment. It is not uncommon for a person with a severe visual impairment to "listen" to newspapers or to "great books" on audiotapes. Another example is the manner in which information is presented in learned lectures regarding such topics as "the birth of the universe" or the "evolution of humans." This information can be captured on audiotape and played back for memory purposes.

As discussed in Chapter 6, it should be possible for deaf individuals to develop critical and reflective thinking skills via the use of ASL, even though they might not develop the ability to read and write in English. Essentially, these individuals need to be exposed to the same amount and diversity of learned, complex information, especially as it is preserved on videotapes in ASL. In many ASL/English bilingual program, the optimal goal is the development of literate thought in both languages—ASL and English. However, one of the major reasons for such programs is to guarantee the development of literate thought in at least one language, namely American Sign Language, because many deaf individuals should be able to acquire this language as their first language. With competency in one language, deaf students can have access to school-based curriculum and other important cultural knowledge of mainstream society. We are supportive of this issue, as can been seen in our ASL/English bilingual minority-language immersion model discussed in Chapter 6.

Although the first question addressed above needs to be researched
ʰer, the second question—regarding the sufficiency of literate thought—
ᵛ difficult to assess scientifically. At first glance, the answer should

be obvious: Many nonliterate deaf individuals, particular those who know ASL, are functioning well in the mainstream of U.S. society. It can be argued that these individuals might perform much better if they have or have had access to complex information during their school years and during their participation in the wider society. Accessibility, in this sense, means having access to information presented in or preserved via the use of American Sign Language.

The second question cannot be addressed fully in this chapter. In fact, the answer to this question depends on one's philosophical (perhaps, metatheoretical) position. For example, if one ascribes to the high status of English and English text-based literacy in a society such as the United States, then proficiency in English text-based literacy is critical for gaining access to higher education, scientific, and industrial occupations, and the learned professions (Adams, 1990; Anderson et al., 1985). From another perspective, critical theorists would argued that this "valued position" is oppressive, particularly for those capable individuals who, for whatever biological or environmental reason, are unable to function adequately in a technological, information intensive society (e.g., see discussion of critical theory in Gibson, 1986). In any case, the answer to the second question depends, in part, on the outcome of the ongoing debate on whether the possession of high-level text-based literacy skills is the hallmark or an epiphenomenon of an advanced civilization—one that possesses scientific and technological prowess (e.g., see discussions in Olson, 1989; Wagner, 1986).

FINAL REMARKS

For teachers and clinicians to better understand the problem of English literacy in deaf students, both groups need to have a fairly extensive knowledge of language instruction and language assessment. These issues were covered in Chapter 7 and Chapter 8, respectively. In this last chapter (Chapter 9), we attempted to provide some final insights regarding the development of language, text-based literacy, and literate thought in individuals with severe to profound hearing impairment.

One conclusion that can be drawn from the work in the language and communication development of deaf children is that these children cannot be considered as a single population. This is not a trite restatement of the doctrine of individual differences. Rather, it is a recognition that the development of language in a deaf child is inextricably related to the form of communication which is used initially and consistently with the child. In addition, language development is also dependent upon the representativeness or completeness of the form and its processing constraints.

In sum, additional research is needed on the execution of the communication systems by teachers, clinicians, and parents and the reception of such systems by deaf individuals. The persistent issue has been the development of a language at as early an age as possible. The existence of these several possible approaches to language development presents the persons who are primarily responsible for a deaf child's language development with the dilemma of choosing one in the absence of any clear directions from research of their relative effectiveness. In addition, there is a growing doubt that the development of adequate English levels in both conversational and written forms might not be a feasible goal for some, perhaps a large minority of, students with severe to profound impairment. It should still be possible for these individuals to develop a high level of literate thought, particularly through the use of American Sign Language. In any case, it is safe to conclude that there is not, and may never be, a "true path" to language development for all deaf students.

FURTHER READINGS

Beveridge, W. (1980). *Seeds of discovery: The logic, illogic, serendipity, and sheer chance of scientific discovery.* New York: Norton.

Kuhn, T. (1970). *The structure of scientific revolutions* (2nd ed.). Chicago, IL: University of Chicago Press.

Medawar, P. (1984). *The limits of science.* New York: Harper & Row.

Searle, J. (1983). *Intentionality: An essay in the philosophy of mind.* New York: Cambridge University Press.

A P P E N D I X

TOPICS AND
QUESTIONS

For each chapter in the text, the Appendix contains a list of chapter top-ics to guide students' reading and understanding of the chapter. Each topic is described briefly. The Appendix also contains comprehension questions for students to answer. The answers to the comprehension questions can be found in the *Student's Study Guide* (Singular Publishing Group, Inc.).

CHAPTER 1: OVERVIEW OF LANGUAGE AND DEAFNESS

Chapter Topics

- *Function of language*
  Language has several functions or uses. Some of the functions of language include the communication of ideas, social interaction, a tool for thought, expression of identity, emotional expression, re-cording of information, special effects, and the control of reality.

- *Structure of language*
  The structure of language refers to the various components, whose names and descriptions are influenced by the prevailing linguistic theories. The language components are phonology, morphology, syntax, semantics, and pragmatics.

- *Perspectives on deafness*
  Language theories, research, and interventions/practices are influenced by philosophical perspectives on deafness. There are two broad perspectives that affect descriptions of deafness: clinical and cultural.

- *Communication systems*
  There are two modes, or communication philosophies: oralism and total communication (TC). Although the TC philosophy permits the use of American Sign Language (ASL) as one approach, ASL has not been widely used in classroom settings. Thus, it might be the case that there is or should be a third communication philosophy—the use of American Sign Language.

- *American Sign Language*
  ASL is a visual-gestural language, which contains both manual and nonmanual aspects. ASL, like other sign languages, does not involve the use of speech sounds.

Comprehension Questions

1. What is the most commonly recognized function of a language? List at least five other language functions. Which language function is strongly related to pragmatics, one of the components of a language?
2. Describe briefly both the language-dominates-thought position and the thought-dominates-language position.
3. Relative to the structure of language, there are five language components discussed in the chapter. Describe briefly each language component.
4. List the prosodic features associated with the phonological system of a language. Why are these features important?
5. Describe the following terms:
   a. inflectional morphology
   b. derivational morphology
6. Describe briefly the two major categories of syntactic relations.
7. List and discuss a few tenets of the two broad philosophical perspectives on deafness.
8. Relative to communication systems, there is often some confusion between language-teaching and language-representation. Discuss the differences between these two terms.

9. What are three common features of all oral approaches?
10. Label the following terms as belonging to oralism or manually coded English.
    a. cued speech
    b. acoupedic
    c. Rochester method
    d. SEE systems
    e. signed English
    f. aural
    g. multisensory
11. List the manual English codes, starting with the most representative code of English and ending with the least representative code of English. What determines the placement of a code on a continuum from most representative to least representative?
12. Identify the signed system within the manually coded English framework.
    a. The use of a sign is based on its entry (i.e., boldface type) in a dictionary of standard English.

    _____

    b. The selection or use of a sign is based on a two-out-of-three rule involving sound, spelling, and meaning.

    _____

    c. This method entails the use of finger spelling and speech simultaneously.

    _____

    d. The form of signing does not adhere to a clear-cut set of principles, save the following of an English word order.

    _____

13. Describe briefly American Sign Language. What are manual and nonmanual features?

CHAPTER 2: LANGUAGE ACQUISITION: METATHEORIES, THEORIES, AND RESEARCH

Chapter Topics

- *Metatheory*
  In science, a metatheory is a framework, or perspective, that determines how one should do science. A metatheory ascertains whether a particular discipline is a science or not.

- *Metatheories of psychology*
  The three broad metatheories of psychology are introspectionism, behaviorism, and cognitive science. Each metatheory is distinguished by its approach to the study of the mind, or what is commonly known as the oldest problem in philosophy—the mind/body problem.

- *Theories of language acquisition*
  In this chapter, three broad groups of language acquisition theories are used: behavioristic, linguistic, and interactionist. These broad terms underscore major differences relative to two controversial issues: innateness versus empirical and competence versus performance.

- *Study of language*
  The study of language entails an understanding of three concepts, prescription, description, and explanation. These three terms are not always mutually exclusive. In addition, it is important to relate the study of language to the ongoing debate on the mind/brain problem.

- *Issues in language and deafness*
  Relative to deafness, there are three important issues discussed in this chapter: the interrelationships of theory, research, assessment, and practice; the study of language and deafness; and the development of language in deaf children and adolescents.

Comprehension Questions

1. In science, what is a metatheory?
2. Describe the three general types of metatheorizing. [Note: The fourth type of metatheorizing is considered a weak form.]
3. Describe briefly the three broad metatheories of psychology. Each metatheory is distinguished by its approach to the study of the mind, or what is commonly known as the oldest problem in philosophy—the _____ .
4. Describe briefly the three broad categories of language theories.
5. According to Chomsky, there are three levels of theoretical adequacy. Describe them.
6. Describe the following terms:
   a. performance of speakers
   b. competence of speakers

7. According to Wasow (in Ingram, 1989), what is the difference between child language research and language acquisition research?

8. Describe briefly the following terms:
   a. prescription
   b. description
   c. explanation

9. Searle reasoned that mental events are features of the brain in the same way that liquidity is a feature of water. For Searle, the important concepts are _____ and _____.

10. In the field of deafness, much of the research and practice seems to be _____ .

11. Relative to language development, King (1981) has argued that there are two foci that need to be recognized and researched further. These can be expressed as questions:
    a. _____?
    b. _____?

12. What does the following sentence mean?
    The English language development of deaf students is qualitatively similar to that of hearing students.

13. Relative to theory, the issue of qualitative (or developmental) similarity is related to a "deeper issue." What is the "deeper issue"?

CHAPTER 3: LANGUAGE AND THOUGHT

Chapter Topics

- *Intelligence and cognition*
  These concepts and the relationships between them have been influenced by the prevailing metatheory of an era. At present, there is a move to develop "process-oriented" assessments and to replace the concept of intelligence with that of cognitive processing.

- *Research on intelligence and deafness*
  The chapter discusses the tenets of the three major stages of research on intelligence and deafness. It also highlights the emergence of a fourth stage, which represents a different way of thinking about intelligence or cognition.

- *Thought and language*
  The thinking on the relationship between thought and language has influenced the interpretation of research on intelligence, cognition,

and deafness. The chapter presents the basic tenets of strong, weak, and interactive positions regarding this relationship.

- *Research on cognition and deafness*
  The research on cognition and deaf individuals is examined within the framework of commonly used cognitive models. The findings have contributed to advances in the understanding of language and deafness. Much of the research on cognition and deafness has been influenced by the model of Piaget's and those espoused by information-processing theorists, particularly the stage-of-processing model.

- *Memory research and deafness*
  Research on memory has shown that this entity is important for language and literacy development. Much of the research within the information-processing paradigm has focused on the basic processes in short-term memory (STM). Advances in this area have contributed to a better understanding of the relationship between language and thought.

- *A psychology of deafness*
  This phrase is centered on the question of whether the language development of deaf students is qualitatively similar to that of hearing students. This discussion considers the acquisition of a spoken language such as English.

Comprehension Questions

1. Consider the following question: What is intelligence? What influences the answer to this question?
2. List and briefly describe the major highlights of the three stages of research on intelligence and deafness. To which stage can one attribute the phrase, psychology of deafness, particularly as it relates to qualitative differences in language and cognition?
3. Briefly describe the highlights of the emerging fourth stage of intelligence testing and deafness.
4. Describe briefly the following terms:
   a. strong forms of thought-based hypotheses
   b. weak forms of thought-based hypotheses
   c. linguistic determinism
5. List and describe briefly the major highlights of Piaget's four stages of cognition.

6. Relative to Piaget's stages, observations reveal that deaf children progress typically through the _____ stage and through most of the _____ stage.

7. In agreement with Greenberg and Kusche, the authors of the text argued that differences between deaf and hearing individuals on the higher stages are due mainly to _____ .
Little difference exists between deaf and hearing children on the lower-level stages because progress is dependent on the role of _____ ability.

8. Much of the research within the information-processing paradigm has focused on the basic processes in short-term memory (STM). This line of investigation has attempted to _____ _____ (note: three areas).

9. Describe briefly the following terms:
   a. sensory register
   b. short-term memory
   c. long-term memory
   d. sequential processing
   e. simultaneous processing

10. Research on deafness reveals four different types of coding on either working memory (WM) tasks or during reading. List and describe briefly each type.

11. Consider the following statement as true: Deaf students who use predominantly a phonological-based code in WM tend to be better readers than other deaf students who use predominantly a nonphonological-based code. Why is this true?

12. According to the authors of the text, what does it mean to say that there might be a psychology of deafness relative to the acquisition of spoken and written English?

CHAPTER 4: PRIMARY LANGUAGE DEVELOPMENT

Chapter Topics

- *Development of language*
  For most hearing children, this process appears effortless and relatively simple; however, an in-depth analysis reveals its complex and intricate nature. Despite voluminous research, the exact nature of this language learning process is still being debated. Even the manner in which child language development should be studied abounds with controversies.

- *Prelinguistic development*
  The prelinguistic period, that is, the period prior to the emergence of a child's first words has only recently attracted the attention of linguists. More recently, this period has come within the purview of developmental psychologists and developmental psycholinguists.

- *Linguistic development*
  Prelinguistic development does not simply culminate with the emergence of the first words. In fact, the development of the later stages of this period may parallel the beginning stages of linguistic development. The child's first words generally mark the beginning of linguistic development. Depending on the nature of the linguistic criteria established, different ages may be reported for the emergence of the first words.

- *Comprehension-production issue*
  Central to the analyses of the first words is the comprehension-production issue. The productions of children have received more attention than the corresponding comprehension of words. The paucity of research is not due to a lack of interest, but rather to the difficulty of measuring the comprehension of children.

- *Language development of deaf children*
  Describing the primary language development of a deaf child is much more complicated. It is true that most deaf children in the United States are exposed to English in infancy and early childhood. The description of this exposure needs to consider two issues: (1) the nature of the language input and (2) the nature of the communication mode used, that is, manual or oral.

- *Oral English*
  Oral English refers to the use of cued speech and/or traditional oral-English methods (e.g., unisensory and multisensory approaches).

- *Total communication*
  TC refers to the use of speaking and signing simultaneously in some fashion. The chapter covers approaches such as the Rochester method, seeing essential English, signing exact English, and English-based signing (also known as pidgin sign English).

- *American Sign Language*
  There is general agreement that ASL is a bona fide language, although there seems to be some disagreement on how ASL is used or should be described. Some recent research focuses on comparing the processing of sign languages with that of spoken languages.

More research is needed on how skills can be transferred from a sign language to a spoken language or on important differences between ASL and English that pose problems for late second-language learners.

Comprehension Questions

1. Briefly describe what is meant by the phrase *prelinguistic period*, and list several factors that have contributed to a renewed interest in this area.
2. Describe the following terms:
   a. segmental aspects
   b. suprasegmental aspects
3. Why is the relationship between speech perception and speech production difficult to describe?
4. What milestone marks the beginning of linguistic development?
5. What are the three general conclusions regarding the description of phonological development of young children?
6. Briefly list the units of speech analyses. Which type is related to reading and why?
7. Briefly describe Halliday's mathetic and pragmatic functions of language acts.
8. List the approaches within oral English and manually coded English systems.
9. What role can cued speech play in the development of reading skills?
10. Which manual communication system is considered most representative of the written grammatical structure of English? least representative? What determines the placement on the continuum from least representative to most representative?
11. Which manually coded English system, in its entirety, is widely used in the education of deaf students?
12. The processing of sign languages is said to be similar to that of spoken languages. List some similarities.

CHAPTER 5: READING AND WRITING

Chapter Topics

- *Theoretical models of reading*
  There are two groups of theoretical models that are concerned with reading and, in some cases, writing: reading-comprehension and

literary critical. Reading-comprehension models (bottom-up, top-down, and interactive) are concerned with the decoding and comprehension of the written language of English. Literary critical models are concerned with the context of the application of skills associated with literacy.

- *Factors associated with the reading process*
  The three groups of factors that have been delineated and discussed are text-based (vocabulary, grammar, orthography), reader-based (prior knowledge, metacognition), and context-(or task-)based (tests, setting in which reading is accomplished).

- *Reading achievement and deafness*
  Despite improvements in the construction of tests and the implementation of early intervention, there are two general themes that can be gleaned from the findings. One, the overwhelming majority of 18- to 19-year-old deaf students do not read above a fourth-grade level. Two, this "plateau" has been in existence since the beginning of the formal testing movement.

- *Research on selected text-based factors*
  Much of the reading research on deaf children and adolescents has been conducted on text-based factors such as vocabulary, syntax, and figurative language.

- *Research on selected reader-based and other factors*
  The research on the effects of reader-based and other factors has not been as systematic and extensive as the research on the effects of text-based factors. Three of the most critical—and highly related—reader-based factors are prior knowledge, inferencing, and metacognition.

- *Development of writing*
  Theories and research on writing have been influenced by theories and research on reading. The development of writing has also been affected by the recent thinking on models of instruction. In addition, research on writing has been discussed relative to the type of research inquiry.

- *Product and process views of writing*
  The products of writing refer to items such as spelling, punctuation, capitalization, grammar, and legibility. Within a process view, writing is not merely or only a representation of an individual's

thoughts. Written language is the writer's creation or construction of reality.

- *Research on written language and hearing children*
  Results demonstrate that there is a strong early relationship between oral and written language productions. This reciprocal relationship is deemed important for the later development of advanced reading and writing skills.

- *Research on written language and deaf children*
  The research on the written language of deaf students is discussed relative to two broad areas: the sentence level and multisentence level. At the sentence level, the chapter focuses on data from both free-response and controlled-response studies, influenced by both traditional/structural and generative theories. The more recent studies, focusing on the multisentence level, view writing as a process.

Comprehension Questions

1. The similarity between reading and writing, often termed the _____, has been motivated by both theories of _____ and _____ .
2. List and briefly describe the two overall groups of theoretical models that are concerned with the condition of reading, and in some cases, writing.
3. Describe briefly the major principles associated with the following terms:
   a. bottom-up models
   b. top-down models
   c. interactive models
4. Relative to the processing of words, two types are often debated in the literature. What are the two types?
5. List and briefly describe the three groups of factors that are associated with the reading process.
6. What are the two general themes that can be gleaned from the findings on reading achievement and deafness?
7. Relative to research on text-based reading factors and deafness, describe briefly the major highlights of the following studies:
   a. LaSasso & Davey (1987)
   b. Paul & Gustafson (1991)
   c. The work of Quigley and his associates
   d. Wilbur, Goodhart, & Fuller (1989)
   e. Payne & Quigley (1987)

8. Relative to research on reader-based reading factors and deafness, describe briefly the major highlights of the following studies:
   a. Wilson (1979)
   b. Strassman (1992)
   c. Yamashita (1992)
9. Discuss briefly the following perspectives on writing:
   a. product
   b. process
10. There are a number of problems associated with the use of spontaneous written language productions. Discuss three of the four general problems.
11. List and describe briefly the two broad methods for eliciting written language productions.
12. What were the two predominant findings of the early traditional free-response studies?
13. The research on sentence level, free-response, generative grammar and on sentence level, controlled-response, generative grammar aspects has been discussed relative to four categories. List the four categories.
14. Discuss briefly the results of the good and poor writers in the Gormley and Sarachan-Deily (1987) study relative to three categories: content, linguistic aspects, and surface mechanics.
15. In one sense, focusing on the product of writing only (particularly, lower-level skills) is similar to a _____ approach in reading whereas focusing on the higher-level skills only (as in a process approach) is similar to a strict _____ model.

CHAPTER 6: BILINGUALISM AND SECOND-LANGUAGE LEARNING

Chapter Topics

• *Definitions*
Bilingualism implies the use of two languages; however, this seemingly simple notion has produced a great deal of confusion in the theoretical and research literature. Factors which contribute to the lack of consensus include the notion of language, language competency, language proficiency, and the time frame in which languages are learned.

- *Theoretical models of bilingualism*
  There is a diversity of theoretical models in the literature. This diversity depends on the metatheories, methodologies, and foci of the researchers. The chapter covers two groups of models. The first group seems to be most related to the effects of bilingualism on cognition and academic achievement whereas the second group focuses mainly on the acquisition process.

- *Development of L1 and L2: similar or different?*
  The chapter discusses whether the acquisition of English as a second language is qualitatively similar to the acquisition of English as a first language by hearing individuals. This notion is also examined relative to the acquisition of English literacy, particularly reading.

- *Research on bilingualism, second-language learning, and deafness*
  The information on these issues is organized around five areas: (1) primary bilingual development; (2) effects of ASL on the subsequent development of English; (3) language production and preference of deaf students, including bilingual deaf students; (4) ASL/English instructional programs; and (5) development of L1 and L2 in deaf students, including Spanish deaf students.

- *Bilingual education models*
  In addition to having a variety of theoretical acquisition models, the field of bilingualism has a number of program models. The controversies in this area are due primarily to the philosophies and goals of specific programs. To provide a better understanding of this issue, the chapter discusses type of student and language goals.

- *Bilingual education program for deaf students: a model*
  One L1 immersion model has been described in several publications. This model is based on the theoretical and research data available for hearing minority-language students in L1 immersion programs. The model is also based on reading research with both L1 and L2 students.

Comprehension Questions

1. List four factors that contribute to the lack of consensus about what constitutes bilingualism and second-language learning.

2. Bilingualism is not an all-or-nothing phenomenon. Rather, it is a function of degree depending on at least two factors. What are the two factors?

3. The chapter covers two broad groups of theoretical models on bilingualism. What are the two broad groups?

4. Discuss briefly the major highlights of the following models:
   a. balance theory
   b. interdependence theory
   c. societal factor model
   d. threshold model
   e. vernacular advantage model

5. Describe briefly the following terms:
   a. Selinker's interlanguage
   b. Krashen's language acquisition and language learning concepts

6. According to McLaughlin (1984), is the development of L1 by first-language learners similar to or different from the development of L2 by second-language learners?

7. Relative to the effects of ASL on the subsequent development of English, studies have employed the paradigm of comparing

   _____

   _____ .

8. Describe briefly the "biological predisposition" hypothesis of Gee and Goodhart (1985, 1988).

9. Relative to ASL/English instructional programs, discuss the major highlights of the following studies/projects:
   a. Jones (1979)
   b. Marbury & Mackinson-Smyth (1986)

10. Is the development of English as a second language similar to the development of English as a first language for deaf students? [Use the results of King's (1981) study to answer this question.]

11. Describe briefly the following terms:
    a. majority-language students
    b. minority-language students
    c. language shift
    d. language maintenance
    e. language enrichment

12. The most effective bilingual programs for minority-language students are _____

    _____ .

13. Discuss briefly the five major guidelines of the bilingual minority-language immersion program model for deaf students (Paul & Quigley, 1987b, in press).

CHAPTER 7: LANGUAGE INSTRUCTION

Chapter Topics

- *Teachability/learnability*
  This notion revolves around the question of whether or not language can be "taught." It is also not uncommon to encounter such debates in the fields of reading and writing, including second-language literacy. The notion of learnability refers to the specification of conditions and constraints that contribute to or enable the "learning" of a first or second language.

- *Approaches to language instruction*
  Historically, there have been two major approaches to language instruction, structural and natural, as well as "combinations" of these approaches. In many cases, it is possible to state that structural approaches adhere to the concept of teachability whereas natural approaches adhere to that of learnability.

- *Combined approaches*
  The combined approaches entail the teaching of language in a natural manner via the use of a structured approach. This approach seems to be a balanced approach, "combining" the best features of both natural and structured approaches.

- *Language instruction and best method*
  One of the most controversial and long-standing issues in the teaching of language to deaf children and adolescents is the notion of "best method." It might be that the notion of best method is misguided; the best we can hope for is an understanding of the teacher-learner situations via the use of qualitative research approaches.

- *Instruction of literacy*
  Both reading and writing are interactive processes which entail interactions between the individual and a text whose meaning needs to be constructed. Both reading and writing involve the application of lower-level and higher-level skills.

- *Teachability and guidelines*
  We emphasize two salient guidelines. One, there needs to be a stronger interrelationship among theory, curriculum, instruction,

and assessment. Two, teachers of deaf individuals need more training in language and literacy.

Comprehension Questions

1. Briefly describe the following dichotomy: teachability/learnability.
2. True or False?

    a. _____ Linguistic theories, specifically those motivated
    by Chomsky's thinking, ascribe to the condition of teachability.

    b. _____ The behavoristic approaches epitomize the learn-
    ability of language.

    c. _____ The third broad group of theories—interactionist,
    particularly social-interactionist—represents a "balanced" view of
    language development.

    d. _____ The teachability/learnability dichotomy does not
    apply to reading and writing.

3. The balanced approach to the teachability/learnability issue in
    reading is:

    a. interactive theories
    b. bottom-up theories
    c. top-down theories
    d. literary critical theories
    e. all of the above

4. What is the authors' view on the teachability/learnability issue?

5. Label the following as Structured or Natural.

    a. In general, these approaches adhere to the concept of learn-
    ability. _____

    b. In general, these approaches adhere to the concept of teach-
    ability. _____

    c. Students are required to analyze and categorize the grammati-
    cal aspects of the language. _____

    d. Students demonstrate their understanding by writing sentences
    that correspond to previously taught patterns. _____

    e. Students should be able to discover and internalize rules and
    principles associated with the grammar of English._____

    f. APPLE TREE is an example of the _____ approach.

    g. Often associated with the inquiry method. _____

6. Describe combined approaches.

7. According to King (1984), the _____ approaches
    were most frequently used at all levels (preschool, primary, in-
    termediate, junior high, and high school).

8. Describe the three broad interpretations of the notion of "best method."

9. List and briefly describe the three stages of writing instruction.

10. Describe the authors' two major guidelines relative to the notion of teachability.

CHAPTER 8: LANGUAGE ASSESSMENT

Chapter Topics

- *Direct versus indirect procedures*
  Direct procedures refer to the emphasis on the use of language to communicate or convey information in a natural matter. Indirect procedures refer to the conscious reflections of the language user on the language rules that are required to perform or complete a particular linguistic task.

- *Discrete-point versus integrative measures*
  Discrete-point measures focus on the evaluation of certain important language elements or skills (e.g., vocabulary, syntax, distinctive features). Integrative measures were developed because of debates on the validity of the discrete-point measures. The goal of integrative measures is to obtain a global understanding of the language performance of the individual.

- *Characteristics of assessment*
  Three of the most important characteristics of assessment are reliability, validity, and practicality. Reliability is concerned with the consistency of test results regarding the performances of students. Validity refers to the question of whether a test measures what it is designed to measure. There are several issues relative to practicality, such as the amount of time for test administration, special equipment needs, costs of test materials and scoring procedures, and special arrangement needs.

- *Purposes and types of assessment*
  The selection of a test is influenced markedly by the purpose of the evaluation, and this in turn affects the type of assessment. The type of assessment also determines the method that will be employed to collect the data. Three test types discussed in the chapter are achievement, diagnostic, and proficiency. The differences

among these types can be discussed relative to the variables of time and content.

- *Controlled methods*
  With controlled methods, it is possible to examine certain linguistic structures that might appear infrequently or never appear in a spontaneous language sample. The section discusses advantages and disadvantages of these methods.

- *Free methods*
  Free methods refer to the gathering of information on children's spontaneous use of language through the use of elicitation or prompting procedures such as pictures or video tapes.

- *Language dominance*
  The concept of language dominance seems to be concerned with the degree of bilingualism. That is, researchers attempted to compare the individual's levels of skills in two or more languages.

- *Language proficiency*
  Language proficiency refers to the individual's degree of competence in one language, that is, the relative proficiency in both languages. The current debate on language proficiency seems to center on the question of whether language proficiency is a unitary concept.

Comprehension Questions

1. Describe briefly the following terms:
   a. direct procedures
   b. indirect procedures
   c. discrete-point
   d. integrative
2. List and briefly describe three of the most important characteristics of assessment.
3. If there are two equivalent forms of the same test, the alternate or parallel form procedures can be used to determine _____
   _____ .
4. List and briefly describe the types of validity discussed in the chapter.

5. What influences the selection of a test?
6. Describe briefly the following test types:
   a. achievement
   b. diagnostic
   c. proficiency
7. Discuss the advantages and disadvantages of using controlled methods.
8. List and briefly describe two examples of tests that employ controlled methods.
9. Discuss the advantages and disadvantages of using free methods.
10. List and briefly describe two examples of tests that employ free methods.
11. Describe the following terms:
    a. language dominance
    b. language proficiency
12. Discuss the two major perspectives (i.e., theories) regarding the nature of language proficiency (Oller and Cummins).

CHAPTER 9: CONCLUSION

Chapter Topics

- *How Do*
  The *How Do* question refers to both the acquisition of the conversational form of English and of American Sign Language. It refers to the development and use of language intervention systems with deaf students in infancy, early childhood, and during the school years.

- *How Well*
  In the *How Well* question, we attempt to discuss and compare the development of English literacy skills in deaf students with that of hearing students. Related to these questions is the notion of a critical period for learning a language.

- *Language and Communication Intervention Systems*
  The three broad approaches are oral English, total communication, and American Sign Language. Both oral and TC methods are concerned with the representation and development of the conversational form of English.

Comprehension Questions

1. What were the two broad questions that this chapter attempted to answer?
2. Describe briefly the three ways that have been used to enable deaf students to develop a self-controlling, communication system (i.e., Quigley & Paul, in press).
3. Describe briefly the following terms/categories:
   a. oral methods
   b. total communication
   c. American Sign Language
4. What is meant by the phrase "world of vision versus world of audition?"
5. Describe briefly the following terms:
   a. interactive theories
   b. link between phonemes and graphemes
6. Relative to English literacy, there may be two broad difficulties for deaf and hearing second-language learners: knowledge and processing. Describe each difficulty.
7. Decide whether the following statements are True or False?
   a. _____ Only two of the three broad groups of theories assert that a working knowledge of the language of print is important prior to beginning reading activities.
   b. _____ It is possible to learn about the language of print while reading.
   c. _____ There is no compelling evidence that second-language students can learn to read in the second language via exposure to the print of that target language.
   d. _____ All groups of reading theories assert that bottom-up, or word identification, skills must be taught.
8. Describe literate thought. Is literate thought possible without the ability to read and write adequately? Why or why not?

REFERENCES

Abraham, S., & Stoker, R. (1984). An evaluation of methods used to teach speech to the hearing-impaired using a simulation technique. *Volta Review, 86,* 325–335.

Abrams, M. (Ed.). (1991). *Whole language: A folio of articles from Perspectives in Education and Deafness.* Washington, DC: Gallaudet University, Pre-College Programs.

Acoustical Society of America. (1982). *Specification of hearing aid characteristics.* ANSI S3.22–1982. New York: Author.

Adams, M. (1990). *Beginning to read: Thinking and learning about print. A summary.* Prepared by S. Stahl, J. Osborn, & F. Lehr. Urbana-Champaign, IL: University of Illinois, Center for the Study of Reading, The Reading Research and Education Center.

Akamatsu, C. T. (1982). *The acquisition of fingerspelling in preschool children.* Unpublished doctoral dissertation, University of Rochester, New York.

Akamatsu, C. T., & Armour, V. (1987). Developing written literacy in deaf children through analyzing sign language. *American Annals of the Deaf, 132,* 46–51.

Akamatsu, C. T., & Stewart, D. (1989). The role of fingerspelling in simultaneous communication. *Sign Language Studies, 65,* 361–373.

Allen, T. (1986). Patterns of academic achievement among hearing impaired students: 1974 and 1983. In A. Schildroth & M. Karchmer (Eds.), *Deaf children in America* (pp. 161–206). San Diego, CA: Little, Brown.

Anastasi, A. (1982). *Psychological testing* (5th ed.). New York: Macmillan.

Anderson, J., & Bower, G. (1973). *Human associative memory.* Washington, DC: Winston.

Anderson, M., Boren, N., Caniglia, J., Howard, W., & Krohn, E. (1980). *Apple Tree.* Beaverton, OR: Dormac.

Anderson, R., & Freebody, P. (1979). *Vocabulary knowledge* (Tech. Rep. No. 136). Urbana, IL: University of Illinois, Center for the Study of Reading. (ERIC Document Reproduction Service No. ED 177 480)

Anderson, R., & Freebody, P. (1985). Vocabulary knowledge. In H. Singer & R. Ruddell (Eds.), *Theoretical models and processes of reading* (pp. 343–371). Newark, DE: International Reading Association.

Anderson, R., Hiebert, E., Scott, J., & Wilkinson, I. (1985). *Becoming a nation of readers: The report of the commission on reading.* Washington, DC: U.S. Department of Education, The National Institute of Education.

Anderson, R., & Pearson, P. D. (1984). A schema-theoretic view of basic processes in reading comprehension. In P. D. Pearson, R. Barr, M. Kamil, & P. Mosenthal (Eds.), *Handbook of reading research* (pp. 255–291). White Plains, NY: Longman.

Andrews, J., & Gonzalez, K. (1991). Free writing of deaf children in kindergarten. *Sign Language Studies, 74,* 63–78.

Anisfeld, M. (1984). *Language development from birth to three.* Hillsdale, NJ: Lawrence Erlbaum.

Anthony, D. (1966). *Seeing essential English.* Unpublished master's thesis, Eastern Michigan University, Ypsilanti.

Atkinson, R., & Shiffrin, R. (1971). The control of short-term memory. *Scientific American, 225,* 82–90.

Au, T. (1988). Language and cognition. In R. Schiefelbusch & L. Lloyd (Eds.), *Language perspectives: Acquisition, retardation, and intervention* (2nd ed., pp. 125–146). Austin, TX: Pro-Ed.

Austin, J. (1966). *How to do things with words.* London, England: Oxford University Press.

Baars, B. (1986). *The cognitive revolution in psychology.* New York: The Guilford Press.

Babb, R. (1979). *A study of the academic achievement and language acquisition levels of deaf children of hearing parents in an educational environment using signing exact English as the primary mode of manual communication.* Unpublished doctoral dissertation, University of Illinois, Urbana-Champaign.

Babbini, B., & Quigley, S. (1970). *A study of the growth patterns in language, communication, and educational achievement in six residential schools for deaf students.* Urbana, IL: University of Illinois, Institute for Research on Exceptional Children. (ERIC Document Reproduction Service No. ED 046 208)

Baddeley, A. (1979). Working memory and reading. In H. Bouma (Ed.), *Processing of visible language* (Vol. 1, pp. 355–370). New York: Plenum Press.

Baddeley, A. (1990). *Human memory: Theory and practice.* Hillsdale, NJ: Lawrence Erlbaum.

Baddeley, A., & Hitch, G. (1974). Working memory. In G. Bower (Ed.), *The psychology of learning and motivation, Vol. 8* (pp. 47–90). New York, NY: Academic Press.

Baker, C., & Cokely, D. (1980). *American Sign Language: A teacher's resource text on grammar and culture.* Silver Spring, MD: T.J. Publishers.

Baker, D. (1989). *Language testing: A critical survey and practical guide.* New York: Edward Arnold.

Baker, K., & de Kanter, A. (1981). *Effectiveness of bilingual education: A review of the literature.* Washington, DC: U.S. Department of Education, Office of Planning and Budget.

Baker, L., & Brown, A. (1984). Metacognition skills and reading. In P. D. Pearson, R. Barr, M. Kamil, & P. Mosenthal (Eds.), *Handbook of reading research* (pp. 353–394). White Plains, NY: Longman.

Balow, I., & Brill, R. (1975). An evaluation of reading and academic achievement levels of 16 graduating classes of the California School for the Deaf, Riverside. *Volta Review, 77,* 255–266.

Barr, R., Kamil, M., Mosenthal, P., & Pearson, P. D. (Eds.). (1991). *Handbook of reading research* (2nd ed.). White Plains, NY: Longman.

Bateman, W. (1990). *Open to question: The art of teaching and learning by inquiry.* San Francisco: Jossey-Bass.

Bates, E. (1976). *Language and context: The acquisition of pragmatics.* New York: Academic Press.

Battison, R. (1974). Phonological deletion in American Sign Language. *Sign Language Studies, 5,* 1–19.

Beardsmore, H. (1986). *Bilingualism: Basic principles* (2nd ed.). Clevedon, Avon (England): Multilingual Matters Ltd.

Beck, E. (Ed.). (1980). *John Bartlett's familiar quotations: A collection of passages, phrases, and proverbs traced to their sources in ancient and modern literature.* Boston, MA: Little, Brown.

Beebe, H., Pearson, H., & Koch, M. (1984). The Helen Beebe speech and hearing center. In D. Ling (Ed.), *Early intervention for hearing-impaired children: Oral options* (pp. 15–63). San Diego, CA: College-Hill Press.

Bellugi, U. (1988). The acquisition of a spatial language. In F. Kessell (Ed.), *The development of language and language researchers: Essays in honor of Roger Brown* (pp. 153–185). Hillsdale, NJ: Lawrence Erlbaum.

Bellugi, U., & Klima, E. (1985). The acquisition of three morphological systems in American Sign Language. In F. Powell, T. Finitzo-Hieber,

S. Friel-Patti, & D. Henderson (Eds.), *Education of the hearing-impaired child* (pp. 23–56). San Diego, CA: College-Hill Press.

Bellugi, U., Klima, E., & Siple, P. (1974/1975). Remembering in signs. *Cognition, 3*(2), 93–125.

Bereiter, C. & Scardamalia, M. (1983). Levels of inquiry in writing research. In P. Mosenthal, L. Tamor, & Walmsley, S. (Eds.), *Research on writing: Principles and methods* (pp. 3–25). New York: Longman.

Bereiter, C., & Scardamalia, M. (1987). *The psychology of written composition.* Hillsdale, NJ: Lawrence Erlbaum.

Berko, J. (1958). The child's learning of English morphology. *Word, 14,* 150–177.

Bernhardt, E. (1991). *Reading development in a second language.* Norwood, NJ: Ablex.

Berry, M., & Talbot, R. (1966). *Exploratory test for grammar.* Rockford, IL: Berry & Talbot.

Berry, S. (1981). *Written language syntax test.* Washington, DC: Gallaudet College Press.

Best, B., & Roberts, G. (1976). Early cognitive development in hearing impaired children. *American Annals of the Deaf, 121,* 560–564.

Bialystok, E., & Sharwood-Smith, M. (1985). Interlanguage is not a state of mind: An evaluation of the construct for second-language acquisition. *Applied Linguistics, 6,* 101–117.

Blackwell, P., Engen, E., Fischgrund, J., & Zarcadoolas, C. (1978). *Sentences and other systems.* Washington, DC: Alexander Graham Bell Association for the Deaf.

Blanton, R., Nunnally, J., & Odom, P. (1967). Graphemic, phonetic, and associative factors in the verbal behavior of deaf and hearing subjects. *Journal of Speech and Hearing Research, 10,* 225–231.

Blennerhassett, L. (1990). Intellectual assessment. In D. Moores & K. Meadow-Orlans (Eds.), *Educational and developmental aspects of deafness* (pp. 255–280). Washington, DC: Gallaudet University Press.

Bloom, A. (1981). *The linguistic shaping of thought.* Hillsdale, NJ: Lawrence Erlbaum.

Bloom, D., & Green, J. (1984). Directions in the sociolinguistics study of reading. In P. D. Pearson, R. Barr, M. Kamil, & P. Mosenthal (Eds.), *Handbook of reading research* (pp. 395–421). New York: Longman.

Bloom, L. (1970). *Language development: Form and function in emerging grammars.* Cambridge, MA: MIT Press.

Bloom, L. (1973). *One word at a time: The use of single-word utterances before syntax.* The Hague: Mouton.

Bloom, L., & Lahey, M. (1978). *Language development and language disorders.* New York: Wiley.

Bloom, L., Lightbown, P., & Hood, L. (Eds.). (1975). Structure and variation in child language. *Monographs of the Society for Research in Child Development, 40*(2), 1–97.

Bochner, J., & Albertini, J. (1988). Language varieties in the deaf populations and their acquisition by children and adults. In M. Strong (Ed.), *Language learning and deafness* (pp. 3–48). New York: Cambridge University Press.

Bohannon, J., & Warren-Leubecker, A. (1985). Theoretical approaches to language acquisition. In J. Berko-Gleason (Ed.), *The development of language* (pp. 173–226). Columbus, OH: Merrill.

Bolton, B. (1978). Differential ability structure in deaf and hearing children. *Applied Psychological Measurement, 2*(1), 147–149.

Bond, G. (1987). An assessment of cognitive abilities in hearing and hearing-impaired preschool children. *Journal of Speech and Hearing Disorders, 52,* 319–323.

Booth, P. (1985). The relationship of young children's prior background knowledge to their comprehension of textually explicit, textually implicit, and scriptally implicit questions for expository and narrative passages. *Dissertation Abstracts International, 46,* 1887A.

Borg, W., & Gall, M. (1983). *Educational research* (4th ed.). White Plains, NY: Longman.

Bornstein, H. (1982). Towards a theory of use of signed English: From birth through adulthood. *American Annals of the Deaf, 127,* 26–31.

Bornstein, H., & Saulnier, K. (1981). Signed English: A brief follow-up to the first evaluation. *American Annals of the Deaf, 126,* 69–72.

Bornstein, H., Saulnier, K., & Hamilton, L. (1980). Signed English: A first evaluation. *American Annals of the Deaf, 125,* 467–481.

Bornstein, H., Saulnier, K., & Hamiliton, L. (1983). *The comprehensive Signed English dictionary.* Washington, DC: Gallaudet College Press.

Bowerman, M. (1973). Structural relationships in children's utterances: Syntactic or semantic? In T. Moores (Ed.), *Cognitive development and the acquisition of language* (pp. 197–213). New York: Academic Press.

Bowerman, M. (1988). Inducing the latent structure of language. In F. Kessell (Ed.), *The development of language and language researchers: Essays in honor of Roger Brown* (pp. 23–49). Hillsdale, NJ: Lawrence Erlbaum.

Braden, J. (1984). The factorial similarity of the WISC-R performance scale in deaf and hearing samples. *Personality and Individual Differences, 5,* 403–409.

Bradley-Johnson, S., & Evans, L. (1991). *Psychoeducational assessment of hearing impaired students.* Austin, TX: Pro-Ed.

Brady, S., & Shankweiler, D. (Eds.). (1991). *Phonological processes in literacy: A tribute to Isabelle Y. Liberman.* Hillsdale, NJ: Lawrence Erlbaum.

Bragg, B. (1973). Ameslish—Our American heritage: A testimony. *American Annals of the Deaf, 118,* 672–674.

Braine, M. (1963a). The ontogeny of English phrase structure: The first phase. *Language, 39,* 1–13.

Braine, M. (1963b). On learning the grammatical order of words. *Psychological Review, 70,* 323–348.

Brasel, K., & Quigley, S. (1977). The influence of certain language and communication environments in early childhood on the development of language in deaf individuals. *Journal of Speech and Hearing Research, 20,* 95–107.

Bridwell, L. (1980). Revising strategies in twelfth grade students' transactional writing. *Research in the Teaching of English, 14,* 197–222.

Brown, P., Fischer, S., & Janis, W. (1993). Pragmatic and linguistic constraints on message formulation: A cross-linguistic study of English and ASL. *Journal of Speech and Hearing Research, 34,* 1346–1361.

Brown, P., & Long, G. (1992). The use of scripted interaction in a cooperative learning context to probe planning and evaluating during writing. *Volta Review, 95,* 411–424.

Brown, R. (1958). *Words and things.* Glencoe, IL: Free Press.

Brown, R. (1973). *A first language: The early stages.* Cambridge, MA: Harvard University.

Brumfit, C. (1984). *Communicative methodology in language teaching.* Cambridge, England: Cambridge University Press.

Bruner, J. (1974–1975). From communication to language: A psychological perspective. *Cognition, 3,* 255–287.

Bruner, J., & Bruner, B. (1968). On voluntary action and its hierarchial structure. *International Journal of Psychology, 3,* 239–255.

Bunge, M., & Ardila, R. (1987). *Philosophy of psychology.* New York: Springer-Verlag.

Byrnes, J., & Gelman, S. (1991). Perspectives on thought and language: Traditional and contemporary views. In S. Gelman & J. Byrnes (Eds.), *Perspectives on language and thought: Interrelations in development* (pp. 3–27). New York: Cambridge University Press.

CADS. (1991). Center for Assessment and Demographic Studies. *Stanford achievement test, eighth edition: Hearing-impaired norms booklet.* Washington, DC: Gallaudet University, Gallaudet Research Institute, Center for Assessment and Demographic Studies.

Cairns, H. (1986). *The acquisition of language.* Austin, TX: Pro-Ed.

Caleffe-Schenck, N. (1992). The auditory-verbal method: Description of a training program for audiologists, speech language pathologists, and teachers of children with hearing loss. *Volta Review, 94,* 65–68.

Callanan, M. (1991). Parent-child collaboration in young children's under-standing of category hierarchies. In S. Gelman & J. Byrnes (Eds.), *Perspectives on language and thought: Interrelations in development* (pp. 440–484). New York: Cambridge University Press.

Calvert, D. (1986). Speech in perspective. In D. Luterman (Ed.), *Deafness in pespective* (pp. 167–191). San Diego, CA: College-Hill Press.

Calvert, D., & Silverman, S. (1983). *Speech and deafness.* Washington, DC: Alexander Graham Bell Association for the Deaf.

Caniglia, J., Cole, N., Howard, W., Krohn, E., & Rice, M. (1975). *Apple Tree.* Beaverton, OR: Dormac.

Carnine, D., Silbert, J., & Kameenui, E. (1990). *Direct instruction reading* (2nd ed.). Columbus, OH: Merrill.

Carroll, J. (1961). Fundamental considerations in testing for English language proficiency of foreign students. *Testing.* Washington, DC: Center for Applied Linguistics.

Carrow, E. (1974). *Carrow elicited language inventory.* Austin, TX: Learning Concepts.

Carver, R. (1974). Two dimensions of tests: Psychometric and edumetric. *American Psychologist, 29,* 512–518.

Chalifoux, L. (1991). The implications of congenital deafness for working memory. *American Annals of the Deaf, 136,* 292–299.

Chall, J. (1983). *Stages of reading development.* New York: McGraw-Hill.

Chall, J., Jacobs, V., & Baldwin, L. (1990). *The reading crisis: Why poor children fall behind.* Cambridge, MA: Harvard University Press.

Chang, B., & Gonzales, B.R. (1987). A study of conservation abilities between hearing-impaired and normal hearing students in Taiwan. *Journal of Childhood Communication Disorders, 10*(2), 173–184.

Charrow, V. (1975). A psycholinguistic analysis of deaf English. *Sign Language Studies, 7,* 139–150.

Charrow, V., & Fletcher, J. (1974). English as the second language of deaf children. *Developmental Psychology, 10,* 463–470.

Chilson, R. (1985). Effects of cued speech instruction on speechreading skills. *Cued Speech Annual, 1,* 60–68.

Chomsky, N. (1957). *Syntactic structures.* The Hague: Mouton.

Chomsky, N. (1959). Review of Skinner's *Verbal Behavior. Language, 35,* 26–58.

Chomsky, N. (1965). *Aspects of the theory of syntax.* Cambridge, MA: Massachusetts Institute of Technology.

Chomsky, N. (1975). *Reflections on language.* New York: Pantheon Books.

Chomsky, N. (1980). *Rules and representations.* New York: Columbia University Press.

Chomsky, N. (1981). *Lectures on government and binding.* Dordrecht, Netherlands: Foris.

Chomsky, N. (1988). *Language and problems of knowledge: The Managua lectures.* Cambridge, MA: MIT Press.

Clark, E. (1973). What's in a word? On the child's acquisition of semantics in his first language. In T. Moores (Ed.), *Cognitive development and the acquisition of language* (pp. 65–110). New York: Academic Press.

Clark, E. (1991). Acquisitional principles in lexical development. In S. Gelman & J. Byrnes (Eds.), *Perspectives on language and thought: Interrelations in development* (pp. 31–71). New York: Cambridge University Press.

Clarke, B., & Ling, D. (1976). The effects of using cued speech: A follow-up study. *Volta Review, 78,* 23–35.

Clarke, B., Rogers, W., & Booth, J. (1982). How hearing impaired children learn to read: Theoretical and practical issues. *Volta Review, 84,* 57–69.

Cokely, D. (1983). When is a pidgin not a pidgin? An alternate analysis of the ASL-English contact situation. *Sign Language Studies, 38,* 1–24.

Collins-Ahlgren, M. (1974). Teaching English as a second language to young deaf children: A case study. *Journal of Speech and Hearing Disorders, 39,* 486–500.

Collins, A., Brown, J., & Larkin, K. (1980). Inference in text understanding. In R. Spiro, B. Bruce, & W. Brewer (Eds.), *Theoretical issues in reading comprehension* (pp. 385–407). Hillsdale, NJ: Lawrence Erlbaum.

Conley, J. (1976). Role of idiomatic expressions in the reading of deaf children. *American Annals of the Deaf, 121,* 381–385.

Connor, L. (1986). Oralism in perspective. In D. Luterman (Ed.), *Deafness in perspective* (pp. 117–129). San Diego, CA: College-Hill Press.

Conrad, R. (1979). *The deaf school child.* London, England: Harper & Row.

Conway, D. (1990). Semantic relationships in the word meanings of hearing-impaired children. *Volta Review, 92,* 339–349.

Cook, V. (1991). *Second language learning and language teaching.* New York: Edward Arnold.

Cooper, R. (1967). The ability of deaf and hearing children to apply morphological rules. *Journal of Speech and Hearing Research, 10,* 77–86.

Cooper, R., & Rosenstein, J. (1966). Language acquisition of deaf children. *Volta Review, 68,* 58–67.

Cornett, R.O. (1967). Cued speech. *American Annals of the Deaf, 112,* 3–13.

Cornett, R.O. (1984). Book review: Language and deafness. *Cued Speech News, 17*(3), p. 5.

Cornett, R.O. (1991). A model for ASL/English bilingualism. In S. Polowe-Aldersley, P. Schragle, V. Armour, & J. Polowe (Eds.), *Proceedings of the 55th Biennial Meeting of CAID and the 63rd Annual Meeting of CEASD* (pp. 33–39). New Orleans, LA: Convention of American Instructors of the Deaf.

Corson, H. (1973). *Comparing deaf children of oral deaf parents and deaf parents using manual communication with deaf children of hearing parents on academic, social, and communication functioning.* Unpublished doctoral dissertation, University of Cincinnati, Ohio.

Craig, H., & Gordon, H. (1988). Specialized cognitive function and reading achievement in hearing-impaired adolescents. *Journal of Speech and Hearing Disorders, 53,* 30–41.

Crain, S. (1989). Why poor readers misunderstand spoken sentences. In D. Shankweiler & I. Liberman (Eds.), *Phonology and reading disability: Solving the reading puzzle* (pp. 133–165). Ann Arbor, MI: The University of Michigan Press.

Crandall, K. (1978). Inflectional morphemes in the manual English of young hearing impaired children and their mothers. *Journal of Speech and Hearing Research, 21,* 372–386.

Creaghead, N., & Newman, P. (1985). Articulatory phonetics and phonology. In P. Newman, N. Creaghead, & W. Secord, *Assessment and remediation of articulatory and phonological disorders* (pp. 13–39). Columbus, OH: Merrill.

Crittenden, J. (1993). The culture and identify of deafness. In P. Paul & D. Jackson, *Toward a psychology of deafness: Theoretical and empirical perspectives* (pp. 215–235). Boston, MA: Allyn & Bacon.

Cromer, R. (1974). The development of language and cognition: The cognition hypothesis. In B. Foss (Ed.), *New perspectives in child development* (pp. 184–252). Harmondsworth, Middlesex, England: Penguin Books.

Cromer, R. (1976). The cognitive hypothesis of language acquisition and its implications for child language deficiency. In D. Morehead & A. Morehead (Eds.), *Normal and deficient child language* (pp. 283–333). Baltimore, MD: University Park Press.

Cromer, R. (1981). Reconceptualizing language acquisition and cognitive development. In R. Schiefelbusch & D. Bricker (Eds.), *Early language: Acquisition and intervention* (pp. 51–137). Baltimore, MD: University Park Press.

Cromer, R. (1988a). Differentiating language and cognition. In R. Schiefelbusch & L. Lloyd (Eds.), *Language perspectives: Acquisition, retardation, and intervention* (2nd ed., pp. 91–124). Austin, TX: Pro-Ed.

Cromer, R. (1988b). The cognition hypothesis revisited. In F. Kessel (Ed.), *The development of language and language researchers: Essays in honor of Roger Brown* (pp. 223–248). Hillsdale, NJ: Lawrence Erlbaum.

Cronbach, L. (1960). *Essentials of psychological testing.* New York: Harper & Row.

Crutchfield, P. (1972). Prospects for teaching English Det + N structures to deaf students. *Sign Language Studies, 1,* 8–14.

Cruttenden, A. (1979). *Language in infancy and childhood: A linguistic introduction to language acquisition.* New York: St. Martin's Press.

Crystal, D. (1987). *The Cambridge encyclopedia of language.* New York: Cambridge University Press.

Cued Speech Journal. (1990). *Cued Speech Journal: Journal of the National Cued Speech Association, 4* (C. Boggs, Ed.)

Cummins, J. (1977). Cognitive factors associated with the attainment of intermediate levels of bilingual skill. *The Modern Language Journal, 61,* 3–12.

Cummins, J. (1978). Educational implications of mother tongue maintenance in minority-language groups. *Canadian Modern Language Review, 34,* 395–416.

Cummins, J. (1979). Linguistic interdependence and the educational development of bilingual children. *Review of Educational Research, 49,* 222–251.

Cummins, J. (1980). The entry and exit fallacy in bilingual education. *NABE Journal, 4,* 25–60.

Cummins, J. (1984). *Bilingualism and special education: Issues in assessment and pedagogy.* San Diego, CA: College-Hill Press.

Cummins, J. (1988). Second language acquisition within bilingual education programs. In L. Beebe (Ed.), *Issues in second language acquisition: Multiple perspectives* (pp. 145–166). New York: Newbury House.

Cummins, J. (1989). A theoretical framework for bilingual special education. *Exceptional Children, 56,* 111–119.

Curtis, M. (1987). Vocabulary testing and vocabulary instruction. In M. McKeown & M. Curtis (Eds.), *The nature of vocabulary acquisition* (pp. 37–51). Hillsdale, NJ: Lawrence Erlbaum.

Czerniewska, P. (1992). *Learning about writing: The early years.* Cambridge, MA: Basil Blackwell.

Cziko, G. (1992). The evaluation of bilingual education: From necessity and probability to possibility. *Educational Researcher, 21*(2), 10–15.

Dale, E., & Chall, J. (1948). A formula for predicting readability. *Educational Research Bulletin, 27,* 11–20; 37–54.

Dale, E., & Eicholtz, G. (1960). *Children's knowledge of words.* Columbus, OH: Ohio State University, Bureau of Educational Resources.

Dale, P. (1976). *Language development: Structure and function* (2nd ed.). New York: Holt, Rinehart, & Winston.

Davey, B., & King, S. (1990). Acquisition of word meanings from context by deaf readers. *American Annals of the Deaf, 135,* 227–234.

Davies, A. (1990). *Principles of language testing.* Cambridge, MA: Basil Blackwell.

Davies, A., Criper, C., & Howatt, A. (1984). *Interlanguage.* Edinburgh, Scotland: Edinburgh University Press.

Davis, H. (1978). Anatomy and physiology of the auditory system. In H. Davis & S.R. Silverman, *Hearing and deafness* (4th ed., pp. 46–83). New York: Holt, Rinehart, & Winston.

Deaf American. (1990). *Deaf Amerian, 40*(1–4). [Special Monograph— *Eyes, Hands, Voices: Communication Issues Among Deaf People*].

Deal, R., & Thornton, R. (1985). An exploratory investigation of the comprehension of English through sign English (Siglish) and seeing essential English (SEE I). *Language, Speech, and Hearing Services in Schools, 16,* 267–279.

Dechant, E. (1991). *Understanding and teaching reading: An interactive model.* Hillsdale, NJ: Lawrence Erlbaum.

Deighton, L. (1959). *Vocabulary development in the classroom.* New York: Teachers College, Columbia University, Bureau of Publications.

de Jong, J., & Verhoeven, L. (1992). Modeling and assessing language proficiency. In L. Verhoeven & J. de Jong (Eds.), *The construct of language proficiency: Applications of psychological models to language assessment* (pp. 3–19). Philadelphia, PA: Benjamins.

Delaney, M., Stuckless, E.R., & Walter, G. (1984). Total communication effects—A longitudinal study of a school for the deaf in transition. *American Annals of the Deaf, 129,* 481–486.

Demopoulos, W. (1989). On applying learnability theory to the rationalism-empiricism controversy. In R. Matthews & W. Demopoulos (Eds.), *Learnability and linguistic theory* (pp. 77–88). Boston, MA: Kluwer Academic Publishers.

de Villiers, J., & de Villiers, P. (1978). *Language acquisition.* Cambridge, MA: Harvard University Press.

de Villiers, P., & Pomerantz, S. (1992). Hearing-impaired students learning new words from written context. *Applied Psycholinguistics, 13,* 409–431.

DiFrancesca, S. (1972). *Academic achievement test results of a national testing program for hearing-impaired students-United States, Spring* (Series D, No. 9). Washington, DC: Gallaudet College, Office of Demographic Studies.

Dixon, K., Pearson, P.D., & Ortony, A. (1980, December). *Some reflections on the use of figurative language in children's textbooks.* Paper presented at the annual meeting of the National Reading Conference, San Diego, CA.

Doehring, D., Bonnycastle, D., & Ling, A. (1978). Rapid reading skills of integrated hearing impaired children. *Volta Review, 80,* 399–409.

Dolman, D. (1992). Some concerns about using whole language approaches with deaf children. *American Annals of the Deaf, 137,* 278–282.

Dore, J. (1974). A pragmatic description of early language development. *Journal of Psycholinguistic Research, 3,* 343–350.

Dore, J. (1975). Holophrases, speech acts, and language universals. *Journal of Child Language, 2,* 21–40.

Dore, J., Franklin, M., Miller, R., & Ramer, A. (1976). Transitional phenomena in early language acquisition. *Journal of Child Language, 3,* 13–28.

Duchan, J. (1984). Language assessment: The pragmatics revolution. In R. Naremore (Ed.), *Language science: Recent advances* (pp. 147–180). San Diego, CA: College-Hill.

Durkin, D. (1989). *Teaching them to read* (5th ed.). Boston, MA: Allyn & Bacon.

Eacker, J. (1975). *Problems of philosophy and psychology.* Chicago, IL: Nelson-Hall.

Eagney, P. (1987). ASL? English? Which? Comparing comprehension. *American Annals of the Deaf, 132,* 272–275.

Eilers, R., Oller, D., Bull, D., & Gavin, W. (1984). Linguistic experience and infant perception: A reply to Jusczyk, Shea, & Aslin (1984). *Journal of Child Language, 11,* 467–475.

Eimas, P. (1985). The perception of speech in early infancy. *Scientific American, 252,* 46–52.

Eimas, P., Siqueland, E., Jusczyk, P., & Vigorito, J. (1971). Speech perception in infants. *Science, 171,* 303–306.

Engen, E., & Engen, T. (1983). *Rhode Island test of language structures.* Austin, TX: Pro-Ed.

Erber, N. (1982). *Auditory training.* Washington, DC: Alexander Graham Bell Association for the Deaf.

Erickson, M. (1987). Deaf readers reading beyond the literal. *American Annals of the Deaf, 132,* 291–294.

Erting, C. (1992). Partnerships for change: Creating new possible worlds for deaf children and their families. In *Conference proceedings: Bilingual considerations in the education of deaf students: ASL and English* (pp. 35–45). Washington, DC: Gallaudet University, College for Continuing Education.

Everhart, V., & Marschark, M. (1988). Linguistic flexibility in signed and written language productions of deaf children. *Journal of Experimental Child Psychology, 46,* 174–193.

Ewoldt, C. (1981). A psycholinguistic description of selected deaf children reading in sign language. *Reading Research Quarterly, 17,* 58–89.

Felix, S. (1982). *Psycholinguistische Aspekte des Zwitsprachenerwerbs.* Tubingen, Germany: Gunter Narr Verlag.

Ferguson, C., & Farwell, C. (1975). Words and sounds in early language acquisition: English consonants in the first 50 words. *Language, 51,* 419–439.

Feuerstein, R., Rand, Y., & Hoffman, M. (1979). *The dynamic assessment of retarded performers.* Baltimore, MD: University Park Press.

Feuerstein, R., Rand, Y., Hoffman, M., & Miller, R. (1980). *Instrumental enrichment*. Baltimore, MD: University Park Press.

Fincher-Kiefer, R. (1992). The role of prior knowledge in inferential processing. *Journal of Research in Reading, 15* (1), 12–27.

Fitzgerald, E. (1929). *Straight language for the deaf*. Staunton, VA: The McClure Company.

Flavell, D. (1985). *Cognitive development* (2nd ed.). Englewood Cliffs, NJ: Prentice-Hall.

Fodor, J. (1983). *The modularity of mind: An essay on faculty psychology*. Cambridge, MA: The MIT Press.

Frishberg, N. (1975). Arbitrariness and iconicity: Historical change in ASL. *Language, 51,* 676–710.

Fruchter, A., Wilbur, R., & Fraser, B. (1984). Comprehension of idioms by hearing-impaired students. *Volta Review, 86,* 7–18.

Furth, H. (1964). Research with the deaf: Implications for language and cognition. *Psychological Bulletin, 62,* 145–164.

Furth, H. (1966a). *Thinking without language: Psychological implications of deafness*. New York: Free Press.

Furth, H. (1966b). A comparison of reading test norms of deaf and hearing children. *American Annals of the Deaf, 111,* 461–462.

Furth, H. (1969). *Piaget and knowledge: Theoretical foundations*. Englewood Cliffs, NJ: Prentice-Hall.

Furth, H. (1973). *Deafness and learning: A psychosocial approach*. Belmont, CA: Wadsworth.

Furth, H., Youniss, J. (1965). The influence of language and experience on discovery and use of logical symbols. *British Journal of Psychology, 56,* 381–390.

Fusaro, J., & Slike, S. (1979). The effect of imagery on the ability of hearing-impaired children to identify words. *American Annals of the Deaf, 124,* 829–832.

Gallaudet Research Institute. (1985). *Gallaudet Research Institute Newsletter.* J. Harkins (Ed.). Washington, DC: Gallaudet University Press.

Gamez, G. (1979). Reading in a second language: Native language approach vs. direct method. *The Reading Teacher, 32,* 665–670.

Gannon, J. (1981). *Deaf heritage: A narrative history of deaf America*. Silver Spring, MD: National Association of the Deaf.

Gardner, J., & Zorfass, J. (1983). From sign to speech: The language development of a hearing-impaired child. *American Annals of the Deaf, 128,* 20–24.

Gee, J., & Goodhart, W. (1985). Nativization, linguistic theory, and deaf language acquisition. *Sign Language Studies, 49,* 291–342.

Gee, J., & Goodhart, W. (1988). American Sign Language and the human biological capacity for language. In M. Strong (Ed.), *Language learning and deafness* (pp. 49–74). New York: Cambridge University Press.

Gee, J., & Kegl, J. (1982). Semantic perspicuity and the locative hypothesis: Implications for acquisition. *Journal of Education, 164,* 185–209.

Geers, A., & Moog, J. (1989). Factors predictive of the development of literacy in profoundly hearing-impaired adolescents. *Volta Review, 91,* 69–86.

Gelman, S., & Byrnes, J. (Eds.). (1991). *Perspectives on language and thought: Interrelations in development.* New York: Cambridge University Press.

Genesee, F. (1987). *Learning through two languages: Studies of immersion and bilingual education.* Cambridge, MA: Newbury House.

Gentile, A., & DiFrancesca, S. (1969). *Academic achievement test performance of hearing-impaired students-United States, Spring* (Series D, No. 1.). Washington, DC: Gallaudet College, Office of Demographic Studies.

Gibbs, K. (1989). Individual differences in cognitive skills related to reading ability in the deaf. *American Annals of the Deaf, 134,* 214–218.

Gibson, R. (1986). *Critical theory and education.* London, England: Hodder & Stoughton.

Gilman, L., Davis, J., & Raffin M. (1980). Use of common morphemes by hearing impaired children exposed to a system of manual English. *Journal of Auditory Research, 20,* 57–69.

Giorcelli, L. (1982). *The comprehension of some aspects of figurative language by deaf and hearing subjects.* Unpublished doctoral dissertation, University of Illinois, Urbana-Champaign.

Gleason, J. (1988). Language and socialization. In F. Kessell (Ed), *The development of language and language researchers: Essays in honor of Roger Brown* (pp. 269–280). Hillsdale, NJ: Lawrence Erlbaum.

Gleason, J., Hay, D., & Cain, L. (1989). Social and affective determinants of language acquisition. In M. Rice & R. Schiefelbusch (Eds.), *The teachability of language* (pp. 171–186). Baltimore, MD: Paul H. Brookes.

Gliedman, J., & Roth, W. (1980). *The unexpected minority: Handicapped children in America.* New York: Harcourt Brace Jovanovich.

Goldberg, J., & Bordman, P. (1975). The ESL approach to teaching English to hearing impaired students. *American Annals of the Deaf, 120,* 22–27.

Goodluck, H. (1991). *Language acquisition: A linguistic introduction.* Cambridge, MA: Basil Blackwell.

Goodman, K. (1976). Reading: A psycholinguistic guessing game. In H. Singer & R. Ruddell (Eds.), *Theoretical models and processes of reading* (2nd ed., pp. 497–508). Newark, DE: International Reading Association.

Goodman, K. (1985). Unity in reading. In H. Singer & R. Ruddell (Eds.), *Theoretical models and processes of reading* (3rd ed., pp. 813–840). Newark, DE: International Reading Association.

Gormley, K., & Sarachan-Deily, A. (1987). Evaluating hearing-impaired students' writing: A practical approach. *Volta Review, 89,* 157–170.

Grabe, W. (1988). Reassessing the term "interactive." In P. Carrell, J. Devine, & D. Eskey (Eds.), *Interactive approaches to second language reading* (pp. 56–70). New York: Cambridge University Press.

Grabe, W. (1991). Current developments in second-language reading research. *TESOL Quarterly, 25,* 375–406.

Greenberg, M., & Kusche, C. (1989). Cognitive, personal, and social development of deaf children and adolescents. In M. Wang, M. Reynolds, & H. Walberg (Eds.), *The handbook of special education: Research and practice* (Vol. 3, pp. 95–129). New York: Pergamon.

Greenfield, P., & Smith, J. (1976). *The structure of communication in early language development.* New York: Academic Press.

Gregory, J. (1987). An investigation of speechreading with and without cued speech. *American Annals of the Deaf, 132,* 393–398.

Griffith, P., & Ripich, D. (1988). Story structure recall in hearing-impaired, learning-disabled and nondisabled children. *American Annals of the Deaf, 133,* 43–50.

Griswold, E., & Cummings, J. (1974). The expressive vocabulary of preschool deaf children. *American Annals of the Deaf, 119,* 16–28.

Groht, M. (1958). *Natural language for deaf children.* Washington, DC: The Volta Bureau.

Gustason, G. (1983). *Teaching and learning signing exact English.* Los Alamitos, CA: Modern Signs Press.

Gustason, G., Pfetzing, D., & Zawolkow, E. (1975). *Signing exact English* (Rev. ed.). Los Alamitos, CA: Modern Signs Press.

Gustason, G., Pfetzing, D., & Zawolkow, E. (1980). *Signing exact English.* Los Alamitos, CA: Modern Signs Press.

Halliday, M. (1975). *Learning how to mean: Explorations in the development of language.* London, England: Edward Arnold.

Hanson, V. (1989). Phonology and reading: Evidence from profoundly deaf readers. In D. Shankweiler & I. Liberman (Eds.), *Phonology and reading disability: Solving the reading puzzle* (pp. 69–89). Ann Arbor, MI: University of Michigan Press.

Hanson, V. (1990). Recall of order information by deaf signers: Phonetic coding in temporal order recall. *Memory and Cognition, 18,* 604–610.

Hanson, V., Liberman, I., & Shankweiler, D. (1984). Linguistic coding by deaf children in relation to beginning reading success. *Journal of Experimental Child Psychology, 37,* 378–393.

Hanson, V., & Lichtenstein, E. (1990). Short-term memory coding by deaf signers: The primary language coding hypothesis reconsidered. *Cognitive Psychology, 22,* 211–224.

Harris, P. (1982). Cognitive prerequisites to language. *British Journal of Psychology, 73,* 187–195.

Harrison, A. (1983). *A language testing handbook.* London, England: Macmillan.

Hatcher, C., & Robbins, N. (1978). *The development of reading skills in hearing-impaired children.* Cedar Falls, IA: University of Northern Iowa. (ERIC Document Reproduction Service No. ED 167 960)

Haugen, E. (1956). *Bilingualism in the Americas: A bibliography and a research guide.* Montgomery, AL: University of Alabama Press.

Hayes, P., & Arnold, P. (1992). Is hearing-impaired children's reading delayed or different? *Journal of Research in Reading, 15,* 104–116.

Heider, F., & Heider, G. (1940). A comparison of sentence structure of deaf and hearing children. *Psychological Monographs, 52,* 42–103.

Heimlich, J., & Pittelman, S. (1986). *Semantic mapping: Classroom applications.* Newark, DE: International Reading Association.

Hester, M. (1969). Education of the deaf. In J. Griffith (Ed.), *Persons with hearing loss* (pp. 150–165). Springfield, IL: Thomas.

Hillocks, G. (1986). *Research on written composition: New directions for teaching.* Urbana, IL: National Conference on Research in English.

Hirsh-Pasek, K. (1987). The metalinguistics of fingerspelling: An alternative way to increase written vocabulary in congenitally deaf readers. *Reading Research Quarterly, 22,* 455–474.

Hiskey, M. (1966). *Hiskey-Nebraska test of learning aptitude: Manual.* Lincoln, NE: Union College Press.

Hoffmeister, R., & Wilbur, R. (1980). The acquisition of sign language. In H. Lane & F. Grosjean (Eds.), *Recent perspectives on American Sign Language* (pp. 61–78). Hillsdale, NJ: Lawrence Erlbaum.

Horn, J. (1989). Models of intelligence. In R. Linn (Ed.), *Intelligence: Measurement, theory, and public policy* (pp. 29–73). Urbana, IL: University of Illinois Press.

Houck, J. (1982). *The effects of idioms on reading comprehension of hearing impaired students.* Unpublished doctoral dissertation, University of Northern Colorado (Abstract)

Howe, C. (1981). Interpretive analysis and role semantics: A ten-year mesalliance? *Journal of Child Language, 8,* 439–456.

Huey, E. (1908/1968). *The psychology and pedagogy of reading.* New York: Macmillan. (Reprinted, Cambridge, MA: MIT Press)

Humphries, T., Padden, C., & O'Rourke, T. J. (1980). *A basic course in American Sign Language.* Silver Spring, MD: T. J. Publishers.

Hunt, K. (1965). *Grammatical structures written at three grade levels.* Champaign, IL: National Council of Teachers of English.

Hunt, K. (1970). A syntactic maturity in school children and adults. *Monographs of the Society of Research in Child Development, 35,* No. 134.

Hymes, D. (1974). *Foundations in sociolinguistics: An ethnographic approach.* Philadelphia, PA: University of Pennsylvania Press.

Ingram, D. (1989). *First language acquisition: Method, description, and explanation.* New York: Cambridge University Press.

Iran-Nejad, A., Ortony, A., & Rittenhouse, R. (1981). The comprehension of metaphorical uses of English by deaf children. *Journal of Speech and Hearing Research, 24,* 551–556.

Jakobson, R. (1968). *Child language aphasia and phonological universals* (Trans. by A. Keiler). The Hague: Mouton.

Johnson, D., Moe, A., & Baumann, J. (1983). *The Ginn word book for teachers: A basic lexicon.* Lexington, MA: Ginn.

Johnson, R. (1916). What are the fundamentals? *American Annals of the Deaf, 61,* 92–95.

Johnson-Laird, P. (1988). *The computer and the mind: An introduction to cognitive science.* Cambridge, MA: Harvard University.

Johnson, R., Liddell, S., & Erting, C. (1989). *Unlocking the curriculum: Principles for achieving access in deaf education* (Working Paper 89-3). Washington, DC: Gallaudet University, Gallaudet Research Institute.

Johnston, J. (1985). Cognitive prerequisites: The evidence from children learning English. In D. Slobin (Ed.), *The crosslinguistic study of language acquisition: Vol. 2. Theoretical issues* (pp. 961–1004). Hillsdale, NJ: Lawrence Erlbaum.

Jonas, B., & Martin, D. (1985). Cognitive improvement of hearing impaired high school students through instruction and instrumental enrichment. In D. Martin (Ed.), *Cognition, education, and deafness* (pp. 172–175). Washington, DC: Gallaudet University Press.

Jones, P. (1979). Negative interference of signed language in written English. *Sign Language Studies, 24,* 273–279.

Jordan, I.K., Gustason, G., & Rosen, R. (1979). An update on communication trends at programs for the deaf. *American Annals of the Deaf, 124,* 350–357.

Jordan, I.K., & Karchmer, M. (1986). Patterns of sign use among hearing-impaired students. In A. Schildroth & M. Karchmer (Eds.), *Deaf children in America* (pp. 125–138). Boston, MA: Little, Brown.

Joyce, B., Weil, M., & Showers, B. (1992). *Models of teaching* (4th ed.). Boston: Allyn & Bacon.

Jusczyk, P., Shea, S., & Aslin, R. (1984). Linguistic experience and infant speech perception: A re-examination of Eilers, Gavin and Oller (1982). *Journal of Child Language, 11,* 453–466.

Just, M., & Carpenter, P. (1987). *The psychology of reading and language comprehension.* Boston, MA: Allyn & Bacon.

Kantor, R. (1980). The acquisition of classifiers in American Sign Language. *Sign Language Studies, 28,* 193–208.

Kantor, R. (1982). Communicative interaction: Mother modification and child acquisition of American Sign Language. *Sign Language Studies, 36,* 233–282.

Kaufman, A., & Kaufman, N. (1983). *The Kaufman assessment battery for children.* Chicago, IL: American Guidance Association.

Kelly, L. (1993). Recall of English function words and inflections by skilled and average deaf readers. *American Annals of the Deaf, 138,* 288–296.

King, C. (1981). *An investigation of similarities and differences in the syntactic abilities of deaf and hearing children learning English as a first or second language.* Unpublished doctoral dissertaion, University of Illinois, Champaign-Urbana.

King, C. (1984). National survey of language methods used with hearing-impaired students in the United States. *American Annals of the Deaf, 129,* 311–316.

King, C., & Quigley, S. (1985). *Reading and deafness.* San Diego, CA: College-Hill Press.

Kisor, H. (1990). *What's that pig outdoors: A memoir of deafness.* New York: Hill & Wang.

Klecan-Aker, J. (1988). *Developing a reliable means of coding stories.* Unpublished manuscript, University of Houston.

Klecan-Aker, J., & Blondeau, R. (1990). An examination of the written stories of hearing-impaired school-age children. *Volta Review, 92,* 275–282.

Klecan-Aker, J., & Hedrick, D. (1985). A study of the syntactic language abilities of normal middle school children. *Language, Speech and Hearing Services in the Schools, 16,* 187–198.

Klima, E., & Bellugi, U. (1979). *The signs of language.* Cambridge, MA: Harvard University Press.

Kluwin, T. (1981). The grammaticality of manual representation of English in classroom settings. *American Annals of the Deaf, 126,* 417–421.

Kluwin, T., Getson, P., & Kluwin, B. (1980). The effects of experience on the discourse comprehension of deaf and hearing adolescents. *Directions, 1*(3), 49.

Kluwin, T., & Kelly, A. (1991). The effectiveness of kealogue journal writing in improving the writing skills of young deaf writers. *American Annals of the Deaf, 136,* 284–291.

Krakow, R., & Hanson, V. (1985). Deaf signers and serial recall in the visual modality: Memory for signs, fingerspelling, and print. *Memory and Cognition, 13,* 265–272.

Krashen, S. (1981). *Second language acquisition and second language learning.* Oxford: Pergamon Press.

Krashen, S. (1982). *Principles and practices of second language acquisition.* Oxford: Pergamon Press.

Krashen, S. (1985). *The input hypothesis: Issues and implications.* White Plains, NY: Longman.

Kretschmer, R.E. (1989). Pragmatics, reading, and writing: Implications for hearing-impaired individuals. *Topics in Language Disorders, 9* (4), 17–32.

Kretschmer, R.R., & Kretschmer, L. (1978). *Language development and intervention with the hearing impaired.* Baltimore, MD: University Park Press.

Kretschmer, R.R., & Kretschmer, L. (Eds.). (1988a). Communication assessment of hearing-impaired children: From conversation to classroom. *The Journal of the Academy of Rehabilitative Audiology, Monograph Supplement, Vol. 21.*

Kretschmer, R.R., & Kretschmer, L. (1988b). Communication competence and assessment. In R.R. Kretschmer & L. Kretschmer (Eds.), *Communication assessment of hearing-impaired children: From conversation to classroom* (pp.5–17). *The Journal of the Academy of Rehabilitative Audiology, Monograph Supplement, Vol. 12.*

Kuhn, T. (1970). *The structure of scientific revolutions* (2nd ed.). Chicago, IL: University of Chicago Press.

Kusche, C., & Greenberg, M. (1991). Cortical organization and information processing in deaf children. In D. Martin (Ed.), *Advances in cognition, education, and deafness* (pp. 243–249). Washington, DC: Gallaudet University Press.

Labov, W. (1972). *Sociolinguistic patterns.* Philadelphia, PA: University of Pennsylvania Press.

Laine, C., & Schultz, L. (1985). Composition theory and practice: The paradigm shift. *Volta Review, 87, Learning to write and writing to learn* (pp. 9–20). [Special Issue, R.R. Kretschmer (Ed.)].

Lambert, W. (1972). A social psychology of bilingualism. In W. Lambert (Ed.), *Language, psychology, and culture* (pp. 212–235). Stanford, CA: Stanford University Press.

Lambert, W., & Tucker, G. (1972). *The bilingual education of children: The St. Lambert experiment.* Rowley, MA: Newbury House.

Lamendella, J. (1977). General principles of neurofunctional organization and their manifestation in primary and nonprimary language acquisition. *Language Learning, 27,* 155–196.

Lane, H. (1976). Thoughts on oral advocacy today . . . with memories of the society of oral advocates. *Volta Review, 78,* 136–140.

Lane, H. (1988). Is there a "psychology of the deaf"? *Exceptional Children, 55,* 7–19.

Lane, H., & Baker, D. (1974). Reading achievement of the deaf: Another look. *Volta Review, 76,* 489–499.

Lane, H., & Grosjean, F. (Eds.). (1980). *Recent perspectives on American Sign Language.* Hillsdale, NJ: Lawrence Erlbaum.

LaSasso, C. (1985, June). *1984 national survey of materials and procedures used to teach reading to hearing impaired students: Preliminary results.* Paper presented at the CAID/CEASD National Conference in St. Augustine, FL.

LaSasso, C. (1987). Survey of reading instruction for hearing-impaired students in the United States. *Volta Review, 89,* 85–98.

LaSasso, C., & Davey, B. (1987). The relationship between lexical knowledge and reading comprehension for prelingually, profoundly hearing-impaired students. *Volta Review, 89,* 211–220.

Layton, T., & Holmes, D. (1985). *Carolina picture vocabulary test.* Austin, TX: Pro-Ed.

Layton, T., Holmes, D., & Bradley, P. (1979). A description of pedagogically imposed signed semantic-syntactic relationships in deaf children. *Sign Language Studies, 23,* 137–160.

Lee, L. (1966). Developmental sentence types: A method for comparing normal and deviant syntactic development. *Journal of Speech and Hearing Disorders, 31,* 311–330.

Lee, L. (1969). *Northwestern syntax screening test.* Evanston, IL: Northwestern University Press.

Lee, L. (1974). *Developmental sentence analysis.* Evanston, IL: Northwestern University Press.

Lee, L., & Canter, S. (1971). Developmental sentence scoring: A clinical procedure for estimating syntactic development in children's spontaneous speech. *Journal of Speech and Hearing Disorders, 36,* 315–340.

Lemley, P. (1993). *Deaf readers and engagement in the story world: A study of strategies and stances.* Unpublished doctoral dissertation, The Ohio State University, Columbus.

Lenneberg, E. (1967). *Biological foundations of language.* New York: Wiley.

Levine, E. (1981). *The ecology of early deafness: Guides to fashioning environments and psychological assessments.* New York: Columbia University Press.

Levitt, H. (1989). Technology and speech training: An affair to remember. *Volta Review, 91*(5), 1–6. [N. McGarr, (Ed.), *Research on the use of sensory aids for hearing-impaired people*].

Liberman, I., Shankweiler, D, & Liberman, A. (1989). The alphabetic principle and learning to read. In D. Shankweiler & I. Liberman (Eds.), *Phonology and reading disability: Solving the reading puzzle* (pp. 1–33). Ann Arbor, MI: University of Michigan Press.

Lichtenstein, E. (1983). *The relationships between reading processes and English skills of deaf students.* Unpublished manuscript, National Technical Institute for the Deaf, Rochester, NY.

Lichtenstein, E. (1984). Deaf working memory processes and English language skills. In D. Martin (Ed.), *International symposium on cognition, education, and deafness: Working papers* (Vol. 2, pp. 331–360). Washington, DC: Gallaudet University Press.

Lichtenstein, E. (1985). Deaf working memory processes and English language skills. In D. Martin (Ed.), *Cognition, education, and deafness: Directions for research and instruction* (pp. 111–114). Washington, DC: Gallaudet University Press.

Liddell, S. (1980). *Amerian Sign Language syntax*. The Hague: Mouton.

Liddell, S., & Johnson, R. (1992). Toward theoretically sound practices in deaf education. In *Bilingual considerations in the education of deaf students: ASL and English* (pp. 8–34). Washington, DC: Gallaudet University, College for Continuing Education.

Liedel, J., & Paul, P. (1991). An interactive-interaction bilingual-bicultural program model. In S. Polowe-Aldersley, P. Schragle, V. Armour, & J. Polowe (Eds.), *Conference Proceedings of the 1991 CAID/CEASD Convention* (pp. 106–109). New Orleans, LA: Convention of American Instructors of the Deaf.

Lillo-Martin, D., Hanson, V., & Smith, S. (1991). Deaf readers' comprehension of complex syntactic structure. In D. Martin (Ed.), *Advances in cognition, education, and deafness* (pp. 146–151). Washington, DC: Gallaudet University Press.

Lillo-Martin, D., Hanson, V., & Smith, S. (1992). Deaf readers' comprehension of relative clause structure. *Applied Psycholinguistics, 13*(1), 13–30.

Limbrick, E., McNaughton, S., & Clay, M. (1992). Time engaged in reading: A critical factor in reading achievement. *American Annals of the Deaf, 137*, 309–314.

Lindfors, J. (1980). *Children's language and learning*. Englewood Cliffs, NJ: Prentice-Hall.

Ling, D. (1976). *Speech and the hearing-impaired child: Theory and practice*. Washington, DC: Alexander Graham Bell Association for the Deaf.

Ling, D. (Ed.). (1984). *Early intervention for hearing-impaired children: Oral options*. San Diego, CA: College-Hill Press.

Ling, D. (1989). *Aural habilitation: The foundation of verbal learning in hearing-impaired children* (2nd ed.). Washington, DC: Alexander Graham Bell Association for the Deaf.

Ling, D. (1990). Advances underlying spoken language development: A century of building on Bell. *Volta Review, 92*(4), 7–20. [S. R. Silverman & P. Kricos (Eds.), *A centennial review*].

Ling, D., & Clarke, B. (1975). Cued speech: An evaluative study. *American Annals of the Deaf, 120*, 480–488.

Lipson, M., & Wixson, K. (1991). *Assessment and instruction of reading disability: An interactive approach*. New York: HarperCollins.

Livingston, S. (1983). Levels of development in the language of deaf children: ASL grammatical process, SE structures, and semantic features. *Sign Language Studies, 40*, 193–286.

Livingston, S. (1989). Revision strategies of deaf student writers. *American Annals of the Deaf, 134*, 21–26.

Locke, J., & Locke, V. (1971). Deaf children's phonetic, visual, and dactylic coding in a grapheme recall task. *Journal of Experimental Psychology, 89*, 142–146.

Long, N., Fitzgerald, C., Sutton, K., & Rollins, J. (1983). The auditory-verbal approach: Ellison, a case study. *Volta Review, 85*, 27–30, 35.

Looney, P., & Rose, S. (1979). The acquisition of inflectional suffixes by deaf youngsters using written and fingerspelled modes. *American Annals of the Deaf, 124*, 765–769.

Lou, M. (1988). The history of language use in the education of the Deaf in the United States. In M. Strong (Ed.), *Language learning and deafness* (pp. 75–98). Cambridge, MA: Cambridge University Press.

Lucas, C. (Ed.). (1990). *Sign language research.* Washington, DC: Gallaudet University Press.

Lucas, E. (1980). *Semantic and pragmatic language disorders: Assessment and remediation.* Rockville, MD: Aspen Systems.

Luckner, J., & Isaacson, S. (1990). Teaching expressive writing to hearing-impaired students. *Journal of Childhood Communication Disorders, 13*, 135–152.

Luetke-Stahlman, B. (1983). Using bilingual instructional models in teaching hearing-impaired students. *American Annals of the Deaf, 128*, 873–877.

Luetke-Stahlman, B. (1984). Classifier recognition by hearing-impaired children in residential and public schools. *Sign Language Studies, 42*, 39–44.

Luetke-Stahlman, B. (1988a). The benefit of oral English-only as compared with signed input to hearing-impaired students. *Volta Review, 90*, 349–361.

Luetke-Stahlman, B. (1988b). Documenting syntactically and semantically incomplete bimodal input to hearing-impaired subjects. *American Annals of the Deaf, 133*, 230–234.

Luetke-Stahlman, B. (1991). Following the rules: Consistency in sign. *Journal of Speech and Hearing Research, 34*, 1293–1298.

Luetke-Stahlman, B., & Luckner, J. (1991). *Effectively educating students with hearing impairments.* White Plains, NY: Longman.

Luetke-Stahlman, B., & Weiner, F. (1982). Assessing language and/or system preferences of Spanish-deaf preschoolers. *American Annals of the Deaf, 127*, 789–796.

MacGinitie, W. (1969). Flexibility in dealing with alternative meanings of words. In J. Rosenstein & W. MacGinitie (Eds.), *Verbal behavior of the deaf child: Studies of word meanings and associations* (pp. 45–55). New York: Columbia University, Teachers College Press.

Mackey, W. (1965). *Language teaching analysis.* Bloomington, IN: Indiana University Press.

Macnamara, J. (1966). *Bilingualism and primary education: A study of Irish experience.* Chicago, IL: Aldine.

Mann, L., & Sabatino, D. (1985). *Foundations of cognitive process in remedial and special education.* Rockville, MD: Aspen.

Marbury, N., & Mackinson-Smyth, J. (1986, April). *ASL and English: A partnership.* Paper presented at the American Sign Language Research and Teaching Conference, Newark, CA.

Marmor, G., & Petitto, L. (1979). Simultaneous communication in the classroom: How well is English grammar represented? *Sign Language Studies, 23,* 99–136.

Marr, D. (1982). *Vision.* San Francisco, CA: Freeman.

Marshall, W., & Quigley, S. (1970). *Quantitative and qualitative analysis of syntactic structure in the written language of deaf students.* Urbana, IL: University of Illinois, Institute for Research on Exceptional Children.

Martin, D. (Ed.). (1991). *Advances in cognition, education, and deafness.* Washington, DC: Gallaudet University Press.

Martin, D. (1993). Reasoning skills: A key to literacy for deaf learners. *American Annals for the Deaf, 138,* 82–86.

Martin, D., & Jonas, B. (1987). Cognitive modifiability in the deaf adolescent. In R. Ojala (Ed.), *Proceedings of the Tenth World Congress of the World Federation of the Deaf* (Vol. 1, pp. 277–282). Finland.

Martin, D., & Jonas, B. (1991). Cognitive enhancement of hearing-impaired postsecondary students. In D. Martin (Ed.), *Advances in cognition, education, and deafness* (pp. 335–341). Washington, DC: Gallaudet University Press.

Marton, W. (1988). *Methods in English language teaching: Frameworks and options.* New York: Prentice Hall.

Mason, J., & Au, K. (1986). *Reading instruction for today.* Glenview, IL: Scott, Foresman.

Mason, J., & CSR [Staff of the Center for the Study of Reading]. (1984). A schema-theoretic view of the reading process as a basis for comprehension instruction. In G. Duffy, L. Roehler, & J. Mason (Eds.), *Comprehension instruction: Perspectives and suggestions* (pp. 26–38). White Plains, NY: Longman.

Matthews, P. (1991). *Morphology* (2nd ed.). Cambridge, MA: Cambridge University Press.

Matthews, R. (1989). Introduction: Learnability and linguistic theory. In R. Matthews & W. Demopoulos (Eds.), *Learnability and linguistic theory* (pp. 1–17). Boston, MA: Kluwer Academic Publishers.

Maxwell, M. (1987). The acquisition of English bound morphemes in sign form. *Sign Languae Studies, 57,* 323–352.

Maxwell, M. (1990). Simultaneous communication: The state of the art and proposals for change. *Sign Language Studies, 69,* 333–390.

McAnally, P., Rose, S., & Quigley, S. (1987). *Language learning practices with deaf children.* San Diego, CA: Little, Brown.

McAnally, P., Rose, S., & Quigley, S. (in press). *Language learning practices with deaf children* (2nd ed). Austin, TX: Pro-Ed.

McCartney, B. (1986). An investigation of the factors contributing to the ability of hearing-impaired children to communicate orally as perceived by oral deaf adults and parents and teachers of the hearing impaired. *Volta Review, 88,* 133–143.

McClure, W. (1969). Historical perspectives in the education of the deaf. In J. Griffith (Ed.), *Persons with hearing loss* (pp. 3–30). Springfield, IL: Thomas.

McCormick, S. (1987). *Remedial and clinical reading instruction.* Columbus, OH: Merrill.

McCrone, J. (1991). *The ape that spoke: Language and the evolution of the human mind.* New York: Morrow.

McGill-Franzen, A., & Gormley, K. (1980). The influence of context on deaf readers' understanding of passive sentences. *American Annals of the Deaf, 125,* 937–942.

McIntire, M. (1977). The acquisition of American Sign Language hand configurations. *Sign Language Studies, 16,* 247–266.

McKee, P., Harrison, M., McCowen, A., Lehr, E., & Durr, W. (1966). *Reading for meaning* (4th ed.). Boston, MA: Houghton Mifflin.

McLaughlin, B. (1984). *Second-language acquisition in childhood: Vol. 1. Preschool children* (2nd ed.). Hillsdale, NJ: Lawrence Erlbaum.

McLaughlin, B. (1985). *Second-language acquisition in childhood: Vol. 2. School-age children* (2nd ed.). Hillsdale, NJ: Lawrence Erlbaum.

McLaughlin, B. (1987). *Theories of second-language learning.* Baltimore, MD: Edward Arnold.

Meadow, K. (1968). Early manual communication in relation to the deaf child's intellectual, social, and communicative functioning. *American Annals of the Deaf, 113,* 29–41.

Meadow, K. (1980). *Deafness and child development.* Berkeley: University of California Press.

Medin, D., & Ross, B. (1992). *Cognitive psychology.* New York: Harcourt Brace Jovanovich.

Menyuk, P. (1963). A preliminary evaluation of grammatical capacity in children. *Journal of Verbal Learning and Verbal Behavior, 2,* 429–439.

Menyuk, P. (1968). The role of distinctive features in children's acquisition of phonology. *Journal of Speech and Hearing Research, 11,* 138–146.

Menyuk, P. (1977). *Language and maturation.* Cambridge, MA: MIT Press.

Messerly, C., & Aram, D. (1980). Academic achievement of hearing-impaired students of hearing parents and of hearing-impaired parents: Another look. *Volta Review, 82*, 25–32.

Meyerhoff, W. (1986). *Disorders of hearing.* Austin, TX: Pro-Ed.

Miller, G. (1956). The magic number seven, plus or minus two: Some limits on our capacity for processing information. *Psychological Review, 63*, 81–97.

Miller, G. (1965). Some preliminaries to psycholinguistics. In L. Jakobovits & M. Miron (Eds.), *Readings in the psychology of language* (pp. 172–179). Englewood Cliffs, NJ: Prentice-Hall.

Miller, J. (1981). *Assessing language production in children.* Baltimore, MD: University Park Press.

Mitchell, G. (1982). Can deaf children acquire English? An evaluation of manually coded English systems in terms of the principles of language acquisition. *American Annals of the Deaf, 127*, 331–336.

Modiano, N. (1968). National or mother language in beginning reading: A comparative study. *Research in the Teaching of English, 2*, 32–43.

Moeller, M. (1988). Combining formal and informal strategies for language assessment of hearing-impaired children. In R.R. Kretschmer & L. Kretschmer (Eds.), Communication assessment of hearing-impaired children: From conversation to classroom (pp. 73–99). *Journal of the Academy of Rehabilitative Audiology, 21, Monograph Supplement.*

Mohay, H. (1983). The effects of cued speech on the language development of three deaf children. *Sign Language Studies, 38*, 25–47.

Moog, J. (1988). *Central Institute for the Deaf phonetic inventory.* St. Louis, MO: Central Institute for the Deaf.

Moog, J., & Geers, A. (1979). *Grammatical analysis of elicited language: Simple sentence level.* St. Louis, MO: Central Institute for the Deaf.

Moog, J., & Geers, A. (1980). *Grammatical analysis of elicited language: Complex sentence level.* St. Louis, MO: Central Institute for the Deaf.

Moog, J., & Kozak, V. (1983). *Teacher assessment of grammatical structures.* St. Louis, MO: Central Institute for the Deaf.

Moog, J., Kozak, V., & Geers, A. (1983). *Grammatical analysis of elicited language: Pre-sentence level.* St. Louis, MO: Central Institute for the Deaf.

Moores, D. (1987). *Educating the deaf: Psychology, principles, and practices* (3rd ed.). Boston, MA: Houghton Mifflin.

Moores, D., & Meadow-Orlans, K. (Eds.). (1990). *Educational and developmental aspects of deafness.* Washington, DC: Gallaudet University Press.

Moores, D., & Sweet, C. (1990). Factors predictive of school achievement. In D. Moores & K. Meadow-Orlans (Eds.), *Educational and developmental aspects of deafness* (pp. 154–201). Washington, DC: Gallaudet University.

Morse, P. (1974). Infant speech perception: A preliminary model and review of the literature. In R. Schiefelbusch & L.L. Lloyd (Eds.), *Language perspective: Acquisition, retardation, and intervention* (pp. 19–53). Baltimore, MD: University Park Press.

Muma, J. (1986). *Language acquisition: A functionalistic perspective.* Austin, TX: Pro-Ed.

Myklebust, H. (1960). *The psychology of deafness.* New York: Grune & Stratton.

Myklebust, H. (1964). *The psychology of deafness* (2nd ed.). New York: Grune & Stratton.

Naglieri, J. (1987). *Evidence for the planning, attention, simultaneous and successive cognitive processing theory.* Paper presented at the Annual Convention of the American Psychological Association, New York.

Naglieri, J., & Das, J. (1988). Planning-attention-simultaneous-successive (PASS): A model for assessment. *Journal of School Psychology, 26,* 35–48.

Nagy, W., & Herman, P. (1987). Breadth and depth of vocabulary knowledge: Implications for acquisition and instruction. In M. McKeown & M. Curtis (Eds.), *The nature of vocabulary acquisition* (pp. 19–35). Hillsdale, NJ: Lawrence Erlbaum.

Navarro, R. (1985). The problems of language, education, and society: Who decides. In E. Garcia & R. Padilla (Eds.), *Advances in bilingual education research* (pp. 289–313). Tucson, AZ: University of Arizona Press.

Negin, G. (1987). The effects of syntactic segmentation on the reading comprehension of hearing-impaired students. *Reading Psychology, 8,* 23–31.

Neisser, A. (1983). *The other side of silence: Sign language and the Deaf community in America.* New York: Knopf.

Nelson, K. (1973). Structure and strategy in learning to talk. *Monographs of the Society for Research in Child Development, 38*(1–2).

Neuroth-Gimbrone, C., & Logiodice, C. (1992). A cooperative bilingual language program for deaf adolescents. *Sign Language Studies, 74,* 79–91.

Newport, E., & Ashbrook, E. (1977). The emergence of semantic relations in American Sign Language. *Papers and Reports on Child Language Development, 13,* 16–21.

Newport, E., & Meier, R. (1985). The acquisition of American Sign Language. In D. Slobin (Ed.), *The cross-linguistic study of language acquisition* (pp. 881–938). Hillsdale, NJ: Lawrence Erlbaum.

Nicholls, G., & Ling, D. (1982). Cued speech and the reception of spoken language. *Journal of Speech and Hearing Research, 25,* 262–269.

Nickerson, R. (1986). Literacy and cognitive development. In M. Wrolstad & D. Fisher (Eds.), *Toward a new understanding of literacy* (pp. 5–38). New York: Praeger.

Nolen, S, & Wilbur, R. (1985). The effects of context on deaf students' comprehension of difficult sentences. *American Annals of the Deaf, 130*, 231–235.

Novelli-Olmstead, T., & Ling, D. (1984). Speech production and speech discrimination by hearing-impaired children. *Volta Review, 86*, 72–80.

Nystrand, M., & Knapp, J. (1987). *Review of selected national tests of writing and reading*. Unpublished manuscript, University of Wisconsin, National Center on Effective Secondary Schools, School of Education, Madison.

Odom, P., Blanton, R., & McIntyre, C. (1970). Coding medium and word recall by deaf and hearing subjects. *Journal of Speech and Hearing Research, 13*, 54–58.

Ogden, P. (1979). *Experiences and attitudes of oral deaf adults regarding oralism*. Unpublished doctoral dissertation, University of Illinois, Urbana-Champaign.

Oller, J. (1979). *Language tests at school*. New York: Longman.

Oller, J., & Perkins, K. (1978). *Language in education: Testing the tests*. Rowley, MA: Newbury House.

Oller, J., & Perkins, K. (Eds.). (1980). *Research in language testing*. Rowley, MA: Newbury House.

Olson, D. (1989). Literate thought. In C.K. Leong & B. Randhawa (Eds), *Understanding literacy and cognition* (pp. 3–15). New York: Plenum Press.

O'Neill, M. (1973). *The receptive language competence of deaf children in the use of the base structure rules of transformational generative grammar*. Unpublished doctoral dissertation, University of Pittsburgh, Pennsylvania.

Orlando, A., & Shulman, B. (1989). Severe-to-profound hearing-impaired children's comprehension of figurative language. *Journal of Childhood Communication Disorders, 12*(2), 157–165.

O'Rourke, J. (1974). *Toward a science of vocabulary development*. The Hague: Mouton.

O'Rourke, T.J. (1973). *A basic course in manual communication*. Silver Spring, MD: National Association of the Deaf.

Otheguy, R., & Otto, R. (1980). The myth of static maintenance in bilingual education. *Modern Language Journal, 64*, 350–356.

Owens, R., Haney, M., Giesow, V., Dooley, L., & Kelly, R. (1983). Language test content: A comparative study. *Language, Speech & Hearing Services in Schools, 14*, 7–21.

Padden, C., & Humphries, T. (1988). *Deaf in America: Voices from a culture*. Cambridge, MA: Harvard University Press.

Padden, C., & Le Master, B. (1985). An alphabet on hand: The acquisition of fingerspelling in deaf children. *Sign Language Studies, 47*, 161–172.

Page, S. (1981). *The effect of idiomatic language in passages on the reading comprehension of deaf and hearing students.* Unpublished doctoral dissertation, Ball State University, Indiana (Abstract).

Paul, P. (1984). *The comprehension of multimeaning words from selected frequency levels by deaf and hearing subjects.* Unpublished doctoral dissertation, University of Illinois, Urbana-Champaign.

Paul, P. (1985). Reading and other language-variant populations. In C. King & S. Quigley, *Reading and deafness* (pp. 251–289). San Diego, CA: College-Hill Press.

Paul, P. (1990). Using ASL to teach English literacy skills (invited article). *The Deaf American, 40*(1–4), 107–113.

Paul, P. (1991). ASL to English: A bilingual minority-language immersion program for deaf students. In S. Polowe-Aldersley, P. Schragle, V. Armour, & J. Polowe (Eds.), *Conference Proceedings of the 1991 CAID/CEASD Convention* (pp. 53–56). New Orleans, LA: Convention of American Instructors of the Deaf.

Paul, P. (1993). Deafness and text-based literacy. *American Annals of the Deaf, 138,* 72–75.

Paul, P., Bernhardt, E., & Gramly, C. (1992). Use of ASL in teaching reading and writing to deaf students: An interactive theoretical perspective. In *Conference Proceedings: Bilingual Considerations in the Education of Deaf Students: ASL and English* (pp. 75–105). Washington, DC: Gallaudet University, Extension and Summer Programs.

Paul, P., & Gustafson, G. (1991). Hearing-impaired students' comprehension of high-frequency multimeaning words. *Remedial and Special Education* (RASE), *12*(4), 52–62.

Paul, P., & Jackson, D. (1993). *Toward a psychology of deafness: Theoretical and empirical perspectives.* Boston, MA: Allyn & Bacon.

Paul, P., & O'Rourke, J. (1988). Multimeaning words and reading comprehension: Implications for special education students. *Remedial and Special Education* (RASE), *9*(3), 42–52.

Paul, P., & Quigley, S. (1987a). Some effects of early hearing impairment on English language development. In F. Martin (Ed.), *Hearing disorders in children: Pediatric audiology* (pp. 49–80). Austin, TX: Pro-Ed.

Paul, P., & Quigley, S. (1987b). Using American Sign Language to teach English. In P. McAnally, S. Rose, & S. Quigley, *Language learning practices with deaf children* (pp. 139–166). San Diego, CA: Little, Brown.

Paul, P., & Quigley, S. (1989). Education and hard-of-hearing students. In H. Hartmann & K. Hartmann (Eds.), *Conference proceedings: Hard-of-hearing pupils in regular schools* (pp. 48–60, 173–184). Berlin, Germany: International Organization of Hard-of-Hearing Students.

Paul, P., & Quigley, S. (1990). *Education and deafness*. White Plains, NY: Longman.

Paul, P., & Quigley, S. (in press). American Sign Language/English bilingual programs. In P. McAnally, S. Rose, & S. Quigley, *Language learning practices with deaf children* (2nd ed.). Austin, TX: Pro-Ed.

Paul, P., Stallman, A., & O'Rourke, J. (1990). *Using three test formats to assess good and poor readers' word knowledge* (Tech. Rep. No. 509). Urbana-Champaign, IL: University of Illinois, Center for the Study of Reading.

Payne, J.A. (1982). *A study of the comprehension of verb-particle combinations among deaf and hearing subjects*. Unpublished doctoral dissertation, University of Illinois, Urbana-Champaign.

Payne, J.A., & Quigley, S. (1987). Hearing-impaired children's comprehension of verb-particle combinations. *Volta Review, 89*, 133–143.

Pearson, P.D. (1984). *Reading comprehension instruction: Six necessary changes* (Reading Educ. Rep. No. 54). Champaign, IL: University of Illinois, Center for the Study of Reading.

Pearson, P.D., Barr, R., Kamil, M., & Mosenthal, P. (Eds.). (1984). *Handbook of reading research*. White Plains, NY: Longman.

Pearson, P.D., & Valencia, S. (1986, December). *Assessment, accountability, and professional prerogative*. Paper presented at the 1986 National Reading Conference in Austin, TX.

Perfetti, C. (1985). *Reading ability*. New York: Oxford University Press.

Petitto, L. (1986). *Language vs. gesture: Why sign languages are NOT acquired earlier than spoken languages*. Paper presented at the 1986 Conference on Theoretical Issues in Sign Language Research, Rochester, NY.

Petitto, L. (1988). "Language" in the prelinguistic child. In F. Kessell (Ed.), *The development of language and language researchers: Essays in honor of Roger Brown* (pp. 187–221). Hillsdale, NJ: Lawrence Erlbaum.

Petitto, L., & Marentette, P. (1991). Babbling in the manual mode: Evidence for the ontogeny of language. *Science, 251*, 1493–1496.

Philip, M. (1992). The learning center. In *Conference proceedings: Bilingual considerations in the education of deaf students: ASL and English* (pp. 46–47). Washington, DC: Gallaudet University.

Phillips, J. (1981). *Piaget's theory: A primer*. San Francisco, CA: Freeman.

Piaget, J. (1952). *The origins of intelligence in children*. New York: International University Press.

Piaget, J. (1968). *Six psychological studies*. New York: Vintage Books.

Piaget, J. (1971). *Psychology and epistemology*. New York: The Viking Press.

Piaget, J. (1977). *The development of thought: Equilibration of cognitive structures*. New York: Viking.

Piaget, J. (1980). *Six psychological studies.* Brighton, Sussex, England: Harvester Press.

Piatelli-Palmarini, M. (Ed.). (1980). *Language and learning.* Cambridge, MA: Harvard University Press.

Pinker, S. (1989). *Learnability and cognition: The acquisition of argument structure.* Cambridge, MA: The MIT Press.

Pintner, R., Eisenson, J., & Stanton, M. (1941). *The psychology of the physically handicapped.* New York: Crofts.

Pollack, D. (1984). An acoupedic program. In D. Ling (Ed.), *Early intervention for hearing-impaired children: Oral options* (pp. 181–253). San Diego, CA: College-Hill Press.

Power, D., & Quigley, S. (1973). Deaf children's acquisition of the passive voice. *Journal of Speech and Hearing Research, 16,* 5–11.

Prabhu, N. (1990). There is no best method—why? *TESOL Quarterly, 24,* 161–176.

Pressnell, L. (1973). Hearing-impaired children's comprehension and production of syntax in oral language. *Journal of Speech and Hearing Research, 16,* 12–21.

Priest, J. (1991). *Theories of the mind.* Boston, MA: Houghton Mifflin.

Pugh, B. (1955). *Steps in language development for the deaf: Illustrated in the Fitzgerald Key.* Washington, DC: The Volta Bureau.

Quenin, C., & Blood, I. (1989). A national survey of cued speech programs. *Volta Review, 91,* 283–289.

Quigley, S. (1969). *The influence of fingerspelling on the development of language, communication, and educational achievement in deaf children.* Urbana, IL: University of Illinois, Institute for Research on Exceptional Children.

Quigley, S., & Frisina, R. (1961). *Institutionalization and psychoeducational development of deaf children* (CEC Research Monograph). Washington, DC: Council of Exceptional Children.

Quigley, S., & King, C. (Eds.). (1981–1984). *Reading milestones.* Beaverton, OR: Dormac.

Quigley, S., & Kretschmer, R. (1982). *The education of deaf children: Issues, theory, and practice.* Austin, TX: Pro-Ed.

Quigley, S., & Paul, P. (1984). ASL and ESL? *Topics in Early Childhood Special Education, 3*(4), 17–26.

Quigley, S., & Paul, P. (1986). A perspective on academic achievement. In D. Luterman (Ed.), *Deafness in perspective* (pp. 55–86). San Diego, CA: College-Hill Press.

Quigley, S., & Paul, P. (1989). English language development. In M. Wang, M. Reynolds, & H. Walberg (Eds.), *The handbook of special education: Research and practice* (Vol. 3, pp. 3–21). Oxford: Pergamon.

Quigley, S., & Paul, P. (1990). *Language and deafness*. San Diego, CA: Singular Publishing Group.

Quigley, S., & Paul, P. (in press). Reflections. In P. McAnally, S. Rose, & S. Quigley, *Language learning practices with deaf children* (pp. xxx). Austin, TX: Pro-Ed.

Quigley, S., Paul, P., McAnally, P., Rose, S., & Payne, J. (1990). *The reading bridge: Teacher's guide: Mosaic*. San Diego, CA: Dormac.

Quigley, S., Paul, P., McAnally, P., Rose, S., & Payne, J. (1991). *The reading bridge: Teacher's guide: Patterns*. San Diego, CA: Dormac.

Quigley, S., & Power, D. (1979). *TSA syntax program*. Beaverton, OR: Dormac.

Quigley, S., Power, D., & Steinkamp, M. (1977). The language structure of deaf children. *Volta Review, 79*, 73–83.

Quigley, S., Power, D., Steinkamp, M., & Jones, B. (1978). *Test of syntactic abilities*. Beaverton, OR: Dormac.

Quigley, S., Smith, N., & Wilbur, R. (1974). Comprehension of relativized sentences by deaf students. *Journal of Speech and Hearing Research, 17*, 325–341.

Quigley, S., Steinkamp, M., Power, D., & Jones, B. (1978). *Test of syntactic abilities*. Beaverton, OR: Dormac.

Quigley, S., Wilbur, R., & Montanelli, D. (1974). Question formation in the language of deaf students. *Journal of Speech and Hearing Research, 17*, 699–713.

Quigley, S., Wilbur, R., & Montanelli, D. (1976). Complement structures in the language of deaf students. *Journal of Speech and Hearing Research, 19*, 448–457.

Quigley, S., Wilbur, R., Power, D., Montanelli, D., & Steinkamp, M. (1976). *Syntactic structures in the language of deaf children* (Final Report). Urbana, IL: University of Illinois, Institute for Child Behavior and Development. (ERIC Document Reproduction Service No. ED 119 447)

Raffin, M. (1976). *The acquisition of inflectional morphemes by deaf children using Seeing Essential English*. Unpublished doctoral dissertation, University of Iowa, Iowa City.

Raffin, M., Davis, J., & Gilman L. (1978). Comprehension of inflectional morphemes by deaf children exposed to a visual English sign system. *Journal of Speech and Hearing Research, 21*, 387–400.

Raphael, T., & McKinney, J. (1983). An examination of fifth- and eighth-grade children's question-answering behavior: An instructional study in metacognition. *Journal of Reading Behavior, 15*, 67–86.

Rayner, K., & Pollatsek, A. (1989). *The psychology of reading*. Englewood Cliffs, NJ: Prentice-Hall.

Reagan, T. (1985). The deaf as a linguistic minority: Educational considerations. *Harvard Educational Review, 55*, 265–277.

Reagan, T. (1990). Cultural considerations in the education of deaf children. In D. Moores & K. Meadow-Orlans (Eds.), *Educational and developmental aspects of deafness* (pp. 73–84). Washington, DC: Gallaudet University Press.

Regis, E. (1987). *Who got Einstein's office? Eccentricity and genius at the institute for advanced study.* Reading, MA: Addison-Wesley.

Reich, P. (1986). *Language development.* Englewood Cliffs, NJ: Prentice-Hall.

Reid, K., Hresko, W., Hammill, D., & Wiltshire, S. (1991). *Test of early reading ability-deaf or hard of hearing.* Austin, TX: Pro-Ed.

Restak, R. (1988). *The mind.* New York: Bantam Books.

Rice, M., & Kemper, S. (1984). *Child language and cognition.* Baltimore, MD: University Park Press.

Rice, M., & Schiefelbusch, R. (Eds.). (1989). *The teachability of language.* Baltimore, MD: Paul H. Brookes.

Rittenhouse, R. (1977). *Horizontal decalage: The development of conservation in deaf students and the effect of the task instructions on their performance.* Unpublished doctoral dissertation, University of Illinois, Urbana-Champaign.

Rittenhouse, R. (1987). Piagetian conservation in deaf children. *Journal of Childhood Communication Disorders, 10* (2), 201–206.

Ritzer, G. (1991). *Metatheorizing in sociology.* Lexington, MA: Lexington Books.

Robbins, N. (1983). The effects of signed text on the reading comprehension of hearing-impaired children. *American Annals of the Deaf, 128*, 40–44.

Rodda, M., & Grove, C. (1987). *Language, cognition, and deafness.* Hillsdale, NJ: Lawrence Erlbaum.

Rosenstein, J. (1960). Cognitive abilities of deaf children. *Journal of Speech & Hearing Research, 3*, 108–119.

Rosenstein, J. (1961). Perception, cognition, and language in deaf children. *Exceptional Children, 27*, 276–284.

Rosier, P., & Farella, M. (1976). Bilingual education at Rock Point—Some early results. *TESOL Quarterly, 10*, 379–388.

Ross, M. (1986). *Aural habilitation.* Austin, TX: Pro-Ed.

Ross, M. (Ed.). (1990). *Hearing-impaired children in the mainstream.* Monkton, MD: York Press.

Ross, M., Brackett, D., & Maxon, A. (1982). *Hard of hearing children in regular schools.* Englewood Cliffs, NJ: Prentice-Hall.

Ross, M., & Calvert, D. (1984). Semantics of deafness revisited: Total communication and the use and misuse of residual hearing. *Audiology, 9*, 127–143.

Rubin, A., & Hansen, J. (1986). Reading and writing: How are the first two R's related? In J. Orasanu (Ed.), *Reading comprehension: From research to practice* (pp. 163–170). Hillsdale, NJ: Lawrence Erlbaum.

Ruddell, R., & Haggard, M. (1985). Oral and written language acquisition and the reading process. In H. Singer & R. Ruddell (Eds.), *Theoretical models and processes of reading* (pp. 63–80). Newark, DE: International Reading Association.

Rumelhart, D. (1977). Toward an interactive model of reading. In S. Dornic (Ed.), *Attention and performance VI* (pp. 573–603). New York: Academic Press.

Rumelhart, D. (1980). Schemata: The building blocks of cognition. In R. Spiro, B. Bruce, & W. Brewer (Eds.), *Theoretical issues in reading comprehension* (pp. 33–58). Hillsdale, NJ: Lawrence Erlbaum.

Rumelhart, D. (1985). Toward an interactive model of reading. In H. Singer & R. Ruddell (Eds.), *Theoretical models and processes of reading* (pp. 722–750). Newark, DE: International Reading Association.

Rumelhart, D., McClelland, J., & the PDP Research Group. (1986). *Parallel distributed processing: Explorations in the microstructure of cognition: Vol. 1. Foundations.* Cambridge, MA: MIT Press.

Russell, B. (1948). *Human knowledge: Its scope and limits.* New York: Simon & Schuster.

Russell, W., Quigley, S., & Power, D. (1976). *Linguistics and deaf children.* Washington, DC: Alexander Graham Bell Association for the Deaf.

Sacks, O. (1989). *Seeing voices: A journey into the world of the deaf.* Berkeley, CA: University of California Press.

Salvia, J., & Ysseldyke, J. (1991). *Assessment* (5th ed.). Boston, MA: Houghton Mifflin.

Samuels, S.J., & Kamil, M. (1984). Models of the reading process. In P. D. Pearson, R. Barr, M. Kamil, & P. Mosenthal (Eds.), *Handbook of reading research* (pp. 185–224). White Plains, NY: Longman.

Sapir, E. (1958). *Selected writings of Edward Sapir in language, culture, and personality* (Edited by D. Mandelbaum). Berkeley, CA: University of California Press.

Sarachan-Deily, A. (1982). Hearing-impaired and hearing readers' sentence processing errors. *Volta Review, 84,* 81–95.

Sarachan-Deily, A. (1985). Written narratives of deaf and hearing students: Story recall and inference. *Journal of Speech and Hearing Research, 28,* 151–159.

Schank, R., & Farrell, R. (1988). Memory. In M. McTear (Ed.), *Understanding cognitive science* (pp. 120–133). New York: Halsted Press.

Scherer, P. (1981). *Total communication receptive vocabulary test.* Northbrook, IL: Mental Health and Deafness Resources.

Schirmer, B. (1994). *Language and literacy development in children who are deaf.* New York: Maxwell Macmillan International.

Schlesinger, H., & Meadow, K. (1972). *Sound and sign: Childhood deafness and mental health.* Berkeley: University of California Press.

Schlesinger, I. (1982). *Steps to language: Toward a theory of native language acquisition.* Hillsdale, NJ: Lawrence Erlbaum.

Schmitt, P. (1969). *Deaf children's comprehension and production of sentence transformation and verb tenses.* Unpublished doctoral dissertation, University of Illinois, Urbana-Champaign.

Scholnick, E., & Hall, W. (1991). The language of thinking: Metacognitive and conditional words. In S. Gelman & J. Byrnes (Eds.), *Perspectives on language and thought: Interrelations in development* (pp. 397–439). New York: Cambridge University Press.

Schulze, B. (1965). An evaluation of vocabulary development by thirty-two deaf children over a three-year period. *American Annals of the Deaf, 110,* 424–435.

Schumann, J. (1978). *The pidginization process: A model for second language acquisition.* Rowley, MA: Newbury House.

Scouten, E. (1967). The Rochester method: An oral multisensory approach for instructing prelingual deaf children. *American Annals of the Deaf, 112,* 50–55.

Searle, J. (1969). *Speech acts.* Cambridge, UK: Cambridge University Press.

Searle, J. (1976). A classification of illocutionary acts. *Language in Society, 5,* 1–23.

Searle, J. (1992). *The rediscovery of the mind.* Cambridge, MA: The MIT Press.

Searls, E., & Klesius, K. (1984). 99 multiple meaning words for primary students and ways to teach them. *Reading Psychology: An International Quarterly, 5,* 55–63.

Selinker, L. (1972). Interlanguage. *IRAL, 10,* 209–231.

Selinker, L., Swain, M., & Dumas, G. (1975). The interlanguage hypothesis extended to children. *Language Learning, 25,* 139–191.

Shadbolt, N. (1988). Models and methods in cognitive science. In M. McTear (Ed.), *Understanding cognitive science* (pp. 23–45). New York: Halsted Press.

Shankweiler, D., & Liberman, I. (1989). *Phonology and reading disability: Solving the reading puzzle.* Ann Arbor, MI: The University of Michigan Press.

Shipley, E., Smith, C., & Gleitman, L. (1969). A study in the acquisition of language; free responses to commands. *Language, 45,* 322–342.

Shohamy, E., & Walton, A.R. (1992). *Language assessment for feedback: Testing and other strategies.* Dubuque, IA: Kendall/Hunt.

Silverman, S.R., & Kricos, P. (Eds.). (1990). A centennial review. *Volta Review*, *92*(4).

Silverman-Dresner, T., & Guilfoyle, G. (1972). *Vocabulary norms for deaf children: The Lexington school for the deaf education series, book VII*. Washington, DC: The Alexander Graham Bell Association for the Deaf.

Simmons, A. (1963). *Comparison of written and spoken language from deaf and hearing children at five age levels*. Unpublished doctoral dissertation, Washington University, St. Louis, MO.

Siple, P. (Ed.). (1978). *Understanding language through sign language research*. New York: Academic Press.

Skinner, B.F. (1957). *Verbal behavior*. Englewood, Cliffs, NJ: Prentice-Hall.

Slobin, D. (1979). *Psycholinguistics* (2nd ed.). Glenview, IL: Scott, Foresman.

Smith, F. (1975). *Comprehension and learning: A conceptual framework for teachers*. New York: Holt, Rinehart, & Winston.

Smith, F. (1978). *Understanding reading* (Rev. ed.). New York: Holt, Rinehart, & Winston.

Snyder, L. (1984). Cognition and language development. In R. Naremore (Ed.), *Language science* (pp. 107–145). San Diego, CA: College-Hill Press.

Sommers, N. (1980). Revision strategies of student writers and experienced adult writers. *College Composition and Communication*, *31*, 378–388.

Sperling, G. (1963). A model for visual memory tasks. *Human Factors*, *5*, 19–31.

Sperling, G. (1968). Phonemic model of short-term auditory memory. *Proceedings of the 76th Annual Convention of the American Psychological Association*, *3*, 63–64.

Stanovich, K. (Ed.). (1988). *Children's reading and the development of phonological awareness*. Detroit, MI: Wayne State University Press.

Stein, N., & Glenn, C. (1979). An analysis of story comprehension in elementary school children. In R. O. Freedle (Ed.), *New directions in discourse processing* (Vol. 2, pp. 53–120). Norwood, NJ: Ablex.

Steinberg, D. (1982). *Psycholinguistics: Language, mind, and the world*. White Plains, NY: Longman.

Steinberg, D., & Jakobovits, L. (Eds.). (1971). *Semantics: An interdisciplinary reader in philosophy, linguistics, and psychology*. New York: Cambridge University Press.

Sternberg, R., & Detterman, D. (Eds.). (1986). *What is intelligence? Contemporary viewpoints on its nature and definition*. Norwood, NJ: Ablex.

Stevenson, R. (1988). *Models of language development*. Philadelphia, PA: Open University Press.

Stewart, D. (1985). Language dominance in deaf students. *Sign Language Studies*, *49*, 375–385.

Sticht, T., & James, J. (1984). Listening and reading. In P.D. Pearson, R. Barr, M. Kamil, & P. Mosenthal (Eds.), *Handbook on reading research* (pp. 293–317). White Plains, NY: Longman.

Stoefen-Fisher, J., & Lee, M. (1989). The effectiveness of the graphic representation of signs in developing word identification skills for hearing-impaired beginning readers. *Journal of Special Education, 23*(2), 151–167.

Stokoe, W. (1960). *Sign language structure: An outline of the visual communication systems of the American deaf. Studies in Linguistics Occasional Papers No. 8.* Washington, DC: Gallaudet University Press.

Stokoe, W. (1990). An historical perspective on sign language research: A personal view. In C. Lucas (Ed.), *Sign language research: Theoretical issues* (pp. 1–8). Washington, DC: Gallaudet University Press.

Stokoe, W., Casterline, D., & Croneberg, C. (1976). *A dictionary of American Sign Language on linguistic principles* (Rev. ed.). Silver Spring, MD: Linstok Press.

Strassman, B. (1992). Deaf adolescents' metacognitive knowledge about school-related reading. *American Annals of the Deaf, 137,* 326–330.

Strassman, B., Kretschmer, R.E., & Bilsky, L. (1987). The instantiation of general terms by deaf adolescents/adults. *Journal of Communication Disorders, 20,* 1–13.

Strong, M. (Ed.). (1988a). *Language learning and deafness.* New York: Cambridge University Press.

Strong, M. (1988b). A bilingual approach to the education of young deaf children: ASL and English. In M. Strong (Ed.), *Language learning and deafness* (pp. 113–129). New York: Cambridge University Press.

Strong, M., & Charlson, E. (1987). Simultaneous communication: Are teachers attempting an impossible task? *American Annals of the Deaf, 132,* 376–382.

Stuckless, E. R. (1991). Reflections on bilingual, bicultural education for deaf children: Some concerns about current advocacy and trends. *American Annals of the Deaf, 136,* 270–272.

Stuckless, E. R., & Birch, J. (1966). The influence of early manual communication on the linguistic development of deaf children. *American Annals of the Deaf, 111,* 452–460, 499–504.

Stuckless, E. R., & Marks, C. (1966). *Assessment of the written language of deaf students.* Pittsburgh, PA: University of Pittsburgh, School of Education.

Stuckless, E. R., & Pollard, G. (1977). Processing of fingerspelling and print by deaf students. *American Annals of the Deaf, 122,* 475–479.

Supalla, S. (1986). *Manually coded English: The modality question in signed language development.* Unpublished master's thesis, University of Illinois, Urbana-Champaign.

Swain, M., & Lapkin, S. (1982). *Evaluating bilingual education: A Canadian example*. Clevedon, England: Multilingual Matters, Ltd.

Taylor, I., & Taylor, M. M. (1983). *The psychology of reading*. New York: Academic Press.

Taylor, L. (1969). *A language analysis of the writing of deaf children*. Unpublished doctoral dissertation, Florida State University, Tallahassee.

Templeton, S., & Bear, D. (1992). *Development of orthographic knowledge and the foundations of literacy: A memorial festschrift for Edmund H. Henderson*. Hillsdale, NJ: Lawrence Erlbaum.

Templin, M. (1950). *The development of reasoning in children with normal and defective hearing*. Minneapolis, MN: University of Minnesota.

Thompson, M., Biro, P., Vethivelu, S., Pious, C., & Hatfield, N. (1987). *Language assessment of hearing-impaired school age children*. Seattle, WA: University of Washington Press.

Tierney, R., & Leys, M. (1984). *What is the value of connecting reading and writing?* (Reading Education Rep. No. 55). Champaign, IL: University of Illinois, Center for the Study of Reading.

Tierney, R., & Pearson, P. D. (1983). Toward a composing model of reading. *Language Arts, 60,* 568–580.

Troike, R. (1981). Synthesis of research on bilingual education. *Educational Leadership, 38,* 498–504.

Trybus, R., & Karchmer, M. (1977). School achievement scores of hearing impaired children: National data on achievement status and growth patterns. *American Annals of the Deaf, 122,* 62–69.

Tsui, H., Rodda, M., & Grove, C. (1991). Memory and metamemory in deaf students. In D. Martin (Ed.), *Advances in cognition, education, and deafness* (pp. 315–319). Washington, DC: Gallaudet University Press.

Tulving, E. (1983). *Elements of episodic memory*. Oxford, England: Oxford University Press.

Tulving, E., & Donaldson, W. (Eds.). (1972). *Organization of memory*. New York: Academic Press.

Turner, J. (1991). *The structure of sociological theory* (5th ed.). Belmont, CA: Wadsworth.

Tyack, D., & Gottesleben, R. (1974). *Language sampling, analysis, and training: A handbook for teachers and clinicians*. Palo Alto, CA: Consulting Psychologist's Press.

Tzeng, S-J. (1993). *Speech recoding, short-term memory, and reading ability in immature readers with severe to profound hearing impairment*. Unpublished doctoral dissertation, The Ohio State University, Columbus.

van Uden, A. (1977). *A world of language for deaf children. Part 1. Basic principles: A maternal reflective method* (2nd ed.). Lisse, Netherlands: Swets & Zeitlinger B. V.

Vellutino, F. (1982). Theoretical issues in the study of word recognition: The unit of perception controversy reexamined. In S. Rosenberg (Ed.), *Handbook of applied psycholinguistics* (pp. 33–197). Hillsdale, NJ: Lawrence Erlbaum.

Verhoeven, L. (1992). Assessment of bilingual proficiency. In L. Verhoeven & J. de Jong (Eds.), *The construct of language proficiency: Applications of psychological models to language assessment* (pp. 125–136). Philadelphia, PA: Benjamins.

Verhoeven, L., & de Jong, J. (Eds.). (1992). *The construct of language proficiency: Applications of psychological models to language assessment*. Philadelphia, PA: Benjamins.

Vernon, M. (1967). Relationship of language to the thinking process. *Archives of Genetic Psychiatry, 16*, 325–333.

Vernon, M., & Andrews, J. (1990). *The psychology of deafness: Understanding deaf and hard-of-hearing people*. White Plains, NY: Longman.

Vygotsky, L. (1962). *Thought and language*. Cambridge, MA: MIT Press.

Wagner, D. (1986). When literacy isn't reading (and vice versa). In M. Wrolstad & D. Fisher (Eds.), *Toward a new understanding of literacy* (pp. 319–331). New York: Praeger.

Walter, G. (1978). Lexical abilities of hearing and hearing-impaired children. *American Annals of the Deaf, 123*, 976–982.

Wampler, D. (1972). *Linguistics of visual English*. Santa Rosa, CA: Author. [Booklets]

Washburn, A. (1983). Seeing essential English: The development and use of a sign system over two decades. *Teaching English to Deaf and Second-Language Students, 2*(1), 26–30.

Webster, A. (1986). *Deafness, development, and literacy*. New York: Methuen.

Wechsler, D. (1974). *Manual for the Wechsler intelligence scale for children—revised*. New York: Psychological Corporation.

Whitehead, M. (1990). *Language and literacy in the early years: An approach for education students*. London, England: Chapman.

Whitt, J., Paul, P., & Reynolds, C. (1988). Motivate reluctant learning-disabled writers. *Teaching Exceptional Children, 20*(3), 36–39.

Whorf, B. (1956). *Language, thought, and reality*. Cambridge, MA: MIT Press.

Wiig, E., & Semel, E. (1980). *Language assessment and intervention for the learning disabled*. Columbus, OH: Merrill.

Wilbur, R. (1977). An explanation of deaf children's difficulty with certain syntactic structures in English. *Volta Review, 79*, 85–92.

Wilbur, R. (1987). *American Sign Language: Linguistics and applied dimensions* (2nd ed.). Boston, MA: Little, Brown.

Wilbur, R., Bernstein, M., & Kantor, R. (1985). The semantic domain of classifiers in American Sign Language. *Sign Language Studies, 46,* 1–38.

Wilbur, R., Fraser, J., & Fruchter, A. (1981). *Comprehension of idioms by hearing impaired students.* Paper presented at the American Speech-Language-Hearing Association Convention, Los Angeles, CA.

Wilbur, R., & Goodhart, W. (1985). Comprehension of indefinite pronouns and quantifiers by hearing-impaired children. *Applied Psycholinguistics, 6,* 417–434.

Wilbur, R., Goodhart, W., & Fuller, D. (1989). Comprehension of English modals by hearing-impaired children. *Volta Review, 91,* 5–18.

Wilson, K. (1979). *Inference and language processing in hearing and deaf children.* Unpublished doctoral dissertation, Boston University, MA.

Wixson, K., Bosky, A., Yochum, M., & Alvermann, D. (1984). An interview for assessing students' perceptions of classroom reading tasks. *Reading Teacher, 37,* 346–352.

Wolff, A., & Harkins, J. (1986). Multihandicapped students. In A. Schildroth & M. Karchmer (Eds.), *Deaf children in America* (pp. 55–81). San Diego, CA: College-Hill Press.

Wong Fillmore, L. (1989). Teachability and second language acquisition. In M. Rice & R. Schiefelbusch (Eds.), *The teachability of language* (pp. 311–332). Baltimore, MD: Paul H. Brookes.

Woodward, J., & Allen, T. (1988). Classroom use of artificial sign systems by teachers. *Sign Language Studies, 61,* 405–418.

Wrightstone, J., Aronow, M., & Moskowitz, S. (1963). Developing reading test norms for deaf children. *American Annals of the Deaf, 108,* 311–316.

Yamashita, C. (1992). *The relationships among prior knowledge, metacognition, and reading comprehension for hearing-impaired students.* Unpublished master's thesis, The Ohio State University, Columbus.

Yoshinaga-Itano, C., & Downey, D. (1992). When a story is not a story: A process analysis of the written language of hearing-impaired children. *Volta Review, 95,* 131–158.

Zwiebel, A. (1991). Intellectual structure of hearing-impaired children and adolescents. In D. Martin (Ed.), *Advances in cognition, education, and deafness* (pp. 210–215). Washington, DC: Gallaudet University Press.

INDEX

A

American sign English (Ameslish).
  See English-based signing
American Sign Language (ASL),
    33–35. *See also* Bilingualism;
    Second-language learning
  acquisition ease, 294
  babbling, prelinguistic, 139, 296
  and bilingualism, 189–191, 290–291
  classifier acquisition, 142
  deaf children of deaf parents
    (DCDP), 141
  deaf children of deaf parents
    (DCDP)/deaf children of hearing
    parents (DCHP), 207–208
  and English, 34–35
    -based signing, 32, 208–209, 290
    interference with acquisition, 214
    as second language (ESL)
      education, 209–211, 290–291
    separation from grammar, 212
    written, 211–212
  first signs, 138–140
  handshape acquisition, 140
  and identity expression, 5

as language-intervention system, 290
and language study, 59–60
linguistic sign emergence, 139–140
morphology, 10
  /syntax development, 140–142
"native language of signs," 206–207
negation acquisition, 141
notational system, 9
phonology, 9–10
  early, 138–140
pronominal reference acquisition,
    141–142
as prior knowledge mechanism, 298
semantic-pragmatic development, 143
and signed English (SE), 208
sign formation (cherology), 138–139
and signing exact English (SEE II),
    208–209
spatial-simultaneous property, 85–86
and Total Communication (TC), 290
APPLE TREE (A Patterned Program
    of Linguistic Expansion through
    Reinforced Experiences and
    Evaluations) structured language
    instruction, 232, 234–237
Assessment. *See also* Testing